EXPERIENTIAL THERAPIES FOR EATING DISORDERS

Experiential Therapies for Eating Disorders

Edited by

LYNNE M. HORNYAK
ELLEN K. BAKER

Foreword by Susan C. Wooley

THE GUILFORD PRESS
NEW YORK   LONDON

Library of Congress Cataloging-in-Publication Data

Experiential therapies for eating disorders / [edited by] Lynne M.
  Hornyak and Ellen K. Baker.
        p.   cm.
  Includes bibliographies and index.
  ISBN 0-89862-740-0
  1. Eating disorders—Treatment.   I. Hornyak, Lynne M.   II. Baker,
Ellen K.
  [DNLM: 1. Appetite Disorders—therapy.   WM 175 E96]
RC552.E18E96   1989
616.85′2—dc19
DNLM/DLC
for Library of Congress   88-24518
                                                              CIP

Contributors

Arnold E. Andersen, MD, Department of Psychiatry and Behavioral Sciences, The Johns Hopkins Hospital, Baltimore, Maryland

Simona Aronow, MMT, ADTR, CMA, The Sheppard and Enoch Pratt Hospital, Activity Therapy Department, Baltimore, Maryland

Ellen K. Baker, PhD, Private Practice, Washington, DC

Monica Leonie Callahan, PhD, Private Practice, Bethesda, Maryland

Mari M. Fleming, MA, ATR, MFCC, Private Practice, Berkeley, California

Marylee Hardenbergh, MA, ADTR, CMA, Private Practice, Minneapolis, Minnesota

Carole Meininger Hoage, PhD, Private Practice, Washington, DC

Lynne M. Hornyak, PhD, Private Practice, Washington, DC

M. Katherine Hudgins, PhD, The Center for Experiential Learning, Richmond, Virginia

Ann Kearney-Cooke, PhD, Private Practice, Cincinnati, Ohio

Laura G. Kogan, PsyD, New England Rehabilitation Hospital, Department of Neuropsychology, Woburn, Massachusetts

Clorinda Margolis, PhD, Department of Psychiatry and Human Behavior, Jefferson Medical College, Philadelphia, Pennsylvania

Theresa McGeehan, MA, DTR, ABTEC Unit, Mercy Hospital, Baltimore, Maryland

Andrea Morenoff, MSW, Private Practice, Bethesda, Maryland

Paul Nolan, MCAT, MT-BC, Hahnemann University, Creative Arts Therapies—Music Therapy, Philadelphia, Pennsylvania

Alice Ball Parente, RMT-BC, MEd, Process Theatre, Inc., Sacramento, California

Helen M. Pettinati, PhD, Carrier Foundation, Belle Mead, New Jersey, and University of Medicine and Dentistry of New Jersey–Robert Wood Johnson Medical School, Piscataway, New Jersey

Julia B. Rice, ADTR, Abbott-Northwestern Hospital, Minneapolis, Minnesota

Maria P. P. Root, PhD, Private Practice, Seattle, Washington

Linda Shrier, MSEd, Department of Psychiatry and Human Behavior, Jefferson Medical College, Philadelphia, Pennsylvania

Barbara Sobol, MA, ATR, Private Practice, Washington, DC

Jane L. Sparnon, RD, Dominion Hospital, Falls Church, Virginia

Arlynne Stark, MA, MAS, ADTR, CMA, Goucher College, Dance/Movement Therapy Graduate Program, Baltimore, Maryland

Julie H. Wade, MS, The Medical College of Pennsylvania at EEPI, Philadelphia, Pennsylvania

Camay Woodall, PhD, Department of Psychiatry and Behavioral Sciences, The Johns Hopkins Hospital, Baltimore, Maryland

Foreword

With this book, a growing trend in the treatment of eating disorders comes of age. Assembled here, for the first time, is a description of the striking array of experiential therapies, developed for use with this patient population by therapists in different parts of the country—often, one suspects, with minimal knowledge of the surprisingly parallel work of colleagues. Readers will be struck both by the concordance of themes among these works as well as their originality and diversity.

It should not surprise us that so many are finding unique value in experiential techniques. The fact that eating-disordered patients adopt physical and often complex metaphoric means of expressing their emotional pain suggests the difficulty we are likely to encounter in asking them to articulate the inarticulable. In moving to spatial, kinesthetic, and symbolic expression, we are, in a sense, agreeing to speak the patient's language rather than our own. I will never forget the sense of wonder I felt when, as a therapist with many years' experience treating eating disorders, I first abandoned my native tongue, finding new ways to let patients talk to me. Before me was a new world, dense in meaning and rich in currents of emotion that had long eluded me. With a "voice" in which to speak, my patients had much to say about the pain of becoming a woman crossing thresholds unknown to their mothers; about the burdens and the necessity of caring; about the alienation and isolation they feared would accompany their maturation; about the assaults on their bodies and minds, which filled them with shame and with fear of their own rage; and much much more.

In learning to speak another language I entered their world of uncertainty. Stripped of my words, I had no choice but to be more real, more spontaneous. There was no well-worn script to refer to, only the immediacy of the moment. This, in turn, led me to more innocent, real and profound connections to my patients. One can wonder whether changes in the nature of the therapist–patient relationship contribute to the success of experiential techniques.

This book contains many cautions about the basic knowledge and personal grounding that therapists require to work in this powerful medium. And rightly so, for one often finds oneself in new territory, dependent on intuitions and understandings not linked to a more readily organizable verbal flow. But therapists who prepare themselves to work in these new ways rarely turn back.

The authors of this book were up against a formidable task: conveying in words the power and nature of nonverbal experiences. They have done this well, bringing to life the experiences and illustrating the translation of nonverbal experience back into the words and concepts needed to help patients organize, consolidate, and generalize their experiences.

Experiential work is not for everyone and some may therefore wonder whether they will find this book useful. I think they will. Even without a major shift in style, readers will find small ways to help patients show what they cannot tell. In addition, the contributors report on what they have learned from the new ways of knowing. By analogy, most physicians will never use magnetic resonance imaging, but all can profit from the findings of this new technique for mapping the body. Similarly, we can all profit from the findings of those who have experimented with new ways of mapping human feelings.

Susan C. Wooley, PhD

Acknowledgments

We would like to acknowledge a number of people whose efforts and support were so valuable to us in editing this volume. We thank all of our chapter contributors, not only for their very thoughtful writings, but also for their integrity and perseverance during many months of writing and revising. Many people offered helpful suggestions and critiques at various stages in the development of this volume, including Drs. Candace Detchon, John Doolittle, Millie Goldstone, Susannah Gourevitch, Joe Mallet, and Marla Zipin. We are grateful to several individuals who lent their expertise as readers for chapters in the following areas: Ruthlee Adler, RMT-BC, music therapy; Sharon Chaiklin, DTR, dance therapy; Sandy Geller, ATR, art therapy; Ken Gorelick, MD, poetry therapy; Joe Mallet, PhD, hypnosis; Ruth Shor-Jannati, DTR, dance therapy; and Nancy Schoebel, ATR, art therapy. We are most appreciative of Seymour Weingarten at Guilford Publications, who not only was responsive to our idea for the book, but generously gave of his time and advice as our editor-in-chief. We are grateful to Pearl Weisinger for her diligent efforts as our production editor. We would also like to acknowledge our families and friends, who in direct and indirect ways influenced the development of this book. And in particular, we thank our husbands, John Doolittle (E. K. B.) and Joe Mallet (L. M. H.) for their continual support, encouragement, and understanding.

Contents

Part II   ANOREXIA NERVOSA

1

Introduction

Lynne M. Hornyak
Ellen K. Baker

Why *another* book on eating disorders? Over the last decade, the literature on the diagnosis and treatment of eating disorders has grown considerably. A number of substantial texts are available that address theoretical and treatment issues from psychodynamic, cognitive–behavioral, family, and sociocultural perspectives. However, our interest in producing this book emerged in response to two perplexing questions: What treatment elements are therapeutic? Why do some individuals improve in treatment while others do not?

As clinicians working in this field, we have frequently been confronted with the sense that something else is needed beyond a suitable theory and method, a "something" that has more to do with understanding and engaging with our clients on an *experiential* level. While attending a conference on countertransference issues for therapists working with eating-disordered clients, we became particularly aware that other professionals had similar concerns. At that particular meeting, we had just heard two excellent—and very different—presentations on the therapist's role in treatment. The moderator, William Davis, Ph.D., reflecting on his reactions to the two presentations, commented that he had felt reassured when the first speaker discussed interventions, the "what to do" with clients. He noted that his response to the second presentation, however, was a mixture of excitement and anxiety; the second speaker had addressed the experience of "being with" one's client, and the concept of using that experience to guide the treatment. While the moderator found this speaker's comments to be on the mark, he found it anxiety-provoking not to be certain as to *how* to connect with clients in this manner. The response of the audience to the moderator's comments indicated that he had put into words what many of us were also thinking and feeling and struggling with in our work.

Our interest in and use of experiential methods were major influences in our decision to edit this particular book. Experiential methods seem particularly applicable to eating-disordered clients given the nature of their problems. First, the disorders have a physical, somatic component accompanied by a disturbance in the individual's body image. As aptly stated by Susan Wooley and Ann Kearney-Cooke (1986) in their paper on the treatment of body image disturbance,

> Expressive therapies, such as guided imagery, movement, and art, are useful in uncovering stored feelings and memories of bodily experience, because they deal with the stuff of which body image is made—images and physical sensations—and because their symbolic nature sufficiently obscures meaning to permit greater freedom of expression. (p. 491)

Second, many eating-disordered clients are cut off from their affective and cognitive internal experiences. Successful treatment involves helping these individuals to become aware of, understand, claim, and integrate their inner world. Experiential techniques facilitate this process. Third, eating-disordered clients are typically reluctant to engage with others when this engagement requires revealing their true selves. This reluctance is usually due to feelings of shame, inadequacy, and self-loathing; lack of self-awareness; and/or fears of exposure, rejection, and criticism. While many of our clients seem to crave some type of involvement, they interact in ways, based on their feelings and fears, that make relating in a healthy way difficult. Experiential methods offer a way to "be with" our clients, to understand what they are communicating in a maladaptive way, and to help them learn more satisfying, effective ways of interacting.

In the interest of applying experiential techniques to treating eating-disordered clients, we searched the literature for writings on this specific topic. In addition to a small number of research and treatment outcome articles, we found a body of self-help literature, in which the authors applied creative and experiential methods to eating and body image issues. No text, however, has systematically organized writings on the application of expressive therapies and experiential techniques to the treatment of eating disorders. Therefore, this book was undertaken in response to this need.

We were particularly interested in providing clinicians with useful, practical information presented in a scholarly manner. The chapters are written for practitioners who seek a conceptual understanding of various experiential treatment methods, who may be interested in expanding their skills repertoire, and/or who wish to become more familiar with creative modalities that may complement and enhance the effectiveness of their work.

One of the most difficult tasks in editing this volume was, in fact, to define its substance: "experiential therapy." We found it paradoxical to attempt to define in words phenomena that are experienced nonverbally. It appears that this has been the case for other authors as well. Our review of the literature revealed that more references were made to the need for (Coursey, 1985), functions (Feder & Feder, 1981; Phillips, 1984), and value (McNiff, 1986) of experiential therapies than to a precise definition. For the purposes of this book, we defined "experiential therapy" as treatment techniques, based on psychological principles, that are developed and used with the specific intention of increasing clients' present awareness of feelings, perceptions, cognitions, and sensations; that is, their in-the-moment experience. The method usually involves some degree of action on the clients' part, either physical or imagined. Expressive or creative arts therapies, which utilize art, dance, music, poetry, and drama, are typically included under the rubric of experiential therapy. We also include hypnosis, family sculpting, and structured eating activities.

Given that this type of clinical work can elicit intense emotional reactions for both client and therapist, we asked contributors to discuss factors that they consider when implementing their respective methods. We noted three broad themes, relating to the client, the therapist, and the therapeutic relationship.

For one, the client's capacity—either structurally (e.g., ego strength) or situationally—for experiential work must be taken into account. Intense feelings, often previously less conscious, can surface, and this material can be very useful to the therapy process; however, the therapist must responsibly assess the client's readiness to experience and tolerate affects that may be aroused. Otherwise, the risk of acting out disinhibited feelings in destructive ways, outside the protection of the therapy context, may be heightened. Chapters 5–8 and 14 address the issue of assessing the client's ego strength or self-structure and, specifically, the client's capacity at any point in therapy to benefit from particular experiential interventions.

There are several issues for the therapist to consider when deciding whether to do experiential work. Chapters 7, 9, 11, and 14 speak to the extent and type of training necessary for using various experiential therapies. Most of the methods included in the book involve some degree of formal training and supervised experience. In deciding to use these methods, the therapist must assess whether he or she has sufficient skills, or the interest in and ability to obtain the skills, to use the particular method.

Second, therapists may vary in their degree of comfort in making use of certain techniques, based on their aptitude and their therapeutic style. For example, some therapists may be uncomfortable using methods that require them to be more active or directive with a client.

Third, in cases where the therapist views a particular experiential treatment as beneficial for a client, but lacks the necessary training, the clinician may consider experiential work conducted by an adjunctive therapist. Several chapters (Chapters 10, 11, and 14) describe the use of experiential therapies within a multifaceted treatment program, such as an inpatient eating-disorders setting, where coordination of various treatment efforts is already established. While several chapters present applications in outpatient settings, Chapters 4–7, 9, 11, and 15 discuss specific considerations in the application of specific methods to outpatient treatment. For instance, the independent practitioner may be faced with the practical difficulties of coordinating adjunctive treatment. It seems important to consider realistic concerns, such as cost in time and money, for both client and therapist when deciding whether to implement these methods.

The effects of experiential methods on the therapeutic relationship, including both transference and countertransference issues, must also be considered. Chapters 2, 3, 5, 6, 7, 9, and 11–13 offer observations from clinical experience along these lines. There can be the hope, on both the therapist's and client's parts, that these methods will be extremely successful. These methods can certainly be very powerful and dramatic. The clinical process can be exciting, even exhilarating, for therapist and client alike. It is important to keep in mind, however, that once the feelings are accessed, the clinical task of assisting the client in working through, or integrating, her newly acquired self-awareness remains to be accomplished.

Questions regarding the effectiveness of expressive and experiential therapies in the treatment of eating disorders are difficult to answer objectively. There is limited systematic research available on treatment outcome using these particular approaches. We hope that this volume will stimulate research interest and encourage more practitioners to develop skills in these areas.

This book is divided into two sections, anorexia nervosa and bulimia nervosa. Authors were requested to limit the scope of their chapters to the treatment of one disorder, although many authors have had experience in treating both disorders with their particular therapeutic approach. The decision to structure the book in this manner was a heuristic one, as a tool for providing organization to the content. The reality, however, is that there is considerable controversy in the field regarding the conceptualization of eating disorders. As Striegel-Moore, Silberstein, and Rodin (1936) comment, "a task for the future is to delineate more precisely the commonalities and differences among the eating disorders and to develop a conceptual framework that integrates them" (p. 246).

Our understanding of the relationship between anorexia and bulimia nervosa is still emerging. Some preliminary data suggest that the style of eating behavior, bulimic or restricting, is clinically significant in terms of distinct biological and psychological profiles, as well as in terms of prognostic implications (Johnson & Connors, 1987). However, the distinction is not clear-cut, as some individuals exhibit both patterns of eating at different times, and patients with these disorders have numerous features in common (Fairburn & Garner, 1986). Therefore, there is insufficient empirical evidence to contend that certain techniques apply specifically to treatment of bulimic individuals while others apply specifically to anorexics. As stated above, our decision to make this division is primarily organizational at this point.

Readers may also wonder if these techniques apply to the full range of weight-concerned, dieting clients who present for treatment of an "eating disorder." As Rodin, Silberstein, and Striegel-Moore (1985) point out, weight concerns and dieting have become normative for women today. While not meeting the criteria for a diagnosis of bulimia or anorexia nervosa, some women are troubled enough by their concerns to seek help. Furthermore, some individuals may have been diagnosed as bulimic under the more inclusive criteria of the *Diagnostic and Statistical Manual of Mental Disorders* (DSM-III; American Psychiatric Association [APA], 1980), which did not require excessive behavior designed to control body weight (e.g., vomiting, laxatives, excessive dieting, excessive exercising) or extreme concerns about shape and weight as criteria for this diagnosis (Fairburn & Garner, 1986). DSM-III-R (1987) was published during the time that these chapters were being written. The applicability of techniques described in this book to people with milder eating syndromes, or "weight-preoccupied dieters," cannot be directly addressed at this point. Only Chapter 6 explicitly notes use of an approach with this more broadly defined population.

Based on available research data, Polivy and Herman (1987) proposed that several characteristics seem to differentiate eating-disordered patients from weight-preoccupied dieters. These elements include various ego deficits and perceptual disturbances: specifically, an underlying sense of ineffectiveness, lack of interoceptive awareness, interpersonal distrust, and, to a lesser degree, maturity fears. These may not be treatment issues for weight-concerned, dieting individuals and seem to relate to differences in degree of impairment. On the other hand, there are problematic behaviors and attitudes that eating-disordered patients and weight-preoccupied dieters share in common. These elements include concerns about weight, appearance, body shape, and eating (Polivy & Herman, 1987). We have observed that most contributors to this volume addressed those elements that characterize "true" eating-disordered clients, focusing on the more long-term, difficult aspects of treatment of such clients. However, we propose that interventions presented in this volume that address the more common elements may be useful in therapy with clients who have milder eating problems.

Throughout this book, we will be using female pronouns to refer to clients, since the great majority of eating disorder clients are female. In addition, to avoid repetition in the chapters, this introduction includes the diagnostic criteria for anorexia nervosa and bulimia nervosa, as defined in DSM-III-R (APA, 1987). As mentioned earlier, this book was written during the period of DSM-III's revision, and some chapters may reflect the greater inclusiveness of the earlier criteria.

Bulimia nervosa is defined by the following diagnostic criteria (APA, 1987, pp. 68–69)*:

A. Recurrent episodes of binge eating (rapid consumption of a large amount of food in a discrete period of time).
B. A feeling of lack of control over eating behavior during the eating binges.
C. The person regularly engages in either self-induced vomiting, use of laxatives or diuretics, strict dieting or fasting, or vigorous exercise in order to prevent weight gain.
D. A minimum average of two binge-eating episodes a week for at least 3 months.
E. Persistent overconcern with body shape and weight.

Anorexia nervosa is defined by the following diagnostic criteria (APA, 1987, p. 67)*:

A. Refusal to maintain body weight over a minimal normal weight for age and height, e.g., weight loss leading to maintenance of body weight 15% below that expected; or failure to make expected weight gain during period of growth, leading to body weight 15% below that expected.
B. Intense fear of gaining weight or becoming fat, even though underweight.
C. Disturbance in the way in which one's body weight, size, or shape is experienced, e.g., the person claims to "feel fat" even when emaciated, believes that one area of the body is "too fat" even when obviously underweight.
D. In females, absence of at least three consecutive menstrual cycles when otherwise expected to occur (primary or secondary amenorrhea). (A woman is considered to have amenorrhea if her periods occur only following hormone, e.g., estrogen, administration.)

In this book, the authors have presented their treatment approaches in formats that highlight the interrelationship of theory and practice. First, they elaborate their theoretical framework, providing a conceptual under-

*Reprinted with permission from the *Diagnostic and Statistical Manual of Mental Disorders. Third Edition. Revised.* Copyright 1987 American Psychiatric Association.

standing of each approach. Second, they describe their treatment method in detail, to allow for replication of the techniques. Case examples, altered to protect confidentiality, are included for illustration. Finally, the authors share observations and recommendations for applying their methods based on their clinical experiences as well as the treatment literature.

We hope that this volume will be a useful resource for practicing clinicians treating clients with eating disorders. Just as this volume is a tool, we want to emphasize that the experiential approaches described here are also tools and not ends in themselves. They are valuable when incorporated thoughtfully and skillfully into the context of an ongoing treatment plan and therapeutic relationship.

We and our colleagues have found experiential methods, such as those included in the following chapters, to be effective and energizing resources in working with clients suffering from eating disorders. We hope that by sharing them we can help to promote in our professional sphere an atmosphere of exploration, exchange, and growth—thereby also giving to ourselves what we attempt to give to our clients.

REFERENCES

American Psychiatric Association. (1980). *Diagnostic and statistical manual of mental disorders* (3rd ed.). Washington, DC: Author.

American Psychiatric Association. (1987). *Diagnostic and statistical manual of mental disorders* (3rd ed., rev.). Washington, DC: Author.

Coursey, R. J. (1985, May). *Working with internalized distortions of self and others through experiential techniques.* Workshop conducted at the Maryland Psychological Association Pre-Convention Institute, Ocean City, MD.

Fairburn, C. G., & Garner, D. M. (1986). The diagnosis of bulimia nervosa. *International Journal of Eating Disorders, 5*(3), 403–419.

Feder, E., & Feder, B. (1981). *The expressive arts therapies.* Englewood Cliffs, NJ: Prentice-Hall.

Johnson, G., & Connors, M. E. (1987). *The etiology and treatment of bulimia nervosa.* New York: Basic Books.

McNiff, S. (1986). *Educating the creative arts therapist: A profile of the profession.* Springfield, IL: Charles C. Thomas.

Phillips, E. L. (1984). Expressive arts. In R. J. Corsini (Ed.), *Encyclopedia of psychology* (Vol. 1). New York: Wiley.

Polivy, J., & Herman, C. P. (1987). Diagnosis and treatment of normal eating. *Journal of Consulting and Clinical Psychology, 55*(5), 635–644.

Rodin, J., Silberstein, L. R., & Striegel-Moore, R. H. (1985). Women and weight: A normative discontent. In T. B. Sonderegger (Ed.), *Nebraska symposium on motivation: Vol. 32. Psychology and gender* (pp. 267–307). Lincoln, NE: University of Nebraska Press.

Striegel-Moore, R. H., Silberstein, L. R., & Rodin, J. (1986). Toward an understanding of risk factors for bulimia. *American Psychologist, 41*(3), 246–263.

Wooley, S. C., & Kearney-Cooke, A. (1986). Intensive treatment of bulimia and body-image disturbances. In K. D. Brownell & J. P. Foreyt (Eds.), *Handbook of eating disorders: Physiology, psychology, and treatment of obesity, anorexia, and bulimia.* New York: Basic Books.

I
Bulimia Nervosa

2

Reclaiming the Body: Using Guided Imagery in the Treatment of Body Image Disturbances among Bulimic Women

Ann Kearney-Cooke

A disturbance of body image has long been recognized as a clinical feature of central importance in the development and diagnosis of anorexia nervosa and bulimia. During the last decade, it has become increasingly prominent as an area of scientific study (Bruch, 1962; Fairburn & Cooper, 1984; Strober, 1981). Fairburn, Cooper, and Cooper (1986) argued that concerns about shape and weight constitute the central psychopathological disturbance of eating disorders.

Disturbance in body image is a multidimensional phenomenon, including such issues as body size distortion, dissatisfaction with body size, concern with body shape, and insensitivity to interoceptive cues (Cooper & Taylor, in press; Garner & Garfinkel, 1981). Body size distortion is the extent to which the patient's perception of her size differs from her actual size. Dissatisfaction with body size is the extent to which the patient's ideal body size differs from its actual size (Cooper & Taylor, in press). "Feeling fat" and seeing her body as repulsive and unattractive are examples of a bulimic patient's concerns about shape. Insensitivity to interoceptive cues refers to an individual's inability to accurately identify and articulate a variety of internal states such as hunger, satiety, and their affects. Bruch (1962, 1973) considered the lack of responsiveness to fatigue, cold, and sexual feeling in anorexia nervosa to be examples of this disturbance.

Body image disturbances among bulimic patients have been con-

11

firmed through various research studies. Willmuth, Leitenberg, Rosen, Fondacaro, and Gross (1985) found that, in comparison to control subjects, bulimic subjects of normal weight significantly overestimated the size of their bust, waist, hips, and abdomen. Birtchnell, Lacey, and Harte (1985), in an attempt to relate overestimation of body size to other clinical features of bulimia, found that high body weight was associated positively with overestimation. Touyz, Beumont, Collins, and Cowie (1985) studied body image perception in patients with bulimia and anorexia nervosa, using distortions of body contours on a video monitor. Ninety-five percent of the bulimic patients saw themselves as larger than they actually were, in contrast to 48% of the patients with anorexia nervosa. Further, the bulimic patients wanted to be slimmer and none wanted to be larger than they actually were; in contrast, 29% of the anorexics desired larger physiques. Cooper and Taylor's research (in press) on their own sample of patients revealed that the factors associated with body size dissatisfaction were those reflecting the general level of psychological disturbance rather than the degree of disturbance in eating habits. Beumont and Abraham (1983) reported that bulimic patients' attitudes toward their weight were "less than healthy." They found that bulimia invariably started after a phase of increased concern about weight; also, patients were reluctant to increase their body weight even when it was recommended that a less rigid attitude regarding diet and weight might reduce the tendency toward subsequent gorging.

It is clear that body image is based on the physical self but not synonymous with it. Recently, efforts have been made to explain the disparity between the way a bulimic patient sees herself and the way she actually looks (Cooper & Taylor, in press; Johnson, 1985). I believe that this discrepancy is based on a mental image of the body that has been formed by past experiences and that is capable of overriding the patient's perception of reality. This chapter focuses on the ways in which guided imagery can be used to help patients rework the past experiences that have left them vulnerable to the development of body image disturbances.

Before presenting the specific theme-centered guided imageries used in treatment, I briefly describe the factors that influence female body image development and the role of body image treatment in a multidimensional treatment program; I also provide an introduction to the technique of guided imagery. I conclude with a discussion of follow-up data on 54 patients who participated in the body image component of the Intensive Treatment Program at the University of Cincinnati.

DEVELOPMENT OF FEMALE BODY IMAGE

A clinician cannot confront the body image concerns of the adolescent or adult female who is struggling with an eating disorder without considering the client's body image history. The first body image is formed during childhood; then, the somatic changes of adolescence are superimposed on this image. The following is a description of the factors that may affect body image during various phases of development.

Fisher, Fisher, and Stark (1980) proposed that body image development begins before birth. It involves the parents' preconceived image of what sex they would like the baby to be and what they want the baby to look like. This image is often an ideal one, influenced by the parents' own body image. Fisher et al. (1980) wrote that, when the baby is born, if enough similarities exist between the parents' ideal image and the baby's actual appearance, the parents will welcome the baby into the world. The baby's emotional needs can then be met in a loving environment, which leads to feelings of personal worth; these feelings in turn are the basis of a secure body image. The physical requirements desired by parents seem to be a resemblance to other members of the family and an absence of deformity.

The infant has practically no knowledge of her body and must distinguish it from other objects in her environment through kinesthetic, visceral, and motor sensation. Adequate somatic sensory stimulation, such as rocking, massaging, and water play, are crucial for the development of body image in the infant. Blaesing and Brockhaus (1972) went so far as to say that if an infant does not receive adequate tactile and vestibular stimulation, there will be an impairment of ego development, an increase in the level of anxiety, and a poor foundation for reality testing. Though, initially, the infant is unable to distinguish her body from the rest of the world, by the end of the first year she accomplishes this developmental task.

Erikson (1950) described the toddler stage as ranging from 1 to 3 years of age. Mastery of body and environment are the major tasks of this stage. Toddlers struggle to master motor skills, language skills, and bowel training. The parents' approval or disapproval of the toddler's more autonomous behavior and appearance has a significant effect on the child's developing body image. Depending on the reactions of the parents, the child may perceive her body and its parts as good or bad, pleasing or repulsive, clean or dirty, loved or disliked. If a child is accepted by her family during this period, she will accept her body and not overvalue or devalue it. If she feels that her body fails to meet the expectations of those around her, she will develop feelings of shame, helplessness, and inadequacy.

Critical developments during the preschool period (ages 3 through 6 years) include gender identity, rapid growth of intellectual capacities, and increased psychomotor skills. Sense of balance, spatial orientation, and precision of movement are the aspects of psychomotor development that are particularly relevant to body image during this period. The manner in which the child handles this stage of development will determine how she feels about the sex of her body and how she relates to both sexes throughout her lifetime (Blaesing & Brockhaus, 1972).

Sex typing and sex role identification are major tasks of this stage. In our culture, muscular build, overt physical aggression, competence at athletics, competitiveness, and independence are generally regarded as desirable for boys, whereas dependency, passivity, inhibition of physical aggression, smallness, and neatness are seen as more appropriate for girls. If her body build or behavior does not conform to cultural expectations for her sex, a girl may feel negative about her body at this stage.

Most children engage in some form of modified masturbation during this period. They discover that touching the genital area releases tension and produces pleasurable sensations. If punishment is the reaction of significant others to a child's emerging interest in her own and other people's genitals, her genitals may become a focus of conflict. The feelings of shame and humiliation produced by these negative reactions may lay the groundwork for a distorted image of the genital area.

As the child enters school, the reactions of peers also play a role in her body image development. For the first time, the child enters a group that has no special interest in her. For example, her big ears, which look like her grandmother's, are no longer seen as cute but are now regarded as deviant and are ridiculed. The members of the child's peer group are at an age where they must compete and assert their own ability to survive outside their homes. Often, popularity and leadership are based on appearance. Thus, the child whose bodily appearance is considered unattractive (such as the fat child in our society) is often rejected and ridiculed, and her body image may suffer permanent damage.

Schilder (1950) proposed that an individual develops conscious and unconscious attitudes about his or her body primarily through identification with another person. The mother typically is the primary focus of the daughter's identification; thus mother–daughter transmission of body image is another salient factor in body image development for girls. Today's young women are the first generation to be raised by mothers who reject their own bodies and who are often concerned about the size of their daughters' bodies from the moment of birth (Wooley & Kearney-Cooke, 1986). This phenomenon was illustrated in a *Glamour* survey of body image (Wooley & Wooley, 1984): Mothers who were critical of their own bodies also were more critical of their daughters' bodies. Daughters who reported that their mothers were critical of their bodies showed a poorer body image, a greater use of severe dieting practices, and a higher incidence of bulimia. Through identification with a mother whom they perceived as powerless and contemptuous of her own body, young women learned to regard their own bodies with disgust, possibly contributing to the development of an eating disorder.

The way in which a person responds to the somatic changes of puberty has a significant effect on her body image, her female identity, and her subsequent behavior as an adult woman. The transformation of puberty is a difficult one, complicated by physiological, hormonal, and psychological revisions of earlier conflicts. The adolescent female must cope with physical changes such as developing curves, getting acne, and developing breasts—or not developing breasts. These changes come at a vulnerable time, when the adolescent is preparing to exist independently and survive on her own. In addition, current adolescents belong to the first generation of women expected to live a life like their fathers', reflecting traditional male values of achievement, autonomy, and power. These females learn that the more masculine-looking physique is preferred in this society; the new fullness of body that attends puberty dooms them to a subordinate position in which curves and softness cause them to be devalued.

Body image development also is affected by traumatic events such as sexual abuse or surgery. In a survey of 75 consecutive bulimic patients treated at the University of Cincinnati's Eating Disorders Clinic, more than half the respondents had been sexually abused (Kearney-Cooke, 1988). It makes sense that a disturbance in body image could result from sexual victimization since the body is the site of the original trauma. The feelings of shame and "dirtiness" reported by many victims do not dissipate when the abuse ends; instead, they persist into adulthood and may leave a woman at risk of developing an eating disorder. The intense need to lose weight and to "get rid of the body" may be a defensive way of handling these feelings. Bulimia, then, can become a ritual of self-purification, offering the hope that if the victim's body is "perfect," she will be cared for and will no longer feel ashamed.

Johnson (1987) proposed that, from birth, humans develop feelings of personal mastery by gaining control of our bodies. From the time we are able to reach out and grab things, crawl, walk, gain sphincter control, ride a bicycle, and so on, a massive feedback loop exists between control of body and self-esteem. The more we feel in control of those things going on in our bodies, the greater our feelings of personal mastery in general. In a group of abused women who feel vulnerable around issues of control and power, to whom popular culture says that they can achieve control through thinness, it is not surprising that some attempt to regain a sense of personal mastery through dieting. Unfortunately, restrained eating then leaves them at risk for the development of an eating disorder (Polivy, Herman, Jazwinski, & Olmsted, 1984).

BODY IMAGE TREATMENT AS PART OF A TREATMENT PROGRAM

The body image component of treatment described in this chapter is part of two programs at the University of Cincinnati's Eating Disorders Clinic:

the outpatient program and the intensive treatment program. In the outpatient program, bulimic patients are seen in individual therapy once a week and in body image group therapy once a week for 20 weeks. Each intensive treatment program includes eight patients who are housed in a nearby hotel during their month-long stay and come to the clinic for 6–8 hours of therapy each weekday. During their stay, they live in apartments with kitchens and are responsible for preparing their own meals and managing their own affairs when therapy is not in session.

After a thorough medical examination, these patients follow a regular schedule, which includes body image therapy four days a week from 8:00 to 10:00 A.M., a daily food group from 10:00 to 11:00 A.M., a daily psychotherapy group from 2:00 to 4:00 P.M., two sessions of individual therapy per week, and three educational seminars per week. Families are asked to attend a 2-day multifamily session during the latter half of the second week of the program.

OVERVIEW OF BODY IMAGE TREATMENT

The body image treatment program has three goals: (1) to reconstruct each individual's history of body image development and to work through such key issues as family and body image and the impact of abusive sexual experiences; (2) to help clear up distortions of body image and to assist patients in coming to terms with a realistic weight range for their frame and height; and (3) to help patients face the loss involved in developing a positive body image, in which the body is accepted as a positive source of feelings, physical needs, and information about one's self. Many of the techniques used to treat sexual victimization, shame, mother–daughter transmission of body image, and other body image issues have been described elsewhere (Kearney-Cooke, 1988; Wooley & Kearney-Cooke, 1986; Wooley & Wooley, 1985). This chapter focuses on four new areas that are useful in reworking the psychohistorical material related to body image development.

At this point, it is important to remind the reader that the techniques described in this chapter are only useful where a strong therapeutic alliance has been established. Johnson (1987) proposed that eating-disordered patients have significant interpersonal and intrapsychic problems that interfere with their ability to use human contact. Consequently, they enter into therapy discouraged about the possibility of establishing a meaningful connection. In the past, they turned to inanimate objects such as food or alcohol to take care of themselves; thus, a key therapeutic task is to demonstrate to them that they can have their needs met within a relationship.

I believe that therapists who treat eating-disordered patients must be willing to step out of the role of silent expert and to struggle actively with patients to help them develop a new type of connection with others. In such a connection, feelings of affection, anger, competitiveness, and so on can be experienced within the confines of the relationship without a threat to the relationship. Conflicts between the therapist and patient are out in the open, and the therapist's acceptance and consistency help the patient develop the capacity to tolerate the intense feelings inherent in the therapeutic process. Finally, the therapist must be clear enough about her own boundaries that the eating-disordered patient can test the limits of her dependency needs without destroying the relationship.

My underlying perspective in this work is feminist. The female body is seen not from a phallic-centered deficiency model but as an active body, full of potential for creativity. The power of the female body, as expressed through menarche, pregnancy, and menopause, is honored and celebrated rather than feared and ridiculed. Female aggressiveness is reassessed and seen as a source of life and growth, with the result that women can express their anger, compete, take initiative, and reach their goals. Finally, women's tremendous capacity for connectedness and relatedness is no longer seen as a weakness but as a source of empowerment for all.

Guided Imagery

The past two decades have seen a proliferation of research and reports about the clinical application of guided imagery in the treatment of a wide range of disorders (Crits-Cristoph & Singer, 1981; Schultz, 1978; Singer & Pope, 1978; Turk, 1977). Guided imagery has been found to be a powerful tool in treatment approaches ranging from psychoanalytic psychotherapy (Reyker, 1977) to behaviorism (Wolpe, 1958).

The work of two forerunners in this field is particularly relevant here. Desoille (1969) developed a technique called the guided daydream, which includes six standard situational themes with symbolic value that the therapist can use as starting images. Desoille was influenced strongly by the work of Jung, Freud, and Pavlov; his scenes involve descension and ascension through imaginal space. The patient is asked to descend into the dark, primitive, instinctual imaginal underworld, where she is to confront and dispel her antagonists. Symbolic ascension gives the patient an opportunity to subject her conflicts to the light of higher wisdom and thus to develop more highly evolved coping behaviors. According to Desoille (1969), the guided daydream provides the patient with a device for tapping the anxieties, fears, and hopes that she has accumulated during the course of her life and that influence her ongoing behavior. The patient transfers the imaginal learning to everyday life through extensive writing and discussion with the therapist during the final phases of therapy.

Leuner (1969) developed a method called guided affective imagery, which combines the hypnagogic state with the introduction of ten imagery situations that serve as crystallization points. After introducing an image, the therapist encourages the patient to associate to it in pictures rather than in words, to enable her to develop her own image with its accompanying affective quality. Then the therapist gently asks the patient to give a detailed description of her images. It is Leuner's belief that the imagery evokes intense latent feelings that are relevant to the patient's problems. Leuner (1969) further suggested that this method can be used in conjunction with any theoretical view of personality dynamics that acknowledges subconscious motivation, the significance of symbols, resistance, and the therapeutic importance of the mobilization of affect.

Hutchinson (1983) demonstrated the effectiveness of combining guided imagery with keeping a journal in the treatment of negative body image among adult non–eating-disordered women. Her 7-week treatment consists of weekly 2-hour group meetings that use a comprehensive, progressive series of guided visual–kinesthetic imageries designed to study the physical, historical, and psychological underpinnings of negative body cathexis. Hutchinson wrote that the most important features of imagery as a transformational tool include efficiency and economy in affective arousal; access to preverbal, primary-process material; circumvention of defensiveness and resistance; and creation of new mental patterns.

According to Hutchinson (1983), the process of imagery can be receptive or guided. The latter approach is used in the body image work described in this chapter. The therapist leads group members in a relaxation exercise and then in theme-centered imagery about their bodies. The group then provides a safe place for the revival of relevant emotion along with support to work through these issues.

Guided imagery is an especially powerful tool because body image itself is an image that patients have the potential to change. It is a powerful technique for psychic reconstruction, by which repressed material around the body can be brought to the surface. For women struggling with eating disorders, the symbolic nature of imagery permits greater freedom of exploration in the highly charged area of their bodies.

"Beginnings"

To help patients begin to explore the roots of their feelings about their bodies, the following imagery, called "Beginnings," was developed. The patient is asked to imagine her mother pregnant with her, sitting with the father at a holiday family gathering. She is told that her mother begins to daydream about the baby inside her; the mother imagines the sex she prefers and how she wants this baby to look (color of eyes and hair, small or large, and so on). The father also begins to daydream about the baby;

he imagines the sex he would prefer and how he would like the baby to look. The patient is then told to imagine the delivery room where she was born and to visualize her mother and father in the room (even if the father was not present at the delivery). She is asked to imagine the birth process as she thinks it occurred. Was the labor long or short? Was it a cesarean section, a vaginal delivery, a breech birth? As the baby emerges and the doctor says, "It's a girl," what happens to the father's body? The expression on his face? What is the mother's reaction? How does she respond to the baby? Are the parents happy with the baby's appearance? Finally, the patient is asked to imagine that her mother is in the recovery room, daydreaming about how she would like her daughter to look and what she would like her daughter to be doing at the patient's present age. The patient is then asked to imagine her father doing the same thing.

Perception of Mother's Ideal. In response to this imagery, most patients in the groups imagine that their mothers wanted a daughter. They felt that their mothers were pleased with their appearance as babies but were critical of their bodies as they matured. The following is a typical response:

> I know my mother was happy I was a girl. She always said that female babies were less demanding. She said I was a cute, cuddly baby. . . . But I know the way I look now disappoints her. She wants me to look like she did before she gained weight. . . . She'd hoped I'd be pretty, dress well, and be fairly showy and sought-after . . . that's just not me.

Almost all the patients stated that their mothers did not accept the patients' adult bodies. It seems that as the bulimic daughter matures, grows more independent, and looks more womanly, she receives less acceptance and more criticism about her body from her mother. Possibly, the mother is more accepting of her daughter's body when she is young because the mother can then operate from fantasy; she can imagine her daughter as an extension of herself, who can become what she wished to become. As the child matures and develops a unique self, however, she evokes old conflicts around womanhood for the mother. The mother can no longer regard her daughter as a baby who is free to develop; instead, she sees a daughter who is facing the struggles of becoming a woman and who must make decisions about career, motherhood, marriage, and other issues— the issues about which the mother may feel the most conflict in her own life.

About 15% of the patients reported that they imagined that their mothers liked their adult bodies, but they were concerned that their mothers were envious of their bodies. One patient said,

I feel uneasy whenever my mother comments about what a nice shape I have.
. . . It's the tone of her voice. Sometimes I worry that she is jealous of me. Even
before I was bulimic she used to ask me how I stayed so thin when "the rest of
us" were so fat.

Hence, even when patients felt that their bodies fit the appearance
that they imagined their mothers wished for, they still didn't feel validated by their mothers. Instead, they felt their mothers' anger and feared
that they posed a threat to them. Developing an eating disorder is a way
to be a sick daughter who can never be too much of a threat to her mother.

Perception of Father's Ideal. The father is the prime masculine figure
in most young girls' lives. A father's reactions influence a girl's responses
to her changing body, her femininity, and herself in general. Three common models of father–daughter interaction seem to emerge during the
discussion following the "Beginnings" imagery.

"I have to become the boy he wanted." Many bulimic patients imagine that
their fathers really wanted them to be boys and that they never really
accepted the more feminine aspects of their daughters. One patient made
the following comments after the imagery:

My father would have been more comfortable with a boy. He doesn't quite
know how to react to a girl. He always pushed me to compete against boys because
they provide more competition. I grew up wishing I was a guy because I felt like
girls were weaker, less competitive, and more emotional. My dad refuses to acknowledge or deal with any emotional matters. To him, being a success means
beating over everyone else, and that should make you happy and satisfied. . . .
Work, success, and being number 1 were all that mattered in life. I feel a lot of
hatred towards my dad for putting so much pressure on me all the time and
demanding so much from me, and at the same time not allowing me to feel any
emotion.

These remarks by Carol, a 19-year-old patient who dressed, moved,
and responded as if she were a boy, exemplify a daughter's attempt to
hide her femaleness from a father who felt threatened by her emerging
womanhood. For years Carol tried to please her father by building a strong
masculine identity through mastery of sports and academic achievements
in school. Her need to stay "in control" was played out in her bouts with
anorexia nervosa and bulimia. Her many suicide attempts covered up her
intense rage toward herself and constituted a form of emotional blackmail
against her father. By the time she arrived for treatment, she was ex-
hausted by her efforts to meet her father's demands to be "perfect."

During treatment, Carol was able to see that dieting to make her body
look like a man's was not working. This masculine identity became a protective wall against other people and distracted her from the painful feel-

ings of abandonment and rejection that she had experienced in her relationship with her father. Underneath the facade of strength, Carol felt helpless, dependent, and afraid that she would consume those around her. She was afraid that facing her needs and wants meant losing control forever.

The group honored the strength and power that Carol had developed in her life but encouraged her to find new avenues of self-expression. She saw that her anorexic identity provided her with a false sense of control and that a real sense of power would come from facing the more primitive, undeveloped parts of herself. She was encouraged to find a new source of strength from her feminine core by exploring who she really was when she abandoned the facade.

"I must be his princess." Another type of father–daughter interaction is represented by the remarks of Connie, a 25-year-old bulimic who was depressed, suicidal, and unable to finish college when she came for treatment:

I know my father wanted a girl . . . a beautiful daughter, small, and fine-boned. . . . He's an empire builder and his family is part of the plan. It's important to have a glamorous daughter in his empire. My sister went the academic route and I was the glamorous daughter he showed off at parties and on trips. . . . He always bragged about how classy I was . . . yet I always felt like he looked down upon me.

Connie spent her early teen years enjoying the fruits of her father's successful business—living lavishly, attending the right parties, living the glamorous life that her father glorified. She was admired for being his little princess and felt no pressure to face the demands of adulthood. During her college years, however, her eating disorder worsened and she began to feel trapped.

Her father, a patriarch, used money to control his wife, his children, and his employees. He made all the rules and threatened to cut off the finances of those who disobeyed him. It was becoming clear to Connie that, in exchange for the benefits of the "good life," she had given up her striving to become independent and had to settle for a passive, dependent existence. Rather than facing the struggle of breaking away from her father and working out her identity, she became more and more obsessed with her body and binged five to ten times a day.

As part of her recovery, Connie had to face the father she held within her and acknowledge his inability to validate her as a total person. She had to look at the destructive pattern of her relationships and accept the struggle with her father that would bring emancipation. She had to give up her girlish dependence and face the challenges of adulthood.

"I've got to succeed for him." Another pattern of father–daughter rela-

tionship involves a father who was not successful in the world and who subtly communicated to the daughter that she must succeed for him. The following quote by Susan exemplifies this relationship:

> My father loves women so I imagined he was really happy when the doctor said the baby was a girl. . . . He always joked that he finally got his "Susan Hayward" in his daughter. I was always happy that he was proud of me because things never seemed to go right for him in the business world. The luck never went in his direction and he seemed kind of depressed.
>
> He always wanted me to succeed and really make it in the world . . . yet he always said he wanted me to marry a rich man, have children. . . . It's confusing.

Susan, bulimic for 10 years, had a history of outstanding achievement for her age. She had put so much energy into her work that by age 35 she had risen to a top management position. At about this time, her eating disorder had worsened, and she became depressed. She had numerous affairs with married men but could not seem to develop an intimate relationship. By the time she came for treatment, she felt trapped in a lifestyle controlled by her eating disorder and driven by a compulsion to achieve at work and to perfect her body.

During treatment Susan realized how much of her childhood she had spent in protecting her father from his feelings of inadequacy. To please him, she tried to have a beautiful body and to succeed in her profession; she hoped he would feel less depressed as a result. Though she rebelled internally against her father's values and was angry about his affairs, still she was trying to live up to his fantasies about her. Susan realized how guilty she felt about all the attention he gave her; he put more energy into his relationship with her than with his wife. She saw how, at the expense of cutting herself off from healthier relationships with men, she acted the role of her father's "lover."

"The Lineup"

The following imagery, called "The Lineup," was created to help patients deal more directly with their competitive feelings toward other members of the group regarding weight, fitness, and other issues.

The eight patients are asked to close their eyes, visualize the body of each woman in the room, and decide who has the thinnest body and who has the fattest. Then they are asked to form a lineup in their heads, placing the thinnest woman as number 1 and the fattest person as number 8, with everyone else in between according to their places on the continuum. The patients are asked next to consider where they fit in the lineup and how they feel about their position; they are told to trust any images or memories that may come to them during the imagery. The therapist then sets up eight chairs in the room and asks the patients to line up according to their own places in the fat–thin continuum they saw in the imagery. If any two people think that they belong in the same chair, they are asked to use nonverbal means to decide who will occupy that chair.

This imagery often brings back strong feelings about competition during childhood and adolescence. Patients often tell what it was like to be the last person chosen for teams in gym class or to be ridiculed for having a body that developed too fast or too slow. The sharing by group members permits them to explore the early roots of shame around peers' reactions to their bodies. They spend time in sharing the painful experiences and, at times, in reenacting them to explore them further.

Through sharing and reenactments, the patients begin to let go of their shame. Without that burden, they can look more closely into the political implications of women's competition regarding the body. From early childhood, girls in our society learn from many socialization agents that their appearance is extremely important; whether they are accepted or rejected depends to a large extent on how they look. Because a parallel exists between role and body for women, females learn that they will succeed only if their body looks a certain way. This referent sets up a tremendous emotional charge for women around their bodies that few women are able to escape.

Often, the therapist asks the women in the group to imagine what it would have required 25 years ago to be number 1 in the lineup. The patients then discuss the power they give to the designers of women's clothing, who set standards of female beauty that are impossible for most women to meet. The patients see how quickly the standards change and how trying to keep up with them could take all their time and energy. A more curvaceous look, for example, was in style 40 years ago; then the tubular body became more fashionable; now breasts are coming back into style but with no hips (a biological impossibility for most women). A body can be in fashion one year and out another.

Patients begin to question the goal of a perfect body that is superior to other women's bodies. They see how this goal isolates them and prevents them from developing close relationships with other women, which could yield a sense of connectedness and create a more cohesive sense of self. One bulimic patient expresses her anger at this dilemma in the following way:

This was almost more pain than I could deal with. I immediately blocked it. I'm either first or last. Yes, a part of me likes the last chair and will fight for it and another part hates being there. I do always seem to come up last with attention and affection. I was last with my father . . . his band was more important. Last with mom . . . her needs overshadowed everything. And how can I compete with my [anorexic] sister? So I stay in the back . . . hating myself for settling for it and hating everyone else in front of me. I'm last a lot but I'm also first a lot.

The best pianist in high school and college and everywhere I go, I'm at the top. And I'm resented for being there, but I love being there and I've worked to be there.

I don't feel comfortable in either place . . . my life always works in fucking extremes. And I know everything involves conflict and I hate that more than anything. I'll do anything to avoid it.

This patient has found a way to avoid the conflict. By being bulimic she can stay in the middle and not threaten anyone. Her feelings of shame when she's number 1 stop her from competing; her anger about being last leaves her feeling depressed and powerless. If she is busy bingeing and purging all day, she doesn't have the time to compete in the adult world and face the conflicts inherent in that process. She can focus all her energy on losing weight and can stay busy counting the calories in the piece of bread she just ate, which will distract her from the real issues.

How can we honor women's "relational self" (Steiner-Adair, 1984) and also encourage what Bernay (1986) described as women's use of creative aggression? Bernay defined "creative aggression" as aggression in the service of life, growth, and constructive action, not in the service of destruction. Women are taught to suppress aggression for fear that they will be seen as unfeminine or deviant. Bernay wrote that "women are not taught to test the limits of their achievement, to play with it, have fun with it." It is clear from the discussion that follows "the Lineup" that patients don't feel entitled to win. They are stuck; they are angry if they are in the last seat but ashamed to be in the first seat. They hesitate to go out, struggle, fall down, devise a new strategy, pick themselves up, and learn their limits. To struggle, to stand up for something they believe, would mean accepting that they are separate adults who are relational, competitive, and sexual. They would be compelled to face negative reactions from others as well as the positive feelings that grow out of being an adult. During the struggle for the chairs, patients are challenged to find nonverbal ways to obtain what they believe is theirs.

Patients seem to be liberated by the discussion of this oppressive lineup, which they experience with other women in most areas of their lives. It is an empowering experience to talk with other women about freeing some of the energy that they have used to compete around bodies for other goals. As they work through their early body-shaming experiences and probe their deepest fears about reaching their goals, they tap a rich reservoir of power that was lost through the obsession.

"Goddess of Fertility"

During treatment, patients are instructed to go home and look at their body for 20 uninterrupted minutes. They are asked to make notes during the experience about what they see and how they feel about what they see.

Patients report consistently that they like their faces, arms, and legs. A few even accept their breasts. However, almost all are repulsed by their hips, buttocks, and stomachs. One patient, who was pregnant, pointed out that these are the parts of the body that become fullest during pregnancy; they are striving for a prefertility, prepubescent look.

I have developed a guided imagery, called "Goddess of Fertility," to help patients explore the deeper meanings of their revulsion toward the full, pregnant body. Patients are asked to imagine themselves with the "perfect" body that they wished they had the night before when they did the body-viewing exercise. They are asked to imagine themselves with this flawless body, moving around the room with other members of the group. Then they are instructed to imagine that their hips, buttocks, stomachs, and breasts are expanding—that they are turning into goddesses of fertility. They are to imagine themselves walking slowly through fields; with each step, they become more fertile and more full. They are throwing seeds everywhere, and growth appears wherever the seeds land.

After the imagery is completed, participants are instructed to use materials in the room to create the perfect body they saw in the imagery. For example, patients often take black cloth and tie up their waists or thighs to show they want tighter, leaner body parts. Patients are then told to interact with each other with their perfect bodies and to position themselves so as to convey how close or how distant they feel toward each other. In many groups, patients position themselves far away from other group members. The atmosphere generally is a competitive one, and later most participants report feeling disconnected and isolated from one another.

Patients then are asked to find material to make their bodies look like the goddess of fertility in their imagery. Many patients stuff coats inside their pants and foam rubber in their bras to make themselves look pregnant. Then they are instructed to move around the room, throwing the seeds and feeling the power of their fertility, and to position themselves again so as to convey how close or how distant they feel toward each other. Most patients move toward the center of the room and form a circle; many patients cry.

The therapist then announces that the middle of the room is labeled "the world of womanhood" and the outside circle "the world of prepuberty." Patients are asked to choose the world in which they would like to be at the moment. They are asked to be aware of the advantages and disadvantages of their choice and to consider whether they are protecting or threatening someone with their choice.

In the discussion that follows it becomes clear that it is not the pregnant body *per se* that is so repulsive, but the *meaning* of the womanly body. Mary, a 20-year-old patient, captured the sadness she experienced during the imagery when she stated,

> When we started making ourselves into the goddess of fertility I thought it was fun and I kind of liked the idea of being fertile. Then I started to feel sad. . . . When I am throwing the seeds, I am giving. . . . When I am giving, I end up alone. I started to feel powerful, but then was disgusted and didn't want to be part of the world of womanhood with the other patients in the middle of the room.
>
> Then all I could see was my mother. I started feeling really sorry for her and realized that she is the person I am protecting by staying outside the world of womanhood. I don't want to be like her. I feel sorry for her. By staying little I can stay away from that giving everything to others and losing myself. I am afraid to lose myself, afraid of being dominated, of bottling up inside. All she does all day is give. . . . Maybe that's why I stay so thin. It looks like I don't have any "extra" that people expect me to give.

This response is typical and is heard from many bulimic women who participate in the body image treatment program. These are young women who are bombarded with the message that they can have it all and must be superwomen. When they are asked directly about what it means to be a woman, they reflect the popular messages about being the new, liberated, autonomous women; they insist that they will not end up like their mothers, whom they perceive as powerless. Yet they fail to see that they themselves are victims, struggling with eating disorders in which they are obsessed with their bodies and out of control.

I believe that womanhood, experienced through being with one's mother, is encoded deeply at a feeling level and plays a powerful role in the daughter's basic identity formation and self-concept. Thus, it is crucial in therapy that these feelings be brought to the surface. Consequently, patients see that the issue is not the fat on their thighs but the immobilization caused by their intense fears about what womanhood really means versus popular messages about modern womanhood. Their anger about this dilemma is not expressed toward a cultural system that encourages female powerlessness, nor is it expressed directly at their mothers. Instead, it is diverted toward themselves and toward the female body they share with their mothers (Vetere, 1987).

Dealing with the deep feelings around their mothers often leads to feelings of powerlessness within the group. The two images of womanhood—the self-sacrificing, powerless image with which they grew up and the new superwoman—are both unsatisfactory. The superwoman image stirs feelings of self-hatred in many patients and increases feelings of contempt toward their mothers. These superwomen whom the patients perceive as intelligent, financially productive, and beautiful, at the same time seem emotionally absent and cut off from more feminine aspects of themselves. Although the superwoman image is not as restrictive as the mother's role, it is seen as an exhausting standard by which women are expected to perform all roles well. Because patients do not perceive superwomen's qualities as available to them in a way that encourages the development of their competent, relational selves and the valuing of their femininity, encounters with seeming superwomen result in a further injury to their female spirit.

Thus, for bulimic women, both internal images of womanhood are restrictive and influence their fears of becoming adults. Thomas (1983) pointed out that women are a diverse group with a variety of needs and desires of their own, which have been overshadowed by masculine needs and desires. Bulimic women are faced with a challenge. First, they must deal with the intense feelings about being female that they experienced in the mother–daughter relationship. Next, they must examine the cultural message about the ideal woman, determine what fits them, and discard what does not fit. Finally, they must have the courage to define womanhood creatively in a way that reflects their own unique goals, values, and beliefs.

Loss

The last three sessions of body image treatment are spent in helping patients develop a positive body image and in dealing with the issues that will accompany this change. At this point in treatment, patients have identified the factors that left them vulnerable to the development of body image disturbances. Often, they have cited sexual victimization, the meaning of the female body, competition, and parents' reactions to their bodies as among the factors leading to body hatred and playing a major role in their feelings about their bodies. Many patients realize that their obsession has distracted them from feelings of emptiness. They begin to entertain the idea of putting less energy into their bodies, and they question contemporary impossible, unhealthy cultural ideals of feminine beauty.

In the guided imagery, patients are asked to imagine that they wake up the next morning feeling good about their bodies. They are no longer obsessed with their bodies or critical of body parts. They are asked to visualize going through a normal day aware of what it is like to live with a positive body image. They are instructed to watch what they eat, how they dress, how they move, how they interact with others, and what they do with their free time. At the end of the imagined day, they are asked to think about everything they have gained from being free of body hatred. Then they are asked to imagine what they have lost as a result of getting over their eating disorder and body obsession. Are any relationships threatened? Have they lost an excuse or a distraction from other difficult issues? Must they grieve for lost illusions? Finally, they are asked to choose whatever seems to be the most difficult loss and to grieve for it in a loss ritual.

During the loss ritual, which follows the imagery, each group member passes in turn through a double line of women, announcing what she will lose. Then she lies face down on the floor and is covered with a black cloth. The others gather around her, place their hands on her back, and tell what they think she might lose. Patients name such losses as the refuge that illness provides and excuses for their failures; in compensation, they name such gains as enhanced power and genuineness. With this support from other group members, the patient stands up, says good-bye to each group member, and then leads the group back to the double line so that the next person can take her turn.

In response to the guided imagery, one 24-year-old woman who was struggling with bulimia described what she would lose in the following way:

I will have to face the fact that I am good at what I do, and that scares me. . . . By keeping the obsession I avoid testing my potential. I will have to face my feelings of inadequacy around people. . . . I will lose an excuse for not dating. I always blamed it on my fat. I will lose a way of knowing that people care and are concerned about me. If I stop looking emaciated, people will stop coming up to me, concerned, and asking if I am okay. . . . I will lose a protective mechanism because I used to think about it constantly. I will have to feel some things. The scariest thing of all is that I will no longer be able to avoid finding out who I am.

I believe that women who change their body image must go through a period of grieving for a way of life that was structured around the eating disorder and body obsession. This obsession provided the patient with a sense of direction, which gave structure to her life. This is similar to when a toddler learns to walk; the change is exciting and the child is more independent, but she also experiences a loss. Her parents will not pick her up as much as they did in the past; instead, they will encourage her to practice her new skill. Patients who begin to feel better about their bodies are excited at feeling liberated from body obsession and body hatred, but they also must face new challenges. They must set new goals and develop strategies to meet these goals. Different approaches to handling these challenges are discussed in the group.

In summary, the guided imagery and the loss ritual provide the patient with an opportunity to grieve not only for her present loss but also for the losses she has experienced at different points in her development. This ritual helps her to connect the past with the present and the outer experience to the inner experience of loss; it can enhance her capacity to handle separation. Each patient has a chance to experience the intense feelings around loss in a safe setting, with an outcome of connectedness and transformation. The ritual helps patients to support each other as they begin to accept their bodily features with their inevitable limits; it also helps them to face the feelings of loss and powerlessness that have been hidden by their obsession with their bodies. Through this new paradigm of growth through loss, confidence in the future can be restored.

Effects of Treatment

Promising results using the body image component of treatment were obtained in a 1-year follow-up of 54 of 70 patients who completed an intensive eating-disorders treatment program. Follow-up data were unavailable for 16 patients who either could not be located after 1 year or did not respond. The mean age of patients was 24 years, with an average history of 7 years of bulimia on entering treatment.

Data were collected as patients entered the program, on the last day of the program, and at the 1-year follow-up. The data were concerned with the frequency of binge–purge behavior, body image, and other measures of psychological functioning; however, only body image findings are reported in this chapter.

The Jourard–Secord Body-Cathexis/Self-Cathexis (BC/SC) Scale (Secord & Jourard, 1953) was used for measuring self-esteem and satisfaction with body parts. The questionnaire consists of 46 items related to body parts and body functions, as well as 55 items related to the conceptual aspects of the self. Each item is followed by the numbers 1 through 5, which correspond to a scale ranging from "have strong feelings and wish change could somehow be made" to "consider myself fortunate." Significant differences were found between the pretest ($M = 137.37$) and posttest ($M = 159.40$) scores on the body cathexis test ($t(54) = 7.56$; $p < .0001$) and between the pretest ($M = 137.37$) and the 1-year follow-up data ($M = 160.35$) on the body cathexis text ($t(54) = 8.21$; $p < .0001$).

The Color-A-Person Test, developed by Wayne Wooley (1986), employs an outline drawing of a female body. Subjects color in the body with five colored markers, which represent a range of attitudes from highly positive to highly negative. This test allows the quantification of like or dislike to the whole body or of body regions and lends itself to qualitative interpretation because the renditions often indicate areas of particular stress. The test is scored on a five-point scale, with 1 representing satisfaction and 5 representing dissatisfaction. Significant differences were found between pretest ($M = 4.16$) and posttest ($M = 3.29$) scores on patients' attitudes toward their hips, buttocks, abdomens, and thighs (HBAT; $t(54) = 7.13$; $p \leq .001$) and between pretest ($M = 4.16$) and 1-year follow-up ($M = 2.89$) scores on attitudes toward HBAT ($t(54) = 9.41$; $p \leq .001$).

The data indicate that the body image component within the intensive treatment program caused significant increases in the scores on the BC/SC and the Color-A-Person Test. Furthermore, these increased scores were maintained at 1-year follow-up. Equally important were the patients' reports of changes in their attitudes toward their bodies, spending less time in worrying about their appearance, and pursuing new goals.

The interactional effects of multiple treatment components must be considered in interpreting the data presented above (although I have clinically observed similar results in the outpatient body image program); members of the body image group are subjected to a number of treatments simultaneously during the intensive treatment program, and there is no way to tell the specific effects of any one treatment.

I believe that an exclusive focus on body image would be ineffective in curing bulimia without treatment for the intrapsychic, nutritional, and interpersonal aspects of the disorder. In the same light, treatments that simply modify patients' bingeing behavior without addressing the body image disturbance may risk an unfavorable outcome.

DISCUSSION

Through the body image work described in this chapter, patients learn how to "decode" their endless talk about their body and to use a richer vocabulary for self-expression. For example, "I feel fat when I am with my mother" eventually may be translated into "I get confused about how I am feeling when I am with my mother." This decoding process also helps patients work through the key issues underlying bulimia. For example, many professionals in the field agree that struggles around separation play a role in the development of an eating disorder. Through the guided imagery and ritual around loss, bulimic patients are provided with a new means of handling the loss inherent in separation. The ritual provides patients suffering from bulimia with an opportunity to use the termination of the group and the separation from other members as a new model for ending important relationships. Working through the loss in such a way promotes the patients' capacity to tolerate the feelings of ambivalence that constitute part of the separation—individuation process. Providing a structure for grieving, which is a natural reaction to change and loss, promotes internal structure building and enhances patients' capacity to tolerate the affect evoked by separation and loss. Finally, the ritual provides the patients with an opportunity to engage in self-affirmation instead of in the self-denigrating ritual of dieting that Kim Chernin (1985) describes in *The Hungry Self*.

This therapeutic work helps women to confront the challenge that Chernin and Adrienne Rich (1976) have set for them: to empower themselves by reclaiming ownership of their bodies. Rich (1976) wrote that women either have become their bodies, complying blindly and slavishly with male theories about them, or try to exist in spite of their bodies. Expressive therapies such as guided imagery assist women in reclaiming their bodies by probing their deep memories, feelings, and desires. Imagery cuts through the layers of oppression and pain to reclaim the self that is submerged inside. Underneath the body hatred, low self-esteem, and fear of one's power, there lies a vision. Many women with eating disorders have lost this vision; they have sacrificed personal fulfillment to driven achievement, they have given up the joy of human connectedness for superficial, compliant relationships, and they have lost dignity as the result of the deceptive behavior they engage in as part of their disorder. Connecting patients with their vision renews their sense of excitement and interest in life.

Past research into body image disturbances in bulimia is limited in scope. Most attention is directed toward the development of instruments to measure distortion in body image, body dissatisfaction, and concerns with the body shape rather than the deeper meaning and the social significance of widespread body hatred and body obsession among women. We can no longer allow young women to be obsessed about their bodies as a coping mechanism or a survival skill in an oppressive environment. Therapists must develop clinical interventions that help eating-disordered patients to find their inner vision and gain a more positive body image. The clinical and empirical results described in this chapter suggest that further development of guided imagery as a technique to achieve these goals is warranted.

Acknowledgment

The author thanks Ruth Tucker, MSW, for her help in developing the "Goddess of Fertility" guided imagery.

REFERENCES

Bernay, T. (1986, August). *What do women want . . . and need in today's therapeutic relationship?* Paper presented at the American Psychological Association Meetings, Washington, DC.

Beumont, P. J., & Abraham, S. F. (1983). Episodes of ravenous overeating or bulimia: Their occurrence in patients with anorexia nervosa and with other forms of disordered eating. In P. L. Darby, P. Garfinkel, D. M. Garner, & D. V. Coscina (Eds.), *Anorexia nervosa: Recent developments in research.* New York: Alan R. Liss.

Birtchnell, S. A., Lacey, J. H., & Harte, A. (1985). Body image distortion in bulimia nervosa. *British Journal of Psychiatry, 147,* 408–412.

Blaesing, S., & Brockhaus, J. (1972). The development of body image in the child. *Nursing Clinics of North America, 7* (4), 597–607.

Bruch, H. (1962). Perceptual and conceptual disturbance in anorexia nervosa. *Psychosomatic Medicine, 24,* 187–194.

Bruch, H. (1973). *Eating disorders: Obesity, anorexia nervosa, and the person within.* New York: Basic Books.

Chernin, K. (1985). *The hungry self: Women, eating and identity.* New York: Times Books.

Cooper, P. J., & Taylor, M. J. (in press). Body image disturbance in bulimia nervosa. *British Journal of Psychiatry* (suppl).

Crits-Cristoph, P., & Singer, J. (1981). Imagery in cognitive-behavior therapy: Research and application. *Clinical Psychology Review, 1*(1), 19–32.

Desoille, R. (1969). *The directed daydream.* New York: Psychosynthesis Research Foundation.

Erikson, E. (1950). *Childhood and society.* New York: W. W. Norton.

Fairburn, C. G., & Cooper, P. J. (1984). The clinical features of bulimia nervosa. *British Journal of Psychiatry, 144,* 238–246.

Fairburn, C. G., Cooper, Z., & Cooper, P. J. (1986). The clinical features and maintenance of bulimia nervosa. In K. D. Brownell & J. P. Foreyt (Eds.), *Physiology, psychology and treatment of the eating disorders.* New York: Basic Books.

Fisher, G., Fisher, J., & Stark, R. (1980). The body image. In *Aesthetic plastic surgery* (pp. 1–32). Boston: Little, Brown.

Garner, D. M., & Garfinkel, P. E. (1981). Body image in anorexia nervosa: Measurement, theory and clinical implications. *International Journal of Psychiatry in Medicine, 11,* 263–284.

Hutchinson, M. G. (1983). Transforming body image: Your body, friend or foe? *Women and Therapy, 1,* 59–67.

Johnson, C. (1985). Initial consultation for patients with bulimia and anorexia nervosa. In D. M. Garner & P. E. Garfinkel (Eds.), *Handbook of psychotherapy for anorexia nervosa and bulimia* (pp. 19–51). New York: Guilford Press.

Johnson, C. (1987, October). *The etiology of bulimia: A biopsychological perspective.* Paper presented at the National Conference on Eating Disorders, Columbus, OH.

Kearney-Cooke, A. M. (1988). Treatment of sexual abuse in eating and body image disturbance. *Women and Therapy, 7*(1), 5–22.

Leuner, H. (1969). Guided affective imagery (GAI): A method of intensive psychotherapy. *American Journal of Psychotherapy, 23,* 4–21.

Polivy, J., Herman, C., Jazwinski, L., & Olmsted, M. (1984). Restraint and binge eating. In R. Hawkins, W. Fremouw, & P. Clement (Eds.), *Binge eating: Theory, research, and treatment.* New York: Springer.

Reyker, J. (1977). Spontaneous visual imagery: Implications for psychoanalysis, psychopathology, and psychotherapy. *Journal of Mental Imagery, 2,* 253–274.

Rich, A. (1976). *Of women born: Motherhood as experience and institution.* New York: Bantam Books.

Schilder, P. (1950). *The image and appearance of the human body.* New York: International Universities Press.

Schultz, D. (1978). Imagery and the control of depression. In J. L. Singer & K. S. Pope (Eds.), *The power of human imagination.* New York: Plenum.

Secord, P., & Jourard, S. (1953). The appraisal of body-cathexis: Body-cathexis and the self. *Journal of Consulting Psychology, 17,* 343–347.

Singer, J. L., & Pope, K. S. (1978). *The power of human imagination.* New York: Plenum Press.

Steiner-Adair, C. (1984). *The body politic: Normal female development and the development of eating disorders.* Unpublished doctoral dissertation, Harvard University, Graduate School of Education, Boston.

Strober, M. (1981). The relation of personality characteristics to body image disturbances in juvenile anorexia nervosa: A multivariate analysis. *Psychosomatic Medicine, 43* (4), 323–330.

Thomas, J. (1983, Autumn). Women and mental health ideals. *Forum: A Women's Studies Quarterly, 10*(1), 6–9.

Touyz, S. W., Beumont, P. J., Collins, J. K., & Cowie, I. (1985). Body shape perception in bulimia and anorexia nervosa. *International Journal of Eating Disorders, 4*, 259–265.

Turk, D. (1977). *A multimodal skills training approach to the control of experimentally-induced pain.* Unpublished doctoral dissertation, University of Waterloo, Belgium.

Vetere, V. (1987). *Primal mother, father, culture, and the development of eating disorders.* Unpublished doctoral dissertation, University of Cincinnati.

Willmuth, M., Leitenberg, H., Rosen, J., Fondacaro, K., & Gross, J. (1985). Body size distortion in bulimia nervosa. *International Journal of Eating Disorders, 4*(1), 71–78.

Wolpe, J. (1958). *Psychotherapy by reciprocal inhibition.* Palo Alto, CA: Stanford University Press.

Wooley, O. W. (1986). Body dissatisfaction: Studies using the Color-A-Person body image test. Unpublished manuscript.

Wooley, S. C., & Kearney-Cooke, M. (1986). Intensive treatment of bulimia and body image disturbance. In K. D. Brownell & J. P. Foreyt (Eds.), *Physiology, psychology and treatment of eating disorders.* New York: Basic Books.

Wooley, S. C., & Wooley, O. W. (1984, February). 33,000 women tell how they really feel about their bodies. *Glamour Magazine,* 198–202.

Wooley, S. C., & Wooley, O. W. (1985). Intensive outpatient and residential treatment for bulimia. In D. M. Garner & P. E. Garfinkel (Eds.), *Handbook of psychotherapy for anorexia nervosa and bulimia* (pp.391–430). New York: Guilford Press.

3

Hypnosis, Hypnotizability, and the Bulimic Patient

Helen M. Pettinati
Laura G. Kogan
Clorinda Margolis
Linda Shrier
Julie H. Wade

Treatment of the bulimic patient raises special concerns since the patient is often in poor physical health yet remains overtly or covertly resistant to any treatment that may involve weight gain or significant habit change. Most treatment programs for bulimia target the various manifestations of the disorder, including the patient's resistance to treatment, by utilizing medical, educational, and psychotherapeutic approaches. Within such multifaceted programs, hypnosis has been successfully utilized. This chapter reviews the literature on the use of hypnosis in the treatment of bulimic patients, including descriptions of the specific hypnotherapeutic techniques that have been reported to be useful with this population. Two case studies are presented that illustrate some of the procedures.

HYPNOSIS AS TREATMENT

For centuries, various forms of trance have been used in healing. However, historians generally trace the origin of hypnosis to a Viennese physician, Franz Anton Mesmer, who, in the latter half of the 18th century, treated patients using trance-inducing methods called "animal magnetism." This procedure, later called "mesmerism," has most commonly been depicted as a group of patients sitting around a wooden tub called a "baquet," holding one of a number of protruding metal rods. Patients would

34

spontaneously become unconscious in an hysterical fit around the "ba-quet." When the patients awoke, they were supposedly cured of all ills. There were documented claims of great success with this technique, al-though these were entirely disregarded by a commission, appointed by the king of France in 1784, which condemned the use of animal magnet-ism due to a lack of scientific basis for the method. Nevertheless, Mes-mer's flamboyance and the seemingly magical quality of his cures at-tracted a great deal of attention to the phenomenon of trance-induced healing. Unfortunately, the picture portrayed of 18th-century trance healing has contributed to a continuing mythology of hypnosis that has hindered efforts to understand the nature of hypnotic phenomena. (See Laurence and Perry, 1988, for the history of hypnosis.)

Definition of Hypnosis

Although there exists a plethora of research describing hypnotic phenom-ena, investigators are still struggling to define the nature of hypnosis. E. R. Hilgard (1965a) has noted that it is difficult to verbally describe the specific qualities of mental states; his description, nevertheless, en-compasses some of the most salient characteristics of the hypnotic expe-rience. He described the hypnotized person as being in an altered state of consciousness characterized by changes in the quality and selectivity of attention as well as in the desire and initiative to carry out activities. The subject experiences a heightened suggestibility, "tolerance for persistent reality distortion," and the ability to fantasize and retrieve past memories. Hilgard pointed out that the hypnotized individual, like an actor, may show a particular willingness to adopt the characteristics of a suggested role. She may also spontaneously experience amnesia to all that occurred during the hypnotized state.

A second definition, proposed by Frankel (1976), places additional emphasis on the subject's ability, under hypnosis, to become temporarily absorbed by vivid images and/or intense bodily sensations. Since these ex-periences and feelings can be altered by changing the hypnotic sugges-tion, hypnosis becomes a potentially powerful method of helping an in-dividual to become more aware of her thoughts, feelings, and sensations and more aware of her ability to change these, if she so desires.

Clinical Use of Hypnosis

Hypnosis is a versatile tool that can be employed in a variety of therapeu-tic contexts by psychotherapists of different theoretical orientations. Therefore, to report that a client has been treated with hypnosis, without providing additional information, is no more informative or instructive than to say that "medicine" or "psychotherapy" was employed as a therapeutic modality (Katz, 1980). Frankel (1976) has described two ways that hypnosis is used in the clinical setting. The first is as an aid to symptom removal or relief. This usually involves suggestions for relaxation and for changes in perceptions, attitudes, or behavior. Hypnotically produced alterations in perception may serve to replace symptoms with more tolerable sensations. Such techniques have been used by physicians and psychologists in the treatment of pain, psychosomatic conditions, and addictive and habit disorders. The second use is as an aid to exploration and interpretation of clinically relevant experiences, thoughts, and feelings. Practitioners of insight-oriented therapies have found techniques such as hypnotically induced dreams and age regression (to be defined subsequently) to be useful in the process of uncovering clinically relevant material.

The contemporary literature is replete with reports of using hypnosis as an adjunct to treatment for such diverse problems as migraine headaches, dermatological conditions, hypertension, asthma, obesity, smoking, and alcoholism as well as multiple personality, phobia, and posttraumatic stress disorder (for comprehensive reviews, see Bowers & Kelly, 1979, and Wadden & Anderton, 1982). In evaluating the varied treatments described in this vast literature, it becomes important to distinguish patient variables from treatment variables that may influence the therapeutic outcome. The most important variables to consider in evaluating the success of the treatment are the nature of the disorder; the hypnotic capacity of the patient; the patient's motivation to get better; the therapist's clinical experience and success rate without hypnosis; and the therapist's experience with hypnosis and comfort in employing a variety of hypnotherapeutic techniques.

BULIMIA

Bulimia is generally a difficult disorder to treat successfully, and there is a need for new and innovative strategies. For example, antidepressants have been employed with bulimics to address depressive aspects of the disorder as well as bingeing behavior (Pope & Hudson, 1986). However, the patient's fear of gaining weight can make it very difficult to obtain compliance with medication regimens—many of which cause weight gain. Nonpharmacological approaches are, therefore, enthusiastically sought, and hypnosis may be a welcome addition to a bulimic's treatment plan.

Of special interest is that the classic symptoms of bulimia—eating large quantities of food and then willfully vomiting—have been likened to dissociative experiences. For example, Beumont and Abraham (1983) reported that 75% of the 30 bulimics they studied had experienced dissociative experiences of "depersonalization or derealization" during their binge–purge cycle. Bulimics report feeling that their bingeing and purging behaviors occur automatically, somehow out of their conscious control. The experience of dissociation, which is perhaps similar to what bulimics spontaneously experience during their binge–purge episodes, has been described by E. R. Hilgard (1977a) as the essence of hypnosis. Thus, by actually inducing a dissociative state during the treatment session, the hypnotherapist can help the bulimic patient to gain control over the dissociative processes associated with her disordered eating behavior. Under the therapist's guidance, the bulimic can explore this particular dissociative state of mind and learn, through hypnosis, to control the accompanying bingeing and purging behaviors. In short, given bulimic patients' natural proclivity to dissociate, hypnosis may be a particularly useful tool in effecting therapeutic change with this population. However, because hypnosis has been so little understood by clinicians in the mental health field, its potential as a therapeutic technique has yet to be fully tapped.

HYPNOTIC CAPACITY OF THE PATIENT

Hypnotizability, that is, the individual's capacity to experience hypnosis, is a stable trait within the realm of what is considered "normal" cognitive functioning. Hypnotic capacity varies from person to person; while most people are moderately hypnotizable, only an estimated 10%–15% of the population possess high hypnotic ability (E. R. Hilgard, 1965b; Perry & Laurence, 1980). The hypnotic response of highly hypnotizable individuals is not limited to simple motor suggestions, such as lifting an arm, or to easily achievable states of hypnotic relaxation; it also involves the ability to experience alterations in perceptions, cognitions, and/or memory. During hypnosis, such individuals may be able to see people who are not present, hear voices in a quiet room, or taste food when they are not eating (Orne, 1972). E. R. Hilgard (1977b) described the highly hypnotizable person as having "such vivid imagery that it becomes of hallucinatory intensity and in the extreme, he cannot tell the difference between veridical perception and hallucinated perceiving" (p. 19). The highly hypnotizable person will report a nonvolitional quality to her responses to hypnosis, although the entire hypnotic experience is, in reality, within the control of the hypnotized person.

Researchers have noted that highly hypnotizable individuals display particular aptitudes and behaviors, even when they are not in a hypnotized state. For example, J. R. Hilgard (1970) has found that these individuals rapidly become absorbed in vivid imagery and fantasy and focus intensely upon activities that interest them. This quality might in fact be considered integral to the highly hypnotizable person's cognitive style.

HYPNOTIZABILITY AND PSYCHOPATHOLOGY

Although hypnotizability has been described as an ability within the repertoire of normal cognitive functioning, it appears that individuals manifesting certain psychiatric disorders may be particularly hypnotizable. For example, Frankel and Orne (1976), and subsequently others (Foenander, Burrows, Gerschman, & Horne, 1980; Perry, John, & Hollander, 1982), reported high hypnotizability in phobic patients, a finding that Frischholz, Spiegel, Spiegel, Balma, & Markell (1982) failed to replicate. Patients with multiple personality have also been found to be highly hypnotizable (Bliss, 1983). Such highly hypnotizable groups stand in contrast to other psychiatric patients, for instance, schizophrenics, who have been traditionally considered to possess lower levels of hypnotic capacity (Pettinati, 1986a; Pettinati, Evans, Horne, & Wade, 1986; Spiegel, Detrick, & Frischholz, 1982).

The discrepancies in hypnotizability levels among groups of psychiatric patients have not been clearly understood. Frankel and Orne (1976) proposed that the particular cognitive processes tapped during a hypnotic trance may also be involved in the development and maintenance of phobic symptoms for some individuals. Spiegel and Spiegel (1978) proposed a relationship between high hypnotizability and a certain configuration of personality traits and/or a particular cluster of disorders that are primarily hysterical in nature. Thus, these authors hypothesized that a patient's hypnotizability is not related to the severity of the disorder, but rather to the particular nature of the disorder itself.

HYPNOTIZABILITY AND TREATMENT OUTCOME

High hypnotizability does not guarantee success in hypnotherapy, although some investigators have reported a relationship between high hypnotizability and good outcome with hypnotic treatment (Bowers & Kelly, 1979; Wadden & Anderton, 1982). High hypnotizability, as measured by standardized hypnotizability scales such as the *Stanford Hypnotic Susceptibility Scale* (Weitzenhoffer & Hilgard, 1962) and the *Hypnotic Induction Profile* (Spiegel & Spiegel, 1978), appears to be an important factor that relates to treatment success with hypnosis, but only for some disorders. For example, high hypnotizability has been associated with positive outcomes in hypnotherapy for non–behavior-based conditions (e.g., pain) and psychosomatic conditions (e.g., asthma) (Wadden & Anderton, 1982), although this relationship has been questioned (Frankel, 1981). These results stand in contrast to evaluations of hypnotic treatment for addictive disorders such as obesity, cigarette smoking, and alcoholism, where hypnotizability levels appear unrelated to outcome (Perry, Gelfand, & Marcovitch, 1979; Wadden & Anderton, 1982). However, these results, too, have been disputed (Spiegel & Spiegel, 1978). Since eating disorders have been discussed in the context of their psychosomatic presentation (Katz, 1982; Pettinati, 1986b), it appears that the hypnotic capacity of the bulimic patient may be important in determining treatment outcome when hypnotherapy is used.

HIGH HYPNOTIZABILITY IN BULIMIC PATIENTS

An empirical investigation of hypnotizability in anorexic and bulimic patients found the latter to be highly hypnotizable (Pettinati, Horne, & Staats, 1985). It was hypothesized that this ability related to their capacity for experiencing dissociation. However, we do not propose that dissociation is central to the bulimic disorder; rather, we propose that the bulimic symptoms signify a capacity for dissociation and hence signal that bulimic patients are likely to be highly hypnotizable. A brief summary of the empirical work follows.

Subjects

The sample consisted of 86 female patients who were consecutive admissions to the Eating Disorders Program at the Carrier Foundation, a private, nonprofit psychiatric hospital. Sixty-five of the patients had a DSM-III diagnosis of anorexia nervosa and 21 had a DSM-III diagnosis of bulimia. The anorexic group consisted of 46 purgers (using vomiting and/or laxatives to lose weight) and 19 restrictors (abstaining from food to lose weight).

Procedure

Three standardized hypnosis scales widely used in hypnosis research were employed. The first two, the *Hypnotic Induction Profile* (HIP; Spiegel & Spiegel, 1978) and the *Harvard Group Scale of Hypnotic Susceptibility, Form A* (HGSHS:A; Shor & Orne, 1962), were administered in counterbalanced order within 2 weeks of admission. The *Stanford Hypnotic Susceptibility Scale, Form C* (SHSS:C; Weitzenhoffer & Hilgard, 1962) was administered 3 weeks after the second assessment.

These standardized scales of hypnotic susceptibility measure hypnotizability by inducing hypnosis and then testing the subject's response to various motor and cognitive suggestions. On the SHSS:C, for example, the hypnotic induction techniques include eye fixation, eye closure, and relaxation. Then, a series of suggestions are given, including direct motor suggestions, such as "lower your arm as it feels heavier and heavier"; challenge items, such as suggesting "your arm is stiff . . . as though it were in a splint so the elbow cannot bend" and then asking the subject to "test how stiff and rigid it is; *try* to bend it"; and perceptual alterations or images, such as hallucinating a buzzing mosquito.

Results

The results of our study indicated that the bulimics were more hypnotizable than were the anorexics. Significantly higher hypnotizability scores were found for bulimics compared with anorexics on all three scales (HIP, 1-tailed predictions, $t = 3.02$, $p < .005$; HGSHS:A, $t = 1.86$, $p < .05$; SHSS:C, $t = 3.24$, $p < .005$). The mean SHSS:C score of 7.71 for bulimics was also found to be significantly higher ($p < .0001$, 2-tailed) than the mean of 5.07 reported for the college student sample on which the SHSS:C normative data were based (possible scores range from 0 to 12). That bulimic patients scored higher than anorexics and non–eating-disordered people on a variety of hypnotizability scales administered at different times during their treatment course suggests that bulimics might be more amenable to treatment utilizing a variety of hypnotherapeutic techniques.

To further explore the nature of the bulimics' hypnotizability, we employed an item analysis to examine the bulimics' responses to each of the hypnotic suggestions on the SHSS:C (Pettinati & Wade, 1986). Significantly more bulimics than nonpatient college students responded to six out of the 12 SHSS:C suggestions, including taste hallucination, arm rigidity, the dream, age regression, arm immobilization, and the hallucinated voice. The restrictor anorexics scored similarly to the nonpatients on each of the SHSS:C items. (The purging anorexics responded to more suggestions than the student controls but not as many as the bulimics.)

We further examined our results within the framework of factor analytic work proposed by E. R. Hilgard (1965b). Hilgard previously found that the items of the SHSS:C loaded onto three primary factors. We were particularly interested in the factor termed "positive hallucinations" by Hilgard, which others have described as representative of a cognitive or dissociative dimension (Hammer, Evans, & Bartlett, 1963; Peters, Dhanens, Lundy, & Landy, 1974). We found that the bulimics responded significantly more frequently than the anorexics to the suggestions in this positive hallucinations factor. This finding lent support to the hypothesis that bulimics possess highly developed dissociative capacities and that this talent mediates their high hypnotizability. The practical significance of this finding is that all three of the parts of the positive hallucinations factor—the mosquito hallucination, the taste hallucination, and the hallucinated voice—require the ability to generate good imagery across various sensory modalities. The bulimic's ability to respond to these types of suggestions can guide the therapist in choosing maximally effective techniques to produce therapeutic change.

Treatment Implications

Given that bulimic patients are highly hypnotizable, a greater number and variety of specialized hypnotic techniques are available to help the patient gain control over the cognitive and emotional processes related to her disordered eating behavior. Also, high hypnotizability may have a greater bearing on treatment outcome when the hypnotic techniques employed draw on the particular abilities of the highly hypnotizable individual (Bowers & Kelly, 1979; Kihlstrom, 1985). For example, bulimic patients seem able to generate vivid imagery, and they may show better therapeutic responses if imagery-laden hypnotic techniques are employed that specifically tap these special skills.

HYPNOTIC TECHNIQUES WITH BULIMIC PATIENTS

The hypnotic interventions potentially useful with bulimic patients have been incorporated into psychodynamic and cognitive–behavioral treatment plans. Within a psychodynamic framework, hypnotic techniques may be employed to reveal and work through conflicts and experiences that might be associated with the patient's eating disorder. More behavioral or cognitive techniques include relaxation exercises and suggestions to improve self-esteem, to increase sensitivity to feelings of hunger and satiation, and to correct body image distortion.

In the past decade, although interest has escalated in the medical uses of hypnosis, only a few case reports have been described using hypnotic techniques with anorexic patients (Baker & Nash, 1987; Crasilneck & Hall, 1975; Gross, 1982, 1983, 1984; Kroger & Fezler, 1976; Spiegel & Spiegel, 1978; Thakur, 1980; Torem, 1986), and even fewer have discussed the use of hypnotherapy with bulimics (Thakur & Thakur, 1985; see also Pettinati, 1986b; Pettinati & Wade, 1986). Since there has been no in-depth, critical dialogue among clinicians and researchers interested in using hypnosis with eating-disordered patients, we are limited to reporting a compilation of techniques advocated by individual clinicians and researchers with no clear consensus as to which are most helpful. It is hoped that this review will stimulate discussion among those interested in refining hypnotherapeutic strategies for treating bulimic patients so that such a dialogue may begin.

The following section describes in more detail some of the techniques that have been employed in the treatment of eating disorders. Some of the work described below refers to anorexia but has been selected due to its applicability to bulimia. In fact, many of the anorectic patients described in the literature are likely to have been of the purger type, but this cannot always be determined from the descriptions provided in the original articles.

In reviewing case reports using hypnosis (particularly successful ones!), the reader should keep in mind that hypnosis is usually only one of many therapeutic strategies employed within a multifaceted treatment program. Therefore, it is not possible to credit hypnosis as solely responsible for therapeutic success; rather, as with any other psychotherapeutic strategy, hypnosis must be evaluated within a larger treatment context.

Rapport Session: Control Issues

A prerequisite to employing any hypnotic technique with bulimic patients is overcoming their resistance to hypnotherapy. Since the eating-disordered patient is likely to regard hypnosis as a threat to the control she tries hard to maintain, special sensitivity and skill on the part of the clinician are necessary to address this issue. Some patients are fearful that the hypnotist will force them to eat while in a trance. A frank discussion with the patient regarding her specific fears about hypnosis may allay her anxiety. Several essential elements should be included in this preparatory session.

1. The therapist should first explore and discuss the patient's prior experiences, if any, with hypnosis. If the patient has had any negative experiences, she will be predictably resistant to future hypnosis sessions. Occasionally, the patient's fears are so great that the use of hypnosis should be delayed until concerns can be worked through.

2. Because the media's portrayal of hypnosis generally includes stage shows where people are made to do embarrassing things, the therapist should be prepared to discuss this popular misconception of hypnosis and to reassure the patient that no embarrassing or harmful suggestions will be given.

3. The individual who has had no prior experience with hypnosis may incorrectly liken hypnosis to being "knocked out" as with anesthesia during major surgery. This image is frightening for most bulimics and signifies the ultimate loss of control, short of death itself. The hypnotic experience is actually very different, and the patient needs to realize this so that she can allow herself to profit from the treatment. In fact, the hypnotized person is wide awake and aware of her surroundings. Hypnosis has been likened by experienced, highly hypnotizable individuals to an intense absorption or concentration in which one deliberately and willingly shuts out extraneous noises and events (similar to being absorbed in

a good movie and tuning out conversations in the next room). Thus, the subject is actually fully in control during her hypnotic experience.

4. Finally, it is important to explain that hypnotic skill varies from individual to individual and lies solely within the individual's capabilities. The hypnotist functions only as a guide (as an athletic coach functions for an athlete) and does not in any way tamper with the individual's mind in such a way as to usurp her autonomy. Since hypnotic skill and, therefore, control reside within the hypnotized individual, it has been contended that, "If hypnotherapy is presented as a tool for the patient to gain control over her weight, it might be accepted. Properly presented, self-hypnosis is then eagerly learned by the patients, regardless of the threat to their personal sovereignty, since it is seen as a means of gaining further control" (Gross, 1982, p. 126).

In addition to the above points, other issues can also be addressed in the rapport session, the purpose being to increase the patient's overall comfort with hypnotic procedures.

TECHNIQUES

In hypnotherapy, as in all genres of psychotherapy, choosing an appropriate technique depends on various factors, including, for example, the patient's presenting complaints, the relationship between patient and therapist, the patient's readiness to begin using hypnosis, and the therapist's training. In all cases, the therapist must ensure that a positive rapport with the client has been established and that issues of control have been adequately resolved.

Addressing Underlying Dynamics

Ego-Enhancing Suggestions

When a patient first comes to therapy, it is often valuable to begin by employing exploratory or ego-enhancing techniques that will be experienced as nonthreatening. For example, the therapist might offer the hypnotic suggestion that the patient feel herself as special, that she can take care of herself, or that she can experience her conflicted and painful feelings as part of an integrated whole. Such techniques were used extensively in both case studies described later in this chapter.

Age Regression

This technique involves suggesting to the hypnotized patient that she take an imaginary voyage back to her childhood, while at the same time describing some of her experiences to the therapist. Gross (1983) described using this technique to treat anorexia nervosa, a disorder that he believes, in some cases, to be precipitated by a traumatic event that the patient has pushed out of conscious awareness. Gross speculated that anorexia becomes a method whereby the patient attempts to stop maturing until she is able to overcome this underlying problem or conflict. He suggested that age regression may be helpful in bringing the traumatic event to light, thus enabling the patient to deal with it using more mature coping skills than she had previously employed. To help a patient imagine herself moving backward through the years of her life, a suggestion such as the following might be employed (Gross, 1982): "Now you are watching the movie of your life going backwards from the present time to your childhood. If you see anything that was very upsetting to you, raise your right finger. I will stop the movie and you can tell me about it" (p. 125). If the experience becomes too overwhelming for the patient, the therapist can reassure her that it is only a movie.

With bulimics, it is sometimes useful to use age regression to help the patient to relive the situation surrounding her first episode of bingeing and purging. Age-regression techniques are very helpful in tapping the powerful feelings that surround the disordered eating behavior.

Hypnotic Dreams

This technique involves asking the patient to have a dream while in a hypnotic trance. The hypnotherapist works with the dream material in a manner very similar to that of an analytically oriented therapist. However, because the hypnotherapist can directly suggest that the patient dream about a particular topic, specific memories or conflict-laden material can be targetted for examination during the therapy session.

Addressing Problematic Cognitions and Behaviors

Relaxation

Relaxation therapy is perhaps the most widely used hypnotic technique with all patient populations. The technique involves giving suggestions to promote muscle relaxation and calm feelings. With bulimics, relaxation can often be employed at the start of therapy as a pleasant and nonthreatening introduction to the hypnotic state. Relaxation techniques are often most effective when the therapist draws on relaxing imagery provided by the patient herself. The patient can describe, in her own words, the sights, sounds, and smells that she associates with relaxation. For example, a patient treated by one of the authors (L. S.) noted ocean imagery to be most intensely relaxing for her. When asked for details, she described a memory of lying in bed, listening to the sounds of the waves and watching the patterns of light and shadow cast on her wall by a nearby lighthouse.

In addition to using the patient's own images of relaxation, imagery such as that suggested by Gross in his work with anorexic patients is frequently employed: "The suggestions given to the anorexic patient include seeing herself in a nice scenic place such as a park or beach. While she is relaxed, it is suggested to her that she be in touch with sensations from her muscles, her stomach, her breathing, and her heartbeat. Suggestions are also given for a greater awareness of external stimuli, such as smelling the grass and flowers in the park or smelling the special salty smell of the sea. These suggestions are directed towards better self-awareness from internal and external stimuli, while enjoying a sense of relaxation all over the body" (Gross, 1982, p. 122).

An hypnotic state of relaxation can also be self-induced by a bulimic at moments when she feels she may be in danger of bingeing. Such a use of the technique is described later in the case of A.N. (case 2).

Reinforcing a Healthy Self-Image

Spiegel and Spiegel (1978) employed a hypnotic technique based on the patient's concern for her health and respect for the basic nutritional requirements of her body. The patient is taught to induce self-hypnosis every couple of hours, for a period of approximately 20 seconds, and told to then focus on statements such as the following: "(1) overeating and undereating are insults to body integrity, in effect they become a poison to the body; (2) you need your body to live; (3) to the extent that you want to live, you owe your body this respect and protection" (p. 227).

Modifying Bingeing and Purging Behaviors

Thakur and Thakur (1985) have written specifically about hypnotherapeutic techniques to modify the bingeing–vomiting cycle in bulimics. For example, these therapists suggest images and sensations that are designed to facilitate swallowing, such as imagining coolness in the throat or imagining that the food flows in a single direction from the mouth to the stomach, "like a waterfall." Similar images are used to promote elimination without using laxatives and enemas. To induce a more relaxed state, passive breathing is encouraged by suggesting that the chest is being expanded and contracted by someone else.

Thakur and Thakur have also used hypnotic paradoxical techniques. For example, with a patient who vomits "a great deal," the Thakurs might suggest, during the trance, that she vomit at predetermined times during the day. This suggestion is intended to help the patient feel that she is in control of her vomiting. At the time when she is supposed to vomit, it is hoped that she will realize that vomiting is an ineffective and even ludicrous means of seeking relief. (These authors do not describe precisely how, in the therapy, they facilitate this outcome.) The patient might also be asked to simply visualize bingeing and vomiting for at least 5–10 minutes daily. Patients whose bulimia is more severe or intractable might get even stronger suggestions, such as to actually engage in behaviors designed to elicit disgust, including "storing vomit in their bathroom or living room, carrying a small bottle of vomit in their purse, keeping a vomit bowl on the dinner table, listening to prerecorded vomiting and toilet flushing sounds" (Thakur & Thakur, 1985, p. 10).

Learning Sensitivity to Hunger or Satiety

These techniques are geared specifically toward helping the bulimic to become more aware of her interoceptive cues signaling hunger, fullness, physical discomfort, and/or various emotional states. For example, Kroger and Fezler (1976) used hypnotic techniques to explore the sensations accompanying an empty stomach as a means of helping patients to accurately perceive inner sensations, particularly those of hunger.

Yapko (1986) employed metaphorical suggestions designed to help eating-disordered patients to become aware of their body signals. "Metaphors, such as the temperature drops that signal winter's arrival to seasonal plants and migratory animals, the signals of sexual attraction that stimulate reproduction, and the signals through which animals mark their individual territory, may enhance awareness for the vital role natural signals play when properly noticed and responded to" (p. 231). Yapko noted that developing a greater awareness of interoceptive sensations is especially important for eating-disordered patients who risk an "overcompensatory weight gain" as they begin to eat more normally.

Altering Body Image Distortion

Clinicians have noted that many eating-disordered patients have a distorted body image, viewing themselves as larger and fatter than they actually are. Hypnotic techniques aimed specifically at correcting these distortions have been used as a method of helping patients to develop a more realistic view of themselves. For example, Gross (1982) might ask his patient to draw a picture of herself so that he can estimate the extent to which she overestimates her body size. During the trance, the patient is instructed to touch each part of her body, including her stomach and heart, and particularly to focus on the parts that she most distorts. He might also ask a female patient to specify a healthy, normal-weight woman with whom she can identify and to imagine herself weighing the same amount as the model she has chosen.

Baker and Nash (1987) used imagery and fantasy in hypnosis to help patients become increasingly aware of their body image distortion and to suggest ways in which it might be corrected. During hypnosis, they might ask a patient to draw herself on an imaginary blackboard and then to erase and redraw the elements of the picture that are particularly distorted. Patients often become anxious during this procedure, but relaxation techniques are an effective means of restoring calm. Baker and Nash suggested that this technique will enable the patient to maintain a realistic self-image, even after leaving the trance.

Baker and Nash also used both age-regression and age-progression techniques to help eating-disordered patients to view their bodies more realistically. Age regression might be incorporated into a psychodynamic therapy where it "may be used to uncover the roots of these distortions in malevolent interactions with family members and the associated development of distorted self and object representations" (p. 190). Baker and Nash employed age-progression techniques to suggest to the patient that she will eventually achieve a more realistic self-image. They guide the patient through progressive physical changes or, more symbolically, "through natural images of differentiation, integration, and growth" (p. 191). Baker and Nash supplemented hypnotherapy with an insight-oriented approach in which they meet with their eating-disordered patients individually and in groups.

Training Recognition of Involuntary Dissociative States

Frankel and Orne (1976) have described a technique that involves educating the patient about her particular dissociative capacity. They have achieved positive results when using this didactic approach to hypnotherapy with phobic patients. Their method may also hold promise for bulimic patients who, like phobic patients, display a tendency to spontaneously enter dissociated states as part of their symptom picture.

By experiencing an induced hypnotic trance during the therapy session, the patient may become attuned to the particular experience of a dissociated state, which might involve, for example, illogical or dream-like thinking or the feeling that her behavior is occurring automatically. Such training may help the patient to understand and identify the shift in functioning that takes place before or during symptomatic episodes and thus enable her to cope better with responses to these "dissociated" states.

CONTRAINDICATIONS AND CAVEATS

When the patient and therapist have a good rapport, hypnosis may intensify the positive elements of the transference and thus significantly help the patient in her attempts to gain control over her dissociative processes. However, hypnosis may appear threatening or intrusive to some patients and, as a general rule of thumb, patients with borderline or paranoid tendencies should be more carefully assessed before beginning hypnotherapy. Inexperienced hypnotherapists might do well to avoid using hypnosis with these patients at all and, in fact, to use hypnosis only with patients whom they know well.

A negative transference constitutes a strong contraindication for hypnotherapy with bulimic patients. Employing an authoritative or confrontative style is also contraindicated. As noted above, bulimic patients tend to be very sensitive to control issues, and they must be gradually and gently introduced to hypnotherapy. In a similar vein, direct suggestions to eat should be avoided (Gross, 1982), as these may threaten the patient to such an extent that she will emerge from the hypnotic trance and resist further hypnotherapeutic intervention. Crasilneck and Hall (1975) warned against careless use of hypnosis as a method of prescribing greater food intake or of directly altering eating behavior. Medically, forced food intake could be contraindicated and dangerous in cases where perforation of the stomach or gastrointestinal tract is a possibility. Furthermore, the emotional side effects of weight gain must also be taken into account; for some patients, such a consequence of treatment could be catastrophic.

At present, there have been no systematic studies comparing the techniques we have described. It remains premature, therefore, to endorse or discourage any of these methods (with the exception of discouraging direct suggestions for food intake). However, hypnosis is a powerful tool and should be used, with discretion, only by mental health professionals well trained in the principles and practice of psychotherapy.*

CASE STUDIES

The following case studies illustrate the use of hypnotic techniques in the treatment of two bulimic patients: one in a psychodynamic context and one in a behavioral context. These cases were treated by two of the authors (C.M. and L.S.), both of whom have extensive experience with hypnosis in the treatment of eating-disordered patients.

Case 1

Introduction

P. L. was referred for therapy in 1976, at the age of 19, by a college professor for whom she had written a paper on eating disorders that had

---

*There are two recognized national hypnosis societies that screen members to ensure proper professional credentials: the American Society of Clinical Hypnosis and the Society for Clinical and Experimental Hypnosis. Hypnosis should be used only as one strategy within a professional's repertoire of therapeutic techniques.

revealed her personal struggles with bulimia. When she began therapy, she weighed 112 pounds at 5'4"; her appearance and behavior resembled that of a young adolescent. She was engaging in a daily eating binge followed by ritualistic purging behavior. P. L. was in therapy for 5 years, meeting twice weekly for the first year and once weekly thereafter. Her treatment involved a complete medical and psychological assessment, supportive and psychodynamic psychotherapy, and hypnotic techniques aimed at inducing relaxation and ego integration.

Background

P. L., the elder of two daughters, grew up in a small town. Both of her parents were socially and professionally active in the community. P. L. felt herself to be completely overshadowed by her parents' powerful personalities, and she resented their many activities, which left them little time for her. P. L. also described feeling inadequate and incompetent due to her parents' tendency to compare her with her attractive and athletic younger sister.

P. L. developed eating problems at age 15, following the breakup of a 2-year relationship with her high school boyfriend. Certain that her chubbiness had driven him away, she not only began starving herself but became obsessed with exercise. She had dropped to 87 pounds by the end of her freshman year of college. At that time, she spent a semester abroad and became bulimic, following the example of her roommate. Her therapy began soon after she returned from Europe.

Assessment

A first important step in P. L.'s therapy was a thorough medical assessment to determine how her disordered eating behaviors had affected her health. At the time that she presented herself for treatment, she had been amenorrheic for 2 years. In addition, her dentist had informed her that the enamel coating on some of her teeth had worn thin, which is often caused by acid in vomit, and she had a large sore on her hand from sticking her finger down her throat. Also, her hair was thin and wispy, suggesting a lack of protein in her diet. P.L. was referred to an endocrinological gynecologist who determined that her weight of 112 pounds and her hormone levels were within an acceptable range. In fact, P. L.'s menstrual periods returned spontaneously within a month after beginning therapy. P. L. was pleased to receive such careful medical attention. This apparently contributed to the rapid development of a very positive working alliance with her therapist, who was responsible for the referral to the gynecologist.

The psychological assessment revealed that P. L. was obsessed with food and that much of her daily routine was consumed by ritualistic food-related activity. Because she had not registered for courses in the current semester, she was home alone all day, leaving ample time to engage in disordered eating behaviors. After her parents left for work, about 8 A.M., she would promise herself that she would have a "normal" day. By 10 A.M. she would be in the kitchen eating; a light breakfast would inevitably lead to a binge lasting several hours. Once she had consumed a large portion of the contents of the refrigerator, she would go into the woods behind the house, dig a hole in the ground and vomit into it, crouching in the same position each time. She would then carefully cover the evidence with dirt and leaves, so that nobody would know that she had been there.

Upon returning to the house, she would clean the kitchen and bathroom until both were spotless. She would then go shopping to replace everything that she had eaten. If one store was out of a particular size or brand of food, she drove to another one until exact replacements were obtained. At home, she arranged every detail so that there would be no indication that anything had been eaten. The ketchup bottle was emptied to the previous level, the butter on the butter dish cut at the same angle, the bread, milk, and other food containers opened and arranged so that they appeared to be the same ones left there that morning. All the extra food was put down the garbage disposal. This whole process was usually complete by about 2 P.M.

P. L. was obsessed not only with her own eating habits but also with those of others. She was fascinated by watching other people eating and drinking although she herself seldom ate in the presence of others. She often came to sessions with reports of people she had seen at school or on the street who were "like her." She felt that she could tell if someone was anorexic or bulimic by their appearance—a concave stomach, careful clothes, thin hair, or other nonspecific clues.

Fixated as she was on the vicissitudes of her own and others' eating behavior, P. L. appeared to lack a clear sense of herself and how she might more comfortably function within her world. She seemed unable to integrate her own "good girl" perfectionist qualities with her "bad girl" inadequate feelings. Her vomiting appeared to serve a powerful function in terms of purging unwanted feelings of anxiety, inadequacy, and anger. A primary goal of treatment was to help her to achieve a more stable and integrated sense of herself and to replace eating and purging with more appropriate methods of self-nurturing.

Clinical Course

Hypnosis was employed by the primary therapist as a complement to the ongoing insight-oriented therapy, first as an aid to relaxation and second as a method of helping P. L. to accept, as part of herself, both the "good" qualities she embraced and the "bad" qualities she was striving to reject. Hypnotic techniques were employed approximately 25% of the time throughout the therapy.

Hypnotic Relaxation. Hypnosis was introduced early in therapy as a technique to help P. L. to feel more relaxed during the treatment process and, thus, to facilitate the work of therapy. Within the context of a very positive rapport, P. L. was cooperative and displayed no resistance to hypnotherapy. However, great care was taken to introduce the hypnotic techniques in a noncontrolling manner. Thus, prior to beginning hypnosis, a version of Jacobson's (1938; 1964) didactic relaxation training (systematically learning to relax different muscle groups) was taught as a nonthreatening technique that might appear less intrusive than hypnotic suggestion. P. L. was taught to systematically flex and then release muscles, always associating the relaxed stage with exhalation.

An abbreviated progressive relaxation routine then became the introduction to trance, which was induced by using an image of walking down seven steps into a room where P. L. could feel absolutely safe, "a profound sense of safety and security with no one to please." This technique was used during the last 10–15 minutes of each session for 10–12 sessions. Standard ego-strengthening suggestions (described below) were given along with relaxation imagery suggesting that P. L. "exhale and relax" in specific situations she encountered. For example, in rehearsal imagery, the therapist might say, "See yourself, feel yourself at school on the day of your test. You walk into the classroom and begin to feel the tension in your shoulders. You take a deep breath, exhale and relax. Exhale, exhale, (pause) . . . and relax." These procedures allowed P. L. to become gradually more familiar with hypnosis and to continue to develop trust in the therapeutic relationship. Furthermore, the "exhale and relax" ritual served as a technique that enabled her to generalize the feelings of relaxation to other situations. For example, following an early session, P. L. described the comforting sensation of hearing the therapist's voice talking to her throughout the week.

Hypnosis in the Aid of Ego Integration. Hypnosis was employed to help P. L. integrate the parts of herself she experienced as "good" and those she considered "bad." The basic suggestion "to feel every part of yourself, altogether at once" was elaborated in many ways in and out of trance, experientially and in imagery. The patient was highly hypnotizable and responded well to hypnotic suggestion. The therapist had the impression that P. L. profited from the hypnotic techniques, particularly at the start of treatment when a strong positive transference, enhanced by hypnosis, helped her to let go of symptoms and work through the issues at the core of her eating disorder.

A typical session in which hypnosis was used might begin with the "coin technique" induction. The patient's arm is outstretched with the palm facing up, and a quarter is placed on the edge of her palm opposite the thumb. The usual instructions are as follows: "Stare at the coin with complete attention and detachment. In a moment I will begin counting and your hand will turn and this will guide you into a deeply useful trance state." For P. L., because control was a core issue, suggestions for controlling the trance by letting her hand and arm guide the therapist were added, such as, "I don't know how quickly or how slowly you may need to or want to go into a trance today. But your arm and hand have this knowledge, and so we can both wait to see." Once the hand had started moving, the therapist might say, "It's interesting and comforting to see that you can be in touch with these deeper automatic levels of control."

This induction provided an experiential basis for the suggestion that different parts of P. L. could at times behave independently and yet remain integrated: "As you continue staring at your right hand, moving in this interesting way, I wonder if you can become aware of your left hand, heavy on your lap. Left hand, here, warm and heavy in your lap; right hand, there, all the way out at the end of the arm, moving almost as if it's no longer attached, and yet, knowing, of course, that it is." Talking in this way about the comfortable left hand and the dissociated right hand also symbolically addressed the split between those parts of P. L. that were acceptable to her and those parts that seemed out of control and were, to some extent, dissociated.

Once P. L.'s hand dropped into her lap, further suggestions for integration were given by elaborating the suggestion to feel every part of herself together at once: "And now that the quarter has fallen off and your hand has dropped, relaxed, into your lap, just feel your left hand comfortable in your lap . . . your right hand, comfortable in your lap . . . your left leg on the chair . . . your right leg on the chair . . . the back of your head against the chair . . . your right side, your left side . . . every part of you here, altogether in the chair . . . comfortable, relaxed. And just feel yourself now, every part of yourself . . . feel that part of yourself that feels special to your friend H. . . . and that part that felt disappointed today when he forgot your meeting . . . two parts of the same P. L. . . . both parts of you . . . the same you, and you can feel every part of yourself . . . altogether. Feeling special even when you are disappointed. Still the same you, still special, even when you're also disappointed."

Another powerful technique used to further elaborate and anchor the suggestion of integration was the use of a transitional object. While in a trance, P. L. was given a small smooth shell, from a collection on the therapist's desk, with the following suggestion: "To remember the feeling of being special, even when you're disappointed, all you need to do is look at this shell, feel this shell in your hand, and remember, really, this feeling of being special to yourself . . . special to your friends, special even when you're disappointed. And you can feel both parts of yourself together."

Outcome

Hypnosis was successfully employed throughout the 5-year therapy with P. L. At the end of the first year, the patient was no longer bingeing but she was continuing to vomit once a week. By the third year, she had stopped vomiting and was maintaining a stable weight. She completed her under-graduate degree and reported feeling less anxious. During the last 2 years of treatment, the therapist employed hypnosis primarily as an aid to ego integration. From both the therapist's and the patient's points of view, the therapy was successful in that the patient developed more appropriate means of coping with negative affect and substantially matured in her manner of relating to others. She was no longer obsessed with her own or others' eating habits, although she remained acutely aware of her daily food intake.

The therapist met with P. L. 1 year following the conclusion of the therapy. P. L. was not engaging in any bulimic behaviors and her weight had remained stable. However, she was working as a waitress, although she was aware that it was "unhealthy" for her to be constantly serving food and despite having completed her college degree. This follow-up interview revealed certain relationship and job-related issues that re-mained unresolved and that might have been amenable to further treat-ment. However, her eating disorder remained in remission.

Case 2

Introduction

In the case of A. N., hypnosis was used in a behavioral context focused on changing her disordered eating behaviors. A. N. was a 32-year-old successful executive in a large corporation. She was referred for hypno-therapy by her psychodyamic therapist, whom she had been seeing for 5 years. Although she had worked hard in the insight-oriented therapy, as manifested by significantly improved relationships with men and with her family, she had continued to binge and vomit daily. A key factor in her therapy was that A. N. was eager to eliminate her problematic eating be-haviors via hypnotherapy.

Background

A. N. was the younger of two children. Her father was unemployed and her mother worked as a secretary. Both of A. N.'s parents were extremely thin, while A. N.'s weight vacillated between 105 and 125 pounds; she was

5′2″ tall. A. N. began bingeing and vomiting around the age of 13. At this time, her family situation, particularly her relationship with her father, was highly stressful. Mr. N. clearly communicated his disgust with women and particularly with his own morbidly obese sister, to whom he often compared A. N. In fact, his nicknames for his daughters were "fat pig" for A. N. and "whore" for A. N.'s sister.

Assessment

A behavioral assessment revealed that A. N.'s binges usually began with the thought of eating "just one" cookie. One cookie was too much for A. N., who would react to this infraction of her dietary standard by consuming enough food to justify vomiting as a method of weight control. Her binges generally lasted an entire evening, during which time she consumed large quantities of sweets and carbohydrates. On a typical evening, she would consume a pound of chocolate, a bag of jelly beans, and a package of cookies. It appeared that many of A. N.'s binges were precipitated by stressful family and work-related interpersonal situations, as well as by situations in which she felt under pressure to appear attractive to men. The goal of the therapy was to teach her new ways of managing her anxiety.

Clinical Course

The hypnotic techniques employed were ego-strengthening suggestions, relaxation, and hypnotic behavioral rehearsal, which are discussed below. Again, great care was taken to enable A. N. to feel in control of the hypnotic process. Also, she continued to see the referring psychodynamic therapist weekly throughout the duration of the treatment.

Ego-Strengthening Suggestions. In the second session, A. N. was asked to alternately close and open her eyes as the therapist counted backward from 20 to 1. She was told that her eyes would be comfortably closed at the count of 1, although she was free to close them earlier if they felt heavy. The patient easily went into a trance state. In her initial session with the hypnotherapist, A. N. had defined areas in which she was satisfied with herself, and these phrases were echoed back to her during the hypnotic trance. These ego-strengthening suggestions involved telling her how well she had already used therapy to be more in control of herself and her life and how she would continue to become more and more "her own person." A. N. had also described specific improvements in her family relationships and in her professional life, and these were also repeated to her, in her own words, during the trance. The therapist then gave A. N. the suggestion that she would use hypnosis and self-hypnosis to effortlessly and automatically gain even more control and that she would relax and experience a profound sense of confidence and comfort using hypnotic techniques.

Relaxation. In the next three to four sessions, A. N. was taught to hypnotize herself using the hypnotic techniques described above, and she was given the suggestion to relax at her desk at least once daily. The therapist modified the patient's own image of tension in order to provide her with a relaxing image on which to focus during the trance. A. N. was to imagine a thermometer with red mercury rising (A. N.'s own image); when it reached a certain threshold, she would imagine releasing a valve and feeling the tension drain out of her body as she watched the red line drop. This intervention alone enabled her to reduce her bingeing and vomiting frequency from once daily to once weekly during the first 2 weeks of treatment.

A. N. tended to keep chewing gum and candy in her desk drawer at work. Later in therapy, it was suggested that when she became tempted to reach into this drawer, her hand touching the handle would become a cue to repeat certain predetermined relaxing and ego-strengthening phrases.

Hypnotic Behavioral Rehearsal. A. N.'s binges appeared related to feelings of being "on display" when she went to the beach with the man whom she was dating. She always binged in anticipation of going to the beach as well as after returning. Hypnotic behavioral rehearsal exercises were used to help her prepare for these beach trips as well as for important social functions related to her job. A. N. was asked to imagine herself choosing her outfit, walking into the room, meeting specific people by whom she felt judged or against whom she measured herself, and then eating at a dinner party. These exercises were done in a series of eight sessions over a 2-month period. During this time, A. N. maintained a significantly decreased rate of bingeing, continuing to binge and purge about once every 2 weeks. She had one serious relapse, in which she binged 4 days in a row, following the breakup of the relationship with the man whom she had been dating. Following this breakup, A. N. asked the therapist to provide hypnotic suggestions that would enable her to continue to "take care of herself," to "remember that she is a complete person," and to "get back on track" with respect to controlling her bulimic behaviors. She was able to bring her bingeing and purging back to the previous twice-monthly level although the breakup continued to feel painful to her for several months.

Outcome

After 3 months, the patient appeared to have reached a plateau, and she felt that her bulimic behaviors were sufficiently within her control to justify reducing her therapy sessions to twice monthly and later to once a month. Approximately 1 year later, she continued to have infrequent contact (less than once monthly) with the hypnotherapist. She was still bingeing approximately twice a month and inducing vomiting approximately once a month. However, she reported feeling substantially more in control, finding that she was capable of eating and even overeating without bingeing; also, she no longer planned binges in advance. Due to the decrease in bingeing frequency, her evenings became free for social activities, which she came to enjoy a great deal. From the patient's as well as the therapist's point of view, this treatment was successful, although the bingeing behavior had not entirely been eliminated and A. N. was still very critical of her body shape. Her weight remained stable at approximately 115 pounds; since she felt dissatisfied with this weight, she decided to have liposuction to remove excess fat from her waist and hips. Four months after the liposuction, A. N.'s weight had stabilized at 105 pounds and her shape became more acceptable to her. At that point, she completely stopped bingeing and purging, became engaged to be married, and terminated psychotherapy, continuing to consult with the hypnotherapist on an infrequent basis.

Discussion of the Case Studies

These two cases were selected to demonstrate two somewhat different approaches to using hypnosis therapeutically. In the first case, hypnotic intervention was an integrated part of the psychotherapy. In the second case, hypnosis was employed as a separate, adjunctive behavioral technique. In both cases, the therapist employed three specific hypnotic interventions to reduce the patients' symptomatology. To begin, the therapist used hypnotic relaxation to reduce the anxiety that served as a trigger for bingeing. Second, the therapist provided hypnotic suggestions to reduce symptomatic behavior in specific situations. Finally, positive and supportive suggestions during hypnosis were employed as ego-strengthening techniques. In our experience, these three hypnotic interventions are particularly effective in helping patients to reduce or eliminate bulimic symptomatology.

At the conclusion of both therapies, significant progress had been made by both women, and it was the therapists' clinical impression that these hypnotherapeutic techniques had facilitated the improvement. Obviously, since hypnosis was employed within a larger therapeutic context, in neither case can the outcome be attributed solely to the hypnotic interventions. When evaluating the outcome of any psychotherapeutic endeavor, it is frequently difficult to determine which particular aspects of the treatment have been most directly responsible for a patient's improvement. At present, there is a need for controlled studies to assess the outcome of hypnotherapy with bulimics by systematically controlling such relevant treatment variables as the nature of the disorder, level of hypnotizability, patient motivation, therapist training, and specific techniques employed.

CONCLUSIONS

That bulimics are highly hyphotizable does not negate the fact that these patients are fearful of relinquishing control to a therapist through hypnotherapy. However, when hypnosis is "demythified" and the eating-disordered patient learns that hypnosis can, in fact, help her to regain control and to maintain a healthy weight, she is often eager to use hypnotic techniques as part of the therapeutic program. A skilled clinician, trained in the use of hypnosis and flexible in utilizing a variety of hypnotherapeutic techniques, may find that the addition of hypnotherapy to the bulimic's treatment regimen may facilitate the work of therapy and improve treatment outcome. Those therapists unfamiliar with hypnosis may find that their clients profit from adjunctive hypnotherapeutic treatment provided by a well-trained professional.

Acknowledgement

Supported in part by the Carrier Foundation and the American Society of Clinical Hypnosis. The authors thank Kathleen Meyers, Marie M. Brown, and Joanne Rosenberg for their helpful comments. We also thank Mary Anne Hinz and Christine Makin for their technical assistance.

REFERENCES

Baker, E. L., & Nash, M. R. (1987). Applications of hypnosis in the treatment of anorexia nervosa. *American Journal of Clinical Hypnosis, 29,* 185–193.
Beumont, P. J. V., & Abraham, S. F. (1983). Episodes of ravenous overeating or bulimia: Their occurence in patients with anorexia nervosa and with other forms of disordered eating. In P. L. Darby, P. E. Garfinkel, D. M. Garner, & D. V. Coscina (Eds.), *Anorexia nervosa: Recent developments in research* (pp. 149–157). New York: Alan R. Liss.
Bliss, E. L. (1983). Multiple personalities, related disorders and hypnosis. *American Journal of Clinical Hypnosis, 26,* 114–123.
Bowers, K. S., & Kelly, P. (1979). Stress, disease, psychotherapy, and hypnosis. *Journal of Abnormal Psychology, 88,* 490–505.
Crasilneck, H. B., & Hall, J. A. (1975). *Clinical hypnosis: Principles and applications.* New York: Grune & Stratton.
Foenander, G., Burrows, G. D., Gerschman, J., & Horne, D. J. (1980). Phobic behavior and hypnotic susceptibility. *Australian Journal of Clinical and Experimental Hypnosis, 8,* 41–46.

Frankel, F. H. (1976). *Hypnosis: Trance as coping mechanism.* New York: Plenum Press.

Frankel, F. H. (1981). Reporting hypnosis in the medical context. *The International Journal of Clinical and Experimental Hypnosis, 29,* 10–14.

Frankel, F. H., & Orne, M. T. (1976). Hypnotizability and phobic behavior. *Archives of General Psychiatry, 33,* 1259–1261.

Frischholz, E. J., Spiegel, D., Spiegel, H., Balma, D. L., & Markell, C. S. (1982). Differential hypnotic responsivity of smokers, phobics, and chronic-pain control patients: A failure to confirm. *Journal of Abnormal Psychology, 91,* 269–272.

Gross, M. (1982). Hypnotherapy in anorexia nervosa. In M. Gross (Ed.), *Anorexia nervosa: A comprehensive approach* (pp. 119–127). Lexington, MA: D. C. Heath.

Gross, M. (1983). Correcting perceptual abnormalities, anorexia nervosa and obesity by use of hypnosis. *Journal of the American Society of Psychosomatic Dentistry and Medicine, 30,* 142–150.

Gross, M. (1984). Hypnosis in the therapy of anorexia nervosa. *American Journal of Clinical Hypnosis, 26,* 175–181.

Hammer, A. G., Evans, F. J., & Bartlett, M. (1963). Factors in hypnosis and suggestion. *Journal of Abnormal and Social Psychology, 67,* 15–23.

Hilgard, E. R. (1965a). *The experience of hypnosis.* New York: Harcourt, Brace, World.

Hilgard, E. R. (1965b). *Hypnotic susceptibility.* New York: Harcourt, Brace, World.

Hilgard, E. R. (1977a). *Divided consciousness: Multiple controls in human thought and action.* New York: Wiley.

Hilgard, E. R. (1977b). Controversies over consciousness and the rise of cognitive psychology. *Australian Psychologist, 12,* 7–26.

Hilgard, J. R. (1970). *Personality and hypnosis: A study of imaginative involvement.* Chicago: University of Chicago Press.

Jacobson, E. (1938). *Progressive relaxation* (2nd ed). Chicago: University of Chicago Press.

Jacobson, E. (1964). *Self operations control.* Chicago: National Foundation for Progressive Relaxation.

Katz, J. L.(1982). Three studies in psychosomatic medicine revisited: A tribute to the psychobiological perspective of Herbert Weiner. *Psychosomatic Medicine, 44,* 29–40.

Katz, N. W. (1980). Hypnosis and the addictions: A critical review. *Addictive Behaviors, 5,* 41–47.

Kihlstrom, J. F. (1985). Hypnosis. *Annual Review of Psychology, 36,* 385–418.

Kroger, W. S., & Fezler, W. D. (1976). *Hypnosis and behavior modification: Imagery conditioning.* Philadelphia: J. B. Lippincott.

Laurence, J-R, & Perry, C. (1988). *Hypnosis, will, and memory: A psycho-legal history.* New York: Guilford.

Orne, M. T. (1972). On the simulating subject as a quasi-control group in hypnosis research: What, why, how. In E. Fromm & R. E. Shor (Eds.), *Hypnosis: Research developments and perspectives* (pp. 399–443). Chicago: Aldine Atherton.

Perry, C., Gelfand, R., & Marcovitch, P. (1979). The relevance of hypnotic susceptibility in the clinical context. *Journal of Abnormal Psychology, 88,* 592–603.

Perry, C., John, R., & Hollander, B. (1982, October). *Hypnotizability and phobic behavior.* Paper presented at the meeting of the Society for Clinical and Experimental Hypnosis, Indianapolis, IN.

Perry, C., & Laurence, J. R. (1980). Hypnotic depth and hypnotic susceptibility: A replicated finding. *International Journal of Clinical and Experimental Hypnosis, 28,* 272–280.

Peters, J. E., Dhanens, T. P., Lundy, R. M., & Landy, F. J. (1974). A factor analytic investigation of the Harvard Group Scale of Hypnotic Susceptibility, Form A. *International Journal of Clinical and Experimental Hypnosis, 22,* 377–387.

Pettinati, H. M. (1986a, September). *Hypnotizability and psychopathology.* Invited address presented at the Annual Meeting of the Society for Clinical and Experimental Hypnosis, Chicago.

Pettinati, H. M. (1986b). Hypnosis and patients with eating disorders: Mind over body? *Hypnos, 13,* 175–183.

Pettinati, H. M., Evans, F. J., Horne, R. L., & Wade, J. H. (1986, September). *Comparing hypnotic response by schizophrenic patients to other psychiatric inpatients.* Paper presented at the Annual Meeting of the Society for Clinical and Experimental Hypnosis, Chicago.

Pettinati, H. M., Horne, R. L., & Staats, J. M. (1985). Hypnotizability in patients with anorexia nervosa and bulimia. *Archives of General Psychiatry, 42,* 1014–1016.

Pettinati, H. M., & Wade, J. H. (1986). Hypnosis in the treatment of anorexic and bulimic patients. *Seminars in Adolescent Medicine, 2,* 75–79.

Pope, H. G., & Hudson, J. I. (1986). Antidepressant drug therapy for bulimia: Current status. *Journal of Clinical Psychiatry, 47,* 339–345.

Shor, R. E., & Orne, E. C. (1962). *Harvard Group Scale of Hypnotic Susceptibility, Form A.* Palo Alto, CA: Consulting Psychologists Press.

Spiegel, D., Detrick, D., & Frischholz, E. (1982). Hypnotizability and psychopathology. *American Journal of Psychiatry, 139,* 431–437.

Spiegel, H., & Spiegel, D. (1978). *Trance and treatment: Clinical use of hypnosis.* New York: Basic Books.

Thakur, K. S. (1980). Treatment of anorexia nervosa with hypnotherapy. In H. T. Wain (Ed.), *Clinical hypnosis in medicine* (pp. 147–153). Chicago: Year Book Medical.

Thakur, A., & Thakur, K. (1985). *Hypnotherapy for bulimia.* Unpublished manuscript.

Torem, M. S. (1986). Dissociative states presenting as an eating disorder. *American Journal of Clinical Hypnosis, 29,* 137–144.

Wadden, T. A., & Anderton, C. H. (1982). The clinical use of hypnosis. *Psychological Bulletin, 91,* 215–243.

Weitzenhoffer, A. M., & Hilgard, E. R. (1962). *Stanford Hypnotic Susceptibility Scale, Form C.* Palo Alto, CA: Consulting Psychologists Press.

Yapko, M. D. (1986). Hypnotic and strategic interventions in the treatment of anorexia nervosa. *American Journal of Clinical Hypnosis, 28,* 224–232.

4

The Use of In-Session Structured Eating in the Outpatient Treatment of Bulimia Nervosa

Carole Meininger Hoage

Since bulimia nervosa entered into the limelight as a significant psychological and health problem, many different therapies have been proposed for its treatment. These include such widely differing techniques as traditional insight-oriented psychotherapy; pharmacotherapy; group psychotherapy and support groups; family therapy; cognitive therapy for distorted thinking about food, body, and self; art and dance therapy to increase self-awareness and freer expression of emotions; and behavior therapies such as eating habit control and exposure with response prevention. This variety of treatments, in part, reflects a struggle to understand a relatively newly defined disorder. It also reflects the complexity of bulimia nervosa, a problem that entwines itself around many areas of functioning, including health, affect, thoughts, and relationships.

From one perspective, bulimia nervosa appears to be similar to substance abuse disorders in that it is both an addictive habit in its own right and an expression of underlying psychological conflict or distress. That is, bulimia nervosa is not just the result of problematic and self-perpetuating dieting habits. It happens to individuals who may also have difficulties with affect, identity, self-esteem, and/or impulse control. These are individuals who therefore may be especially vulnerable to our culture's unrealistic weight and appearance standards. There may also be a genetic predisposition to bulimia nervosa, as there is with substance disorders, although that issue is still being debated (Hudson, Laffer, & Pope, 1982; Hudson, Pope, Jonas, & Yurgelun-Todd, 1983).

This chapter discusses some of the contributions that behavior therapy has made to the many types of *in vivo* and experiential techniques currently in use for the treatment of bulimia nervosa. In particular, the focus is on techniques that involve in-session structured eating. Techniques such as these that directly target eating and purging behavior are primarily concerned with the addictive aspect of bulimia nervosa and can be extremely helpful in obtaining a reduction in overt symptomatology. These techniques can be used in conjunction with psychotherapy that targets underlying issues, such as self-esteem or problem-solving deficits, or that targets concurrent problems, such as relationship difficulties.

In-session structured eating techniques, while emerging largely from the behavioral therapies, have many features in common with experiential techniques. In-session structured eating brings feelings and thoughts about food and body into the session, where assistance with identifying them is available and management strategies can be tried. After all, these negative and/or anxious feelings and thoughts lead to the problematic behaviors of bulimia nervosa in the first place.

The most typical problem behaviors for individuals with bulimia nervosa are bingeing and vomiting. Other associated problem behaviors may include diuretic or laxative use and abuse, chronic dieting, excessive exercising, and self-deprecating thoughts leading to depression and low self-esteem. As the disorder progresses, the client's own problematic strategy for controlling bingeing and vomiting is usually to restrict food intake, on the assumption that rigid dieting will prevent bingeing and subsequent purging. However, this strategy appears only to lead to increased difficulty because of resulting psychological and physiological deprivation (Herman & Polivy, 1980). Thus, a self-perpetuating cycle is set up in which bingeing and purging lead to increasingly restrictive dieting, which in turn leads to further bingeing and purging.

Dieting behaviors used by individuals with this disorder often involve trying to avoid "unsafe" foods. The result is an unrealistic eating pattern in which any one or more of the following problematic situations could occur.

1. Total caloric intake is too low for body comfort and adequate energy, thus cravings and subsequent bingeing occur.
2. Protein or carbohydrate intake is too low, resulting in cravings, which may lead to bingeing.
3. Even if total caloric and nutrient intake are adequate, so many foods become forbidden that regular eating and socializing patterns are disrupted significantly, leaving the individual unable to lead a flexible lifestyle with respect to food.

Thus, it is important for the individual with bulimia nervosa not only to eliminate bingeing and purging behaviors but also to become more flexible and adaptable in the management of food intake.

EXPOSURE PLUS RESPONSE
PREVENTION: THEORY

Rosen and Leitenberg (1982) developed a highly effective treatment for bulimia nervosa using *in vivo* techniques that focused on reducing bingeing by eliminating vomiting behavior. They used a method developed for the treatment of obsessive–compulsive disorders (Foa & Goldstein, 1978). In these disorders, cleaning and checking rituals serve to decrease anxiety. Treatment involves exposing the individual to the anxiety-producing object or situation and preventing the responsive ritual behavior. What occurs is an initial increase in anxiety, which is then followed, after continued exposure, by a decrease in anxiety. This is called exposure plus response prevention (ERP). Rosen and Leitenberg (1982) proposed that the vomiting or purging behaviors of individuals with bulimia nervosa served the same anxiety reduction function and thus could also be effectively treated by using ERP. Their technique involves having the client eat typical binge foods (pasta, sweets, high-fat foods, etc.) in the treatment session. Following this, the response of vomiting is prevented by staying with the individual until the urge is under control. Initially this process may require 2-hour sessions because anxiety does not usually decrease until the second hour. Results of this method showed that most subjects experienced a highly significant reduction in both bingeing and purging behaviors, which was maintained at follow-up (Leitenberg, Gross, Peterson, & Rosen, 1984; Rosen & Leitenberg, 1982). Thus, targeting the eating and purging behaviors directly and bringing these behaviors into the therapy sessions appeared to have significant validity.

The important assumption of the Rosen and Leitenberg (1982) model is that, for the individual with bulimia nervosa, vomiting is a powerful way to reduce anxiety about weight gain after overeating. Rosen and Leitenberg suggest that once vomiting occurs, the amount of overeating actually increases. Thus, the use of vomiting is thought to actually encourage more frequent and larger binges. My clinical experience suggests that, for the majority of individuals with bulimia nervosa, this is accurate. Most of my clients report that initially they vomited infrequently—perhaps once a week to once a month. However, over time, vomiting—and bingeing—gradually increased to a high level, up to many times per day for some individuals. Furthermore, clients report that the size of individual binges also increases over time. Early in the disorder, they report vomiting when they felt either intellectually or physically uncomfortable with the types or amounts of food eaten. However, once vomiting became a habitual response to overeating, the decision to vomit would be made in advance of eating. Individuals would then feel free to eat very large quantities either out of desire or because a large quantity of food makes it much easier to bring the food back up. Based on this type of information, Rosen and

Leitenberg (1982) demonstrated that restricting the availability of vomiting resulted in a decrease in bingeing/overeating behavior.

EXPOSURE PLUS RESPONSE
PREVENTION: TECHNIQUE

In the methodology outlined for ERP (Leitenberg *et al.*, 1984; Rosen & Leitenberg, 1982, 1985), clients are treated in individual sessions. First, a baseline period occurs in which clients record daily food intake, vomiting episodes, and urge to vomit after eating or drinking. Thereafter, treatment sessions are scheduled approximately three times per week. Binge foods are divided into three types (large meals, "junk food," and pasta dishes), and each type of food is targeted for six sessions. Clients purchase and bring food to the sessions and are instructed to eat until a "strong urge to vomit" occurs. The therapist stays in session with the client until the urge to vomit is under control and requests that the client avoid vomiting for at least $2\frac{1}{2}$ hours after the session to allow digestion of the food that is eaten.

Clinical Use of Individual ERP

This method of treatment, as mentioned previously, has the potential for very significant inroads into bulimic behavior in a relatively short period of time. In one study, four out of five subjects significantly eliminated or reduced bingeing and purging within 9–10 weeks (Leitenberg *et al.*, 1984). In my own clinical experience, I have had similar success. Mastery of the urges to binge and vomit in turn appears to have very positive effects on self-esteem and general sense of well-being. Clients almost unanimously report that the most helpful aspect of this treatment is the actual in-session experience of eating "forbidden" foods and discovering that, thereafter, anxiety levels do eventually decrease to a manageable level.

While ERP is probably one of the most powerful treatments available for individuals with bulimia nervosa, there are some difficulties that may be encountered, particularly for the private practitioner or therapist functioning within a clinic or outpatient hospital setting.

Cost

Since most therapists bill by the treatment hour, the cost of these sessions can be high. Six therapy hours per week (three sessions per week, 2 hours per session) are needed for 6 weeks of the treatment phase of ERP. Of course, the total cost is probably far less than the cost of long-term psychotherapy. However, this type of treatment does require a large outlay of money in a short period of time, which for many clients is not possible, especially if their financial situation has been adversely affected by their disorder.

Time

This type of treatment requires a large quantity of both therapist and client time. If done on an individual basis, up to 6 hours of time per week for 6 weeks must be allotted, preferably around lunch or dinner time. This can be impractical for many therapists. Further, to have two clients in individual ERP simultaneously means that a therapist must find 12 hours of therapy time per week for these procedures, which is not often possible unless one's case load is very low. Likewise, many working clients may find it difficult to free up the amount of time required.

Repetitiveness

In my experience, this type of session can be repetitive for the therapist who specializes in eating disorders and has many clients with bulimia nervosa in active treatment. While therapist interest level should not be the primary factor in treatment decisions, it is important since therapist enthusiasm and energy undoubtedly affect treatment outcome.

Modifications to the Technique of Individual ERP

For psychotherapists with more traditionally structured practices who contract with bulimic clients to work on problematic areas of behavior other than the bulimia, modified use of ERP may be helpful.

As one possibility, ERP can be used on an as-needed basis with individuals who are making progress normalizing eating without the use of ERP. Certain types of food (e.g., sweets) or situations (e.g., eating out) may present as roadblocks to continued progress in treatment. It is possible to schedule, for example, three ERP sessions just for a particular stuck point. These sessions, in combination with homework assignments of continued practice, may be sufficient. As an example, for one of my clients, eating any dessert led to purging behavior even though considerable progress had been made with other types of food. We agreed that she would bring sweets to three sequential sessions (which we temporarily lengthened to 2 hours) and eat these until she had a strong urge to vomit. After those sessions, she felt less anxious about eating sweets because she realized both that she did not have to eat a huge portion of sweets to be satisfied and that her anxiety about the food did drop within an hour or so. She agreed to continue practice at home by eating sweets twice a week for a month with the agreement that she would not purge afterwards.

ERP sessions can also be used on an as-needed basis to practice certain types of meals. For some bulimic individuals, the problem might not be the types of foods eaten but rather the type of meal. They often make rules that certain meals are forbidden or that between-meal snacks are never allowed. Thus, breakfast, lunch, or dinner sessions may be scheduled, or between-meal snacks may be practiced in sessions.

Another variation in the ERP technique is for the therapist to eat with the client. This provides modeling of appropriate eating. This can be especially helpful if the therapist is the same sex as the client. The structured eating can be done in a restaurant or cafeteria as well as in the office. Whether or not a therapist uses this variation depends largely on the comfort of the therapist in eating with the client as well as the practicality of scheduling sessions near mealtimes and the availability of food facilities.

Where ERP is possible only on a limited basis (e.g., once a week) or not at all, one option is to train a family member, spouse, or friend to work with the client in homework ERP sessions. This individual should have nondisordered eating habits and be a stable, positive influence in the client's life. Of course, the client must also be willing to involve this person in the treatment. At least one session with both the client and the support individual is necessary for training in the techniques to be used.

GROUP EXPOSURE PLUS RESPONSE PREVENTION

A cost-effective alternative to individual ERP or other individual in-session structured eating is the use of ERP in a group. Some of the impracticalities of doing individual ERP in an outpatient clinic situation originally forced me to consider using ERP in a group. At that time, no model for this existed, so a structure for group ERP was developed and then made the subject of a research study (Hoage & Gray, 1984) described below.

The Technique of Group ERP

The challenge in developing a model for group ERP was to create a method of group eating that would give a similar effect to individual ERP. In a pilot study, each group member was asked to bring her own food to the sessions. This became problematic because, in some instances, members failed to bring the appropriate food; in others, members would arrive without any food at all and want to purchase it on group time. We realized then that group ERP might be somewhat more anxiety producing than individual ERP because it required public eating. Individuals with bulimia nervosa do not feel comfortable eating in front of other people and compare themselves in terms of body size, portion size, type of food, etc.

We decided on a group schedule of foods, with most of the food provided by the group leaders. This had the advantage of everyone eating the same food, with greater control by the leaders over the use of appropriate foods. A sample food schedule is shown below.

Week 1
    Session 1: Snack* (low anxiety level)
    Session 2: Bread and butter
Week 2
    Session 3: Sandwich
    Session 4: Sandwich
Week 3
    Session 5: Pizza
    Session 6: Pizza
Week 4
    Session 7: Fast food
    Session 8: Fast food
Week 5
    Session 9: Sandwich* and potato chips with dip
    Session 10: Sandwich* and buttered popcorn
Week 6
    Session 11: Sandwich* plus dessert
    Session 12: Sandwich* plus dessert
(*Provided by participants)

As with individual ERP, at each session, members are asked to eat until they experience a strong urge to vomit. In order to define this for the participants, we ask each individual to imagine a subjective anxiety scale (subjective units of distress, SUDs) of 0 through 100, where 0 is defined as no anxiety at all about the food being eaten and 100 is defined as as much anxiety as could possibly be imagined about that food. Then we ask the participants to eat to 75 on that scale, a point at which we believe most bulimic individuals would choose to purge. The one exception to this expectation is during the first session, when group members are asked only to eat a snack that they know will produce little anxiety. This is done because we have found that anxiety levels are often very high during the first session due to meeting the group and the prospect of public eating.

Group meetings are scheduled at dinner time and are 2 hours in length so that adequate time is available for the urge to vomit to decrease. As with individual ERP, members are asked to abstain from vomiting for at least $2\frac{1}{2}$ hours after the session. Other rules or guidelines for the group include the following:

1. Members agree not to leave the group therapy room during sessions to go to the bathroom unless they take along an escort. This is a rule that evolved from the pilot study, and we have found that this rule greatly alleviates group anxiety.
2. Participants agree to pay for all sessions whether or not they attend.
3. Smoking is not allowed.
4. Attendance at all sessions is strongly encouraged.

Individuals who know in advance that they will not be able to attend all sessions are asked to wait for a later group.

Most groups have had between four and eight members. Groups larger than eight do not appear to allow sufficient attention to individual group members.

Additional Group Treatment Components

In order to make group ERP as effective as possible, other cognitive and behavioral components were added. Group eating takes 30–40 minutes at the beginning of the group. The remainder of the group is devoted to the other interventions listed below.

Self-Monitoring

Throughout the 6-week group, members are asked to monitor food and liquid intake, binge and/or purge episodes, and thoughts and feelings associated with those episodes. Self-monitoring forms, filled out for a sample client, can be seen in Figures 4-1 and 4-2.

Education

Several sessions at the beginning of the group are devoted to education about nutritional principles with special attention to normalizing the eating pattern. A minimum of three meals a day using healthy but nondietetic foods is encouraged. Appropriate weight control techniques are emphasized, including noncompulsive exercise. In addition, members are educated about body changes that might occur during recovery from bulimia nervosa such as rehydration, temporary bloating or gastrointestinal discomfort, and weight normalization.

Cognitive Restructuring

As has been noted (Crisp, 1967; Fairburn, 1985; Russell, 1979), individuals with bulimia nervosa have dysfunctional thoughts about their bodies,

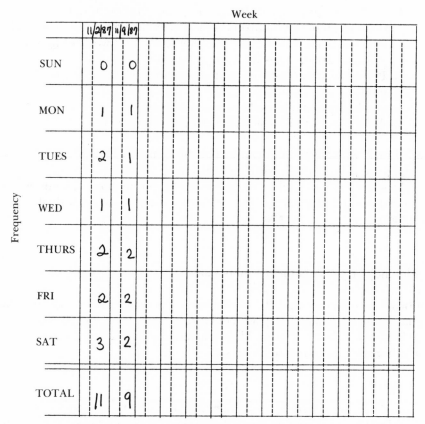

Figure 4-1. Sample record of binge–purge episodes.

their weight, and, often, themselves. These thoughts appear to play an important role in perpetuating bulimic behavior, both by depressing or demoralizing the individual so that energy to change is decreased and by sanctioning purging. Examples of typical negative thinking follow:

Body. "Until I get my body just right, I can't be happy." "Having a beautiful body is the only way a man will ever love me." "I'm a fat pig."

Weight and purging. "I've blown it by overeating and I can't afford to gain weight, so I'll purge." "Since I'm going to purge anyway, I might as well eat as much as I can before I do."

Self. "I have no self-control." "I hate myself."

The middle four sessions of the group are spent teaching participants to monitor their thoughts and then to restructure those that are dysfunctional. In the group sessions, restructuring exercises are sometimes done by the group as a whole; additional homework assignments are done individually.

Problem Solving

The last four to five sessions focus on helping participants identify their most difficult situations or time periods with respect to bingeing and purging. These situations are broken down into identifiable components, then alternative behavioral solutions to problems are discussed. For example, a client who binges most days while fixing dinner for her family might identify that this is a difficult time because she is hungry, she feels hassled by her kids, and she is usually worrying about all the things she meant to do that day but did not achieve. These are three specific problems that can then be addressed by problem-solving techniques.

Date	Food & Drink/Amount Meal (M), Snack (S), or Binge (B)	P?	Mood	Thoughts	Comments
11/16	Bowl of cereal with banana Coffee – 1 Cup (M)	no	Good		
	1 C Chicken soup 2 lemon candies Diet Coke – 16 oz. (M)	no			Did not feel satisfied
	2 slices cake (big) 1 bowl ice cream (B)	yes			I overdid it. – A birthday at the office.
	Pizza – 3 slices 2 beers Chips peanuts (B)	yes		Discouraged	Went out with people from the office.
	Yogurt, low-fat (S) Diet gingerale – 8 oz.	no		Really hungry before I went to bed.	

Figure 4-2. Sample record of food and liquid intake.

Results of Research on Group ERP

Eight bulimic women, vomiting a minimum of five times per week for at least a year, participated in the initial ERP group. This group met twice a week for a total of 12 sessions. At the end of the 6 weeks of treatment, highly significant reductions in bingeing and vomiting behaviors were reported by all but one subject, substantiated by significantly lower depression and bingeing scores. When contacted for follow-up at 6 months and 1 year after treatment, six of eight participants were averaging less than one binge–purge episode per week, one subject had relapsed, and one subject continued unchanged. A group of waiting list controls reported essentially no change in binge–purge frequency. A second ERP group of six bulimic women showed very similar results. ERP done in a group thus appears to be a viable alternative to individual ERP (Hoage & Gray, 1984).

Advantages of Group ERP

Using a group to do ERP provides all the usual advantages of group therapy (Yalom, 1975). Particularly helpful for many individuals with bulimia nervosa is the decrease in isolation that comes from being a part of a cohesive group. Support from others, and an opportunity to help others in return, appears to have significant positive effects. In addition, hope is drawn from seeing others improve, and there is a chance to get feedback about how one is perceived, both interpersonally and in terms of body image.

Furthermore, there are specific advantages to doing ERP in a group. First, in addition to the previously discussed aspects of group ERP being less expensive, time-consuming, and repetitive, this method facilitates comfort with eating in front of others. As mentioned previously, public eating is difficult for many individuals who have bulimia nervosa because they worry about how much they are eating compared with others. Thoughts about this can be elicited and can be a topic of group discussion and cognitive restructuring exercises.

Second, group ERP allows for modeling of appropriate eating behavior. In our groups, the therapists eat with the group members, and their task is to eat approximately normal portions of foods. Seeing others who are comfortable with reasonable portions of potential binge foods allows more anxious members to reconsider their internal rules about these foods.

Third, in contrast to many group therapy situations, between-session contact appears to be helpful for group members. Phone numbers are shared, and group members use each other for support and extra ERP practice. This also helps to reduce the isolation felt by many individuals with bulimia nervosa. Supportive contacts made in some groups have continued past the end of the group.

Modifications to the Techniques of Group ERP

Recently, I varied the structure of an ERP group by having the group meet formally once a week for 10 weeks (see Figure 4-3 for format). I had found that twice-weekly groups were impractical for some individuals, especially for those with time constraints or limited financial resources. However, because it seemed that reducing the number of ERP sessions below 12 might also reduce the effectiveness of the method, a contract was made with group members for them to practice one additional time each week between sessions. Members could choose to practice with another member of the group or with a friend or family member.

While advantageous in terms of time, this method did not seem to have the same degree of effectiveness as the twice-weekly group. Because the practice sessions took place at the sole initiation of the members, there were occasions when individuals avoided the practice, feeling anxious about it. Thus, some practice sessions never occurred. The momentum of a group

BULIMIA PSYCHOTHERAPY GROUP

Wednesday, 2/18/87–4/29/87

6:10 p.m.

Session #	Date	Food (SUDs)	Other
1	2/18	Snack *(you bring)* (50)	Overview of Program Record Keeping Food Budget Meal Stabilization & Effects of Deprivation Body Change with Recovery
2	2/25	Muffins/Croissants (75)	Eating Habit Control Nutrition Exercise
3	3/4	Sandwich (75)	Weight/Food Histories
4	3/18	Sandwich & Chips (75)	Cognitions #1
5	3/25	Pizza (75)	Cognitions #2
6	4/1	Pizza (75)	Cognitions #3
7	4/8	Sandwich *(you bring)* & Buttered Popcorn (75)	Alternatives to Bingeing/Problem Solving
8	4/15	Sandwich *(you bring)* & Dessert (75)	Alternatives to Bingeing/ Problem Solving
9	4/22	Sandwich *(you bring)* & Dessert (75)	Alternatives to Bingeing/ Problem Solving
10	4/29	Eat Out (75)	Wrap-up

Figure 4-3. Schedule for ten-session bulimia nervosa psychotherapy group. SUDs = subjective units of distress.

meeting twice a week instead of once may also be important. However, since this difference in methodology has not been the subject of a formal research study, it is difficult to know what the important factors are. Also, many individuals in the 10-session group did reduce bingeing and purging very significantly, some to zero episodes per week.

Another variation my colleagues and I have tried is to use group eating in the context of ongoing support groups. These support groups were open to all individuals in a hospital-based outpatient eating-disorders clinic so the groups were heterogeneous. Typically, the groups were predominantly made up of individuals with bulimia nervosa; however, some members were of a different subtype, such as laxative abusers or bingers who did not purge. Each session was 1½ hours in length with the first 30 minutes devoted to eating. Groups were held close to dinner time; members agreed in advance to bring typical dinner food and, if possible, food that might arouse some anxiety for them. "Dietetic" dinners (e.g., yogurt or a plain salad) were discouraged. Group rules included an agreement not to purge for 2½ hours after the group. These groups were led by either one or two therapists and generally had no more than six to eight members. The content of the group discussion after the food was eaten was determined by group members.

The goals of this type of support group are to decrease the isolation of individuals with eating disorders and to allow the practice of changed eating behavior in a somewhat public setting. This type of group can be a helpful adjunct in a clinical setting that primarily does individual psychotherapy. It has the additional advantage that it can be used with a group that is heterogeneous in its diagnostic composition. However, this type of group is not a substitute for either group or individual ERP since ERP procedures are not closely followed.

GENERAL TREATMENT ISSUES

As we have come to realize, individuals who present themselves for treatment for bulimia nervosa are a diverse group. It was hoped at first that one type of treatment might help all individuals with this problem; however, it is now clear that diagnostic and treatment-responsive subgroups exist (Ford, 1985; Johnson & Connors, 1986).

Diagnostic and Related Issues

The most amenable individual for ERP appears to be someone whose bulimic behavior involves bingeing followed by vomiting, who is dependable and highly motivated, whose weight is roughly in the normal range, and who can tolerate the possibility of a weight gain in the service of recovery. For those who do not fall into this category, preparatory individual psychotherapy may be necessary. Readiness is an important factor that must not be underestimated.

Other disorders concurrent with the bulimia nervosa can affect a client's ability to cooperate with and benefit from ERP. Examples include alcohol or drug use or abuse; severe depression; and characteristics associated with a borderline personality disorder such as impulsivity, a chaotic life situation, and laxative or diuretic abuse.

For clients who are alcoholic, considerable work may be necessary before treatment of the bulimic symptomatology can be attempted. It is not advisable to attempt ERP with someone who uses alcohol in an abusive or addictive fashion. Rather, any alcohol problem should have primacy in terms of attention. This is in part because alcohol appears to potentiate bulimic symptoms by releasing the inhibitions to binge behavior. Thus, becoming sober may in itself reduce the frequency of bingeing and purging. In addition, alcohol abusers tend not to be as dependable or responsible as is necessary for participation in this type of treatment.

For the severely depressed individual, overall motivation and energy level are low. Since ERP requires both motivation and energy, ERP treatment should be postponed until the depression is lessened by psychotherapy, antidepressant medication, or, in severe cases, hospitalization.

For those individuals who have a borderline personality disorder, impulsiveness and lifestyle chaos may undermine initial treatment efforts. This type of individual is usually quite demanding of attention and thus is probably best seen in individual psychotherapy until greater stability is achieved. At that point, individual or group ERP may be helpful.

ERP was developed specifically to treat individuals who binge and then purge by vomiting. However, many individuals with bulimia nervosa use other or additional methods of purging. Some use laxatives, diuretics, diet pills, enemas, compulsive exercise, or fasting instead of, or in addition to, vomiting. An important question is whether these individuals can be treated with ERP. So far I have tried ERP with individuals whose primary method of purging is vomiting if other methods are used only occasionally. I have not used ERP with individuals who use diuretics or laxatives daily. For a laxative or diuretic abuser, the actual ingestion of the pills usually occurs many hours after a perceived binge, so the time sequence is very different from bingeing and vomiting. In addition, if an individual who uses a high daily dose of laxatives or diuretics stops abruptly, withdrawal effects can be so frightening or severe as to warrant hospitalization. This is not usually true for vomiting.

For individuals who binge and then compulsively exercise or fast, ERP may be helpful if the individual will agree to avoid these behaviors before ERP sessions. I have put a few of these individuals into ERP groups with reasonable success. However, purging and nonpurging clients sometimes have difficulty perceiving themselves as similar in the seriousness of their problems. This sometimes results in the nonpurgers participating less fully in the group.

Some individuals who participate in ERP treatment for bulimia nervosa may be in concurrent treatment with antidepressant or other medication. The only problem with this situation, in my experience, is that it is difficult for the client (and the therapist) to decide whether to attribute the reduction in symptoms to the medication or to the ERP techniques. An attribution that the client's own work in treatment is responsible for success is desirable because it motivates the client to use ERP techniques after treatment ends. This is less of a problem if it is clear that the antidepressant medication is being given primarily to treat depression rather than binge–purge behavior. However, for those clients who are being treated with antidepressants or other medication on a trial basis, it may be helpful to wait to initiate ERP until after the medication trials are either completed or a satisfactory dosage is found and sustained over a period of months.

Combining Therapies

Individuals being seen in long-term individual psychotherapy by other psychotherapists are often referred for either individual or group ERP. These individuals should be screened for readiness using the guidelines outlined earlier in this chapter. One or two individual preparatory sessions are important to explain the rationale for ERP treatment and to answer questions. Occasional consultation with the referring psychotherapist during ERP treatment is important to coordinate efforts and insure that any client problems with ERP techniques are openly addressed.

Group versus Individual ERP

One important consideration is whether group or individual ERP is ever contraindicated. In my experience, if someone seems appropriate for ERP, there are two factors that might suggest individual rather than group treatment. The first is the individual's preference. Some individuals—usually not many—have a strong aversion to anyone else knowing about their problem. While many individuals are initially reluctant to consider group, after some discussion of their concerns they quickly express a willingness to give it a try. However, others are adamant that they want no one else to know about their disorder or that they would feel too embarrassed to participate in a group. These individuals should be seen individually. In the ERP groups I have run, only one individual was so uncomfortable with a group that she requested to change her treatment after the first session.

Another situation in which individual treatment is indicated is when the client is extremely needy in terms of attention. To put such a person into a group is to risk having her either dominate the group or drop out.

CASE STUDY

As mentioned previously, for some clients, bulimia nervosa is only one of several difficulties for which they seek treatment. In such cases it may be inadvisable to put the client into an ERP group until some individual work has been done and treatment needs are prioritized. In one case, a 35-year-old married housewife and mother of three sought treatment not only for her bulimia nervosa but also for marital difficulties and career uncertainties. Initial individual treatment focused on her bingeing and vomiting behavior and on pressing marital problems. It was decided that in addition to her individual psychotherapy, she and her husband would attend sessions on a regular basis to work out the marital issues. (Some therapists may feel more comfortable referring this part of the therapy to another therapist who specializes in marital issues.) After about 5 months of treatment, significant progress had been made on the marital concerns. In addition, vomiting had been reduced from approximately 14 times per week to eight times per week as the result of nutritional education, monitoring of food intake, and some problem-solving. At this point, the client was interested in focusing more directly on reducing binge–purge behavior and joined an ERP group. Individual and marital psychotherapy were suspended during this time since the group met twice weekly and the client had both time and financial constraints. During the 6-week ERP period, she further reduced her vomiting to an average of two times per week. After the group was over, she resumed weekly individual sessions and occasional marital sessions for 8 more months, reducing purging to less than one episode per month, firming up gains made in marital work, and deciding on a career plan for when her children were in school. Thus, ERP was a part of a multifaceted treatment approach.

CONCLUSION

Exposure plus response prevention and related structured eating techniques can be powerful tools in the treatment of bulimia nervosa. Eating difficulties are at the heart of the symptom cluster associated with bulimia nervosa, and ERP and related techniques address bingeing and purging behaviors directly and with significant effect. The power of these techniques is largely derived, I believe, from the evocation in the session of the intense feelings and thoughts about food and body that drive individuals to binge and purge. ERP and adjunctive behavioral strategies then assist individuals in managing and alleviating anxiety, confronting negative thoughts, and developing stronger problem-solving skills. Therapist preferences, as well as financial and time considerations, can determine whether group or individual ERP is utilized, although, in the ideal world, individual ERP may be preferable because it can be tailored to specific client needs. It is extremely important to screen potential participants carefully to determine readiness for ERP treatment. It is also important to assess other psychological difficulties that may need to be treated prior to or concurrently with the bulimia nervosa. ERP can be integrated into long-term treatment at a point when motivation to reduce bingeing and purging is high and when other difficulties are under reasonable control.

More research is needed on this promising treatment approach, especially as to whether group ERP is as powerful as individual ERP. It is also important for us to understand more about which types of clients with bulimia nervosa profit the most from this treatment and which are not responsive. I hope that other practitioners will continue to use and refine these versatile and helpful techniques.

REFERENCES

Crisp, A. H. (1967). The possible significance of some behavioral correlates of weight and carbohydrate intake. *Journal of Psychosomatic Research, 11,* 117–131.

Fairburn, C. G. (1985). Cognitive-behavioral treatment for bulimia. In D. M. Garner & P. E. Garfinkel (Eds.), *Handbook of psychotherapy for anorexia nervosa and bulimia* (pp. 160–192). New York: Guilford Press.

Foa, E. B., & Goldstein, A. (1978). Continuous exposure and complete response prevention in the treatment of obsessive–compulsive neurosis. *Behavior Therapy, 9,* 821–829.

Ford, K. A. (1985). *The heterogeneity of bulimia.* Unpublished doctoral dissertation, The American University, Washington, DC.

Herman, C. P., & Polivy, J. (1980). Restrained eating. In A. S. Stunkard (Ed.), *Obesity* (pp. 208–225). Philadelphia: W. B. Saunders.

Hoage, C. M., & Gray, J. J. (1984, November). *Exposure with response prevention in the treatment of bulimia in a group.* Paper presented at the Association for the Advancement of Behavior Therapy Convention, Philadelphia.

Hudson, J. I., Laffer, P. S., & Pope, H. G. (1982). Bulimia related to affective disorder by family and response to dexamethasone suppression test. *American Journal of Psychiatry, 139,* 685–687.

Hudson, J. I., Pope, H. G., Jonas, J. M., & Yurgelun-Todd, D. (1983). Family history study of anorexia nervosa and bulimia. *British Journal of Psychiatry, 142,* 428–429.

Johnson, C., & Connors, M. (1986). *The etiology and treatment of bulimia nervosa.* New York: Basic Books.

Leitenberg, H., Gross, T., Peterson, T., and Rosen, T. C. (1984). Analysis of an anxiety model and the process of change during exposure plus response prevention treatment of bulimia nervosa. *Behavior Therapy, 15,* 3–20.

Rosen, J. C., & Leitenberg, H. (1982). Bulimia nervosa: Treatment with exposure and response prevention. *Behavior Therapy, 13,* 117–124.

Rosen, J. C., & Leitenberg, H. (1985). Exposure plus response prevention treatment of bulimia. In D. M. Garner & P. E. Garfinkel (Eds.), *Handbook of psychotherapy for anorexia nervosa and bulimia* (pp. 193–209). New York: Guilford Press.

Russell, G. F. M. (1979). Bulimia nervosa: An ominous variant of anorexia nervosa. *Psychological Medicine, 9,* 429–448.

Yalom, I. D. (1975). *The theory and practice of group psychotherapy* (2nd ed.). New York: Basic Books.

5

Family Sculpting with Bulimic Families

Maria P. P. Root

Developmentally, bulimia is a disorder in which the individual does not establish an age-appropriate degree of psychological independence from her family-of-origin (Root, Fallon, & Friedrich, 1986). The reason for this difficulty is complex and usually determined by a combination of individual, social, and familial factors. The developmental impasse within the family system is characterized by suppressed affect, particularly anger, grief, and dependence, emotions that may conflict with cultural and familial prescriptions of ideal behavior.

For many bulimics, these feelings are unresolved in the family-of-origin. As an individual approaches the age of leaving home, feelings of anger, loss, and dependence are heightened. In the bulimic family, a combination of mixed messages about leaving home, proscriptions against the expression of intense feelings, and difficulty resolving conflict create a developmental impasse; the bulimic cannot move into young adulthood as she remains tied to her family by needing their approval, acceptance, and permission to be expressive. Their developmental impasse is innocently built by repeated comments such as "forget the past," "look at the bright side," "other people have it worse," "do as I say, not as I do," "nobody will love you like we do," "she's been the perfect child," or "kids grow up too fast these days."

In this chapter, family sculpting, an experiential technique derived from a combination of Satir's work, psychodrama, and Perls's gestalt therapy, is discussed. Family sculpting provides a "show me" versus "tell me" intervention to heighten affect and facilitate its expression. The use of family sculpting allows affective expression at a nonverbal level, the level to which one attends if there is any incongruence between verbal and nonverbal communication (Watzlawick, Beavin, & Jackson, 1967). Because family sculpting's power as an intervention derives from its nonverbal nature, vignettes and case studies are emphasized in this chapter to illustrate how the technique may be used and its effect upon clients. Consequently, the description of technique is relatively brief compared with the amount of illustrative case material.

BULIMIC FAMILY SYSTEMS

Bulimia is a developmental disorder that expresses the dysfunctional interaction among individual qualities, social proscriptions, family tradition, and family translation of social proscriptions. The process of "growing up" has become increasingly complicated as it necessitates an integration and resolution of numerous social, intellectual, and technological pressures on adolescents and young adults—the results of our quickly evolving technological society. Consequently, parents have an increasingly difficult role in steering their children through the tasks necessary to be psychologically independent from them. The teenagers and young adults, like their parents, are unable to strike a functional balance between autonomy and closeness in their relationships. Thus, while the bulimic is the symptomatic member, or identified patient, in the family, there is a conceptual assumption that, in a broader context, her symptoms indicate the family's difficulty in negotiating family life cycle stages (Root *et al.*, 1986). The symptoms serve a homeostatic function in that the family continues in familiar patterns. Thus, families in which bulimia originates are referred to as "eating-disordered families."

Empirical studies of eating-disordered families demonstrate that heterogeneity in these environments is the rule rather than the exception (Kog, Vandereycken, & Vertommen, 1985; Strober, 1981; Strober & Humphrey, 1987), supporting the perspective that bulimia is multidetermined and complex (Garfinkel & Garner, 1982). Fallon and Root (1986) and Root *et al.* (1986) introduced and described three different family environments that organize the heterogeneity observed among bulimics around the difficulties they have in promoting psychological independence: "the Perfect Family," "the Overprotective Family," and "the Chaotic Family." These family types are briefly described in their pure forms, but in clinical practice they often appear in recognizable combinations such as "the Perfect–Overprotective Family," "the Perfect–Chaotic Family," and "the Overprotective–Chaotic Family."

The Perfect Family

The Perfect Family is similar to the idealized all-American family and embodies many positive qualities. The family is usually intact. The children feel loved and generally report a closeness to the family. The dysfunction of the family is noted most in its prohibition of negative feelings, minimization of interpersonal problems, and promotion of fairy-tale endings to these problems. Achievement is valued highly; for young women, qualities to achieve success may be in direct conflict with traditional female gender roles, which are also highly valued socially and familially. Upon closer inspection, many Perfect Families' closeness is a sign of enmeshment or stifling of individuality, which threatens the family's identity. An imbalance between autonomy and closeness prevents the teenager from moving into adulthood.

The Overprotective Family

The Overprotective Family also provides a positive environment, at least in early childhood. The most positive quality about this family type is the safe and secure physical and psychological environment it provides for the young child. The major dysfunction associated with this family type lies in the parents' inability to change the rules for independent behavior in a timely, age-appropriate manner to support the child's need for increased autonomy as she moves into adolescence. These families do so much in providing for their children that the children feel indebted and guilty for being angry and wanting to grow up. With too few opportunities to learn by trial and error, children from overprotective families leave prematurely at any age, feeling incompetent and ill-equipped to deal with the world.

The Chaotic Family

The Chaotic Family is more indigenous to bulimic than anorexic families. Unlike the Perfect and Overprotective Families, it is difficult to appreciate the positive influence of this family environment on a child's growth. This family is characterized by inconsistent rules, explosiveness, and multiple problems among its members. The family environment encourages a precocity that lacks role models for limit setting, resulting in an inconsistent, changeable balance between autonomy and closeness that severely interferes with the development of trust in self and others.

Similarities and Differences

There are similarities across the three family types, but they manifest themselves at different times in development and with different content.

For instance, individuation is impeded across all family types, whether it be by the uniformity sought by the Perfect Family, the protectiveness of the Overprotective Family, or the lack of consistency in the Chaotic Family.

These family structures become rigidly closed systems to outsiders (individuals without blood ties and or different from them) when their rules of functioning are threatened (which creates tremendous problems in starting new families). The Perfect Family shuts strangers out both by exceedingly high and rigid expectations and an intolerance for differentness. The Overprotective Family has an implicit assumption that no one is good enough for their child. The Chaotic Family's internal organization is marked by an inconsistent rules structure. This inconsistency allows the family to create convenient rules to enable them to exclude anyone who threatens them. The developmental periods during which this closed quality emerges may start at birth within the Chaotic Family, emerge in mid-childhood within the Overprotective Family, and emerge in mid-adolescence within the Perfect Family.

Across the three family types, there is an emphasis on food and/or appearance (Johnson & Flach, 1985; Schwartz, Barrett, & Saba, 1984). This emphasis may be what determines the appearance of bulimic symptoms rather than other psychosomatic symptoms such as asthma or other gastrointestinal problems.

Finally, common to bulimic families is an incongruence between nonverbal and verbal communication around feelings toward one another, especially anger, grief, and dependency. The way in which the bulimic family isolates or excludes either a family member or an outsider is often nonverbal. The incongruence between verbal and nonverbal communication impedes the bulimic's trust in her perceptions and feelings; repeated experiences lead to a fragile sense of identity and self-esteem.

The three bulimic family types described above also share dysfunctional qualities associated with psychosomatic families (Minuchin, Rosman, & Baker, 1978) and alcoholic families (Elkin, 1984; Stanton & Todd, 1982). All of these families are typically rigid, enmeshed, and overprotective; also, they have difficulty resolving conflict and often pull children into the middle of marital conflict (triangulation; Minuchin et al., 1978). Parents may be inappropriately dependent on their children. In Perfect Families, there may be too much dependence on children to affirm their parents' identities. In Overprotective Families, there may be a psychological dependence on the child for companionship. In Chaotic Families, there is often a physical dependence as well as an emotional dependence on the child for responsibilities that may include caretaking of parents who have multiple social and occupational problems. All forms of dependency make it difficult for the individual to have permission to be psychologically independent, a necessary internal condition for successfully leaving home.

The dysfunction associated with bulimic families are significant enough to derail the family's ability to launch their child into psychological independence (Root et al., 1986). The therapist, then, is challenged to help the family allow their child to grow up. The combination of three of the dysfunctional patterns can render traditional verbal therapeutic interventions ineffective: (1) the conflict between verbal and nonverbal communication in bulimic families; (2) the closed nature of the family system when it is threatened; and (3) the family's ability to appear to function better than it actually does.

FAMILY SCULPTING

Family sculpting is a powerful, nonverbal intervention that can circumvent the impasse outlined above (Duhl, Kantor, & Duhl, 1973). It allows the therapist as well as the family and/or clients to discover their feelings, understand their conflict, and validate the tension the bulimic responds to within the family system. Because it is a nonverbal technique, how and when to use family sculpting is shown below through case material and subsequent interpretation. In effect, the elucidation of technique to the reader may unfold in a similar way as it does to family members who are asked to do the sculpture, react, and verbally process their experiences.

Origins

Family sculpting is an intervention that has origins in at least three traditions; the interventions derived from these traditions employ physical movement to discover feelings and highlight nonverbal communication. Virginia Satir, the first prominent woman associated with the family therapy movement, developed nonverbal communication games with families to encourage members to explore their positions of relating to one another (Satir, 1964, 1972). She choreographed scripts and postures to highlight both verbal and nonverbal communication. From these interactions, people accessed their feelings and defined new ways of relating directly and respectfully.

Family sculpting often looks like the translation of gestalt therapy and interventions developed by Fritz Perls (Perls, 1969, 1976) into a family therapy context. While gestalt therapy conceptually originates as an intrapsychically based theory, the interventions are consistent with system-based theories. Gestures, postures, and physical actions are exaggerated, repeated, or developed to help individuals express affect and access memories that are ordinarily preconscious.

Lastly, psychodrama (Moreno, 1946) is a technique most commonly used in a group context. People can simultaneously act out feelings or themes. From these physical dramas emerge old memories and feelings which are subsequently processed.

Rationale

All three types of intervention described above share certain assumptions essential for understanding *how* family sculpting can support traditional verbal therapy for family-of-origin work with bulimics. First, people communicate powerfully in nonverbal ways. Second, this communication is often preconscious. Third, because we are taught to process and subsequently defend ourselves verbally and rationally, we are less ridgidly defended at the level of nonverbal communications. We may nonverbally express feelings of which we are otherwise unaware.

There are two levels at which change occurs within the bulimic family system. There is first-order change, which represents at least a superficial change. For example, a client significantly decreases her bingeing and purging behavior subsequent to establishing a consistent pattern of eating meals; a client stops bingeing and purging when she starts a new romantic relationship; or a family follows recommendations to have family meetings every other night to discuss concerns. All of these changes represent significant changes but, nevertheless, the therapist (and often the client or family) feels uncertain that the changes will last. This uncertainty by the therapist reflects the very nature of first-order change—it does seem to be significant change at the level that created the need for such a desperate symptom in the first place. The difficulty with bulimic families, especially the Perfect and Overprotective Families, is that they may leave therapy after first-order changes only to need help a few months later because of relapse. A worse and even more common scenario is that the bulimic relapses but does not tell the family because of guilt or fear of disappointing them.

Second-order change needs to occur for the therapist to have confidence that the core dysfunctional impasse, difficulty launching the child into adulthood, is resolved. For example, does the family give permission and acknowledgment, at both verbal and nonverbal levels, of anger, disappointment, and hurt? Can the bulimic be both close to her family and independent without feeling guilty or disloyal? Second-order change reflects a change in the basic unspoken rules of the family.

Goals

Family sculpting has three goals for bulimic family systems. One is to challenge the family's unspoken rules of relating and expressing feelings. The second *goal* is to provide a way to show and emphasize the conflict and tension in the family in a concrete, three-dimensional "picture." In working toward the latter goal, power differentials, age-inappropriate rules, dysfunctional alliances, and emotional cutoffs (disengagement) can be exposed and subsequently worked on. A nonverbal intervention such as family sculpting makes it difficult for family members or the bulimic client in a group context to use well-practiced defenses of rationalization and intellectualization. Finally, family sculpting can be used as a "corrective" technique toward a third goal, to explore new patterns of relating.

CREATING THE SCULPTURE

Family sculpting lends itself to use in both the outpatient and inpatient setting. The inpatient setting allows more intensive family work, and sculptures may frequently include family members. Subsequent or alternative sculptures may use staff members as parental figures and other family members. Use of staff members may help the patient and staff work out interactions that may be obstacles in their current treatment.

Directions

The therapist needs no props other than people; thus, the work can be done in either a family or group context. Furniture in the room may be rearranged and objects used to create a scenario. If there is a particular object around which much emotion is centered, the bulimic or family may be requested to bring it in to heighten the affect generated in the sculpture.

The author strongly feels that family sculpting is most useful when a three-generation history has been obtained, that is, the client and her siblings, the parents and their siblings, and the grandparents and their siblings. Such a history can be provided through sharing of family photographs or construction of a genogram, a schematic for recording family relationships (McGoldrick & Gerson, 1985). With such a history, one is able to interpret hints of alliances, enmeshment, triangulation, and emotional cutoffs more accurately.

In general, the therapist asks the client to create a sculpture with directives such as, "Show me a picture of how you feel in your family," "Show me how people relate to one another in your family," "Arrange people in order of their importance in the family," "Recreate a typical scene from your childhood of which you have a strong memory," or "Show me what happened last night." If the client is unable to start the sculpture with these directions, the therapist provide directions such as, "Show me where your mom is," "Is she standing, sitting, or lying down?" and "What expression does she have on her face?" The therapist can also help shape the sculpture by offering observations of feelings the client has shared about her family in the past. For example, "Your mom looks happy. I'm surprised because when you talk about her you suggest she's very unhappy." Additionally, the therapist can suggest themes, such as, "Show me how people relate when someone is angry (or hurting, or grieving)."

The therapist can also direct the client by suggesting she recreate periods in her life; for example, "Show me a scene from a period in your life when you were the happiest," "Show me how people interacted when your dad was drinking heavily," or "Show me how you felt in your family during holidays." No one talks during the sculpting except the therapist and client to create the sculpture, although participating members may ask what postures or facial expressions they should convey.

While the therapist may start out asking the client to create scenes from memory or childhood, he or she may choose to suggest the bulimic is reliving the scene by switching to current tense in grammar. For example, "Chris, create a typical family scene at home during your midteens. Tell Angela (a group member) to look at you like your father would look at you. [Transition.] What is the expression on your mother's face? What is your posture? What are you doing with your hands?"

Family Sculpting in Group Therapy

Family sculpting can be used in bulimic group therapy or general psychotherapy groups. The group context is an important environment for working out family issues because, as Yalom (1975) observes, it recapitulates the experience of being in a family.

In the group setting, the client who is going to create the sculpture supplies the group with descriptions of each family member, her feelings about them, and some brief history of her family, for example, through sharing her family genogram. The therapist, client, and group can collaborate on what might be useful to sculpt. The client then selects group members either by accepting volunteers or by soliciting their participation for the sculpture.

Within the group therapy context, feedback from members allows the client to validate and clarify feelings and issues. Group members may reduce a client's isolation in her family by understanding her feelings even though they were not understood or accepted by her family. Group members can provide feedback that clarifies dysfunctional alliances, rules, or threatening relationships in the family. For example, in one group after a client arranged her sculpture, her temporary stand-in remarked, "I feel creepy about how close your dad is standing to me." Subsequently, the client was able to talk about how uncomfortable she had been with her father's physical closeness. While she did not remember being sexually abused by him, she was able to recognize that her current reactions were guided by a fear that he might sexually approach her. She was able to get validation for her feelings and subsequently deal with her father's covert sexual advances and violation of her physical and psychological space. (In cases where clients have been physically assaulted or violated, the therapist helps negotiate physical boundaries and helps clients understand why being touched or touching others can feel uncomfortable and frightening.)

Family Sculpting with One's Family-of-Origin

Taking a family genogram, suggested earlier, allows the therapist to break the ice with the family and gain their trust. This is particularly important in closed systems because of their tendency to exclude outsiders when they are threatened. The time taken to obtain the family history allows the therapist to assess how much emotional intensity the family may be able to take without retreating from therapy.

The same type of instructions, questions, and directives for sculpting in a group therapy context are appropriate here. Anyone in the family can initiate the sculpture. It can be useful to have family members share their sculptures of the same scene. For example, it was enlightening for one family to discover how differently they reacted to each others' sculptures of a holiday meal around the family dining table. Subsequently, they started to understand how significant the nonverbal gestures, postures, and faces were to the bulimic family member.

Family sculpting is a significant corrective technique in the family-of-origin. Three particularly powerful corrections in bulimic families are removing children from the middle of marital scenes, teaching family members how to comfort one another physically, and defining generation-appropriate alliances.

I recommend against using family sculpting in families where sexual abuse has occurred or is occurring as it may elicit extremely intense emotional reactions in such a way that the victim re-experiences the trauma. The level of denial in some sexually abusive families may not allow therapeutic restructuring of relationships or processing of feelings.

Processing the Sculpture

Because of the bulimic family's tendency to withdraw from and/or have difficulty expressing intense emotions, it is very important that the affect and feelings be processed immediately at an emotional level. While the actual sculpture may take 2–10 minutes to create, an hour may be needed for everyone to share their reactions. Letters to family members, drawings, and/or face-to-face interactions may be appropriate follow-ups to the clients' experiences.

CASE STUDIES

In this section, case studies are offered as a way of demonstrating the rationale for using family sculpting, the goal of the intervention, and the subsequent impact. The case studies selected are typical of bulimic clients' dilemmas and issues. In the first four case studies, family sculpting was used in an outpatient group therapy context. The last two case studies were in a family therapy context.

Marcia

Grief is an emotion that many families, not only bulimic families, have difficulty expressing. The process of grieving, however, is that much more difficult for many bulimics and their families because it includes such intense emotions as sadness, despair, and anger. Death of a parent, particularly before one feels psychologically independent, is always difficult, as was the case for Marcia.

Marcia was 32 when she decided to obtain therapy for her bulimia. Marcia was in 10-week time-limited group therapy for bulimia and in individual therapy. Her goal in the group was to increase her awareness of her feelings and to decrease her bingeing. Every session, Marcia would cry while other people talked, but she was unable to express what she was feeling. In the fifth session, the therapist instructed her, "Marcia, tell us about feeling sad in your family." Marcia immediately started to sob and told the following story.

Marcia was the youngest of three children. She had a sister 4 years older and a brother 2 years older. Her sister seemed to be happy, but she and her brother were "silent messes." She described herself as "bingeing and purging her guts out" while her brother operated in a drugged stupor.

Marcia started bingeing and abusing laxatives when she was 18 years old, shortly after her mother was diagnosed with cancer. At age 20, Marcia was living away from the family while attending college. The family discovered she was bulimic during winter break of her sophomore year in college and insisted she enter individual therapy. Coming from a Perfect Family, Marcia complied with this request for 1 year, and she was able to decrease her binge–purge behavior to twice a month. Two months after she terminated therapy, her mother died. Six months after terminating

therapy her bulimia significantly increased to twice a week. It then gradually became an everyday occurrence over the next 10 years. Marcia, however, never let her family know that she had continued difficulty with her
bulimia. In fact, she tried hard to be the perfect daughter for her father.
She moved back to her hometown shortly after her mother's death and
visited her father at least twice a week.

The therapist directed Marcia to create a family sculpture to help her
understand her tears. Up to this point, despite prompting, Marcia was
not able to talk about feelings in telling her story to the group. The goal
of this intervention was to help Marcia connect her tears to grief and
perhaps guilt associated with her mother's death. The therapist instructed
Marcia, "Show us how your family is when you are together these days.
Choose someone to be your father, sister, and brother. Everyone give
Marcia room to create the scene."

Marcia directed her father to be a pleasant, sensitive man, with a sad
look deep in his eyes, but a proud look for his children. He was seated in
a chair. Next to him Marcia placed an empty chair for her mother, whom
she still felt was present in the family. She placed her brother standing
with his back to the family and her sister reaching out to Marcia, but
blocked by a chair. Marcia sat stiffly, smiling, with her hands clasped in
her lap next to her father. She stated that her posture depicted her efforts to be the perfect daughter.

Marcia was then directed to have another group member be her stand-
in so that she could look at her sculpture. As Marcia looked, she cried
silently but maintained a smile. She said, "It's so sad. . . . There's nothing
I can do to bring my mother back for my father. . . . He misses her so
much. He tells me I remind him so much of my mom. I try to be there
for him. But I resent it sometimes because I can't just be myself, whoever
that is. I have to be a saint . . . and here I am such a hypocrite. If he
only knew . . . [sobbing] I don't want to be perfect anymore. It's killing
me. I'm killing myself. I'm not going to do this anymore! . . . [guiltily]
but I feel so sad because I think Dad is going to be very sad. It might be
like Mom dying all over again." The therapist repeated, "Like mom dying
all over again?" Marcia nodded her head and started to cry louder: "It's
not fair; I wasn't ready for her to die. I didn't take it seriously. Maybe I
would have moved home if I knew she was really going to die." The therapist and group members then leaned in and gave Marcia the support of
physical closeness.

Group members shared their feelings with Marcia; some gave her
hugs. One member asked Marcia if she felt guilty because she was living
away from home when her mother died.

Within the following month and several individual sessions later, Marcia
disclosed to her family that she had been continuously bulimic since her
teens. She also shared that she had struggled with depression ever since

her mother was diagnosed with cancer. After this disclosure, Marcia felt and acted less depressed; she also stopped bingeing and purging. According to her individual therapist, Marcia subsequently cried much less in sessions and was able to recognize her feelings more readily.

The types of changes Marcia made suggest second-order changes. She challenged the rule that she must protect her father. She also discarded behaviors that trapped her in the perfect daughter role; she let her family know she was not functioning well. Also, she assumed a more appropriate generational alliance to her father as his daughter rather than surrogate wife and accepted emotional support from her oldest sister.

Jeannette

Jeannette, 25 years old, had just celebrated her third year of sobriety when she joined an 8-week bulimia treatment group. Growing up in a Chaotic Family, she was the second oldest of six children and designated caretaker of her mother. Her father was absent often during her childhood. Jeannette felt she was a parent to her younger siblings.

One and a half years after getting sober, Jeannette started bingeing and vomiting, behaviors with which she had experimented in high school. Her bulimia started within 1 month of being date-raped. She had gained 15 pounds since being raped. She was bingeing everyday. Jeannette had not considered that her bingeing was related to her feelings about being raped. When the therapist suggested that Jeannette's recovery work would need to include working through her rape, she commented, "The past is past. I can't change that and I'd rather not think about it."

During her first 4 weeks with the group, Jeannette had made many comments about her family being "messed up." During a subsequent session in which clients were sharing their experiences of growing up, Jeannette started to cry. She said she was sensitive and felt sad for other people but could not relate the sadness to herself. The therapist asked her to show the group what it was like growing up: "Jeannette, perhaps you could use members of the group to show us what it was like to grow up in your family. I'm confused at times because your family life seemed very painful, yet you smile when you talk about them. What was a typical family scene?"

The therapist used family sculpting as an intervention to help Jeannette understand her feelings in the group. Verbal feedback about the incongruence between Jeannette's smiling and talking angrily about her family had not had an impact on Jeannette's behavior. The goal of the sculpting was to clarify the conflict to which Jeannette was reacting and to connect her sadness to herself.

Jeannette first told the group that she grew up in a family in which her father, an alcoholic, could not emotionally commit himself to the family. He would enter and exit the family constellation in an unpredictable pattern. From this point, she needed little direction in the sculpture. The scene was vivid for her. She asked someone to be her father and positioned him with one foot out and one foot in the imaginary family room. Jeannette instructed all her siblings to smile. Her oldest sister sat smiling with her eyes closed and hands over her ears to shut out the yelling and noise in the family. Jeannette sat with an imaginary glass behind her and a wastebasket representing a grocery bag on her lap, which virtually hid her body from view. She positioned two other sisters with drinks in their hands and her fourth sister with a bottle of pills. She left her brother out of the sculpture to show his absence in the family. She instructed her mother to lie down behind her. Then she clasped her hands in her lap, then threw them up as she looked at the therapist with a pinched smile and tersely said, "That's it. That's how it was. Pretty, huh?" She started to get up, struggling to keep tears back. The therapist motioned her to stay in position, "Jeannette, not so fast. Let yourself feel . . . don't run."

Jeannette sat in her position for a silent minute during which her facial expression changed from sadness to anger. She said, "I'm not sad, I'm pissed! Look at this shit they left me with! No wonder I can't take care of myself. And I sit and feel sorry for everyone. How about me? I haven't had it so easy, but I just pretend to go on with a smile. [Crying.] This family is a mess and it's not my fault! My life is a mess. They're not going to help me." Jeannette sat with her arms and legs crossed. The therapist asked her if it would be okay for the group to care for her now. Would she let them in? She nodded yes. As group members stepped out of the scene and crouched and sat around her, she doubled over and started to cry. The therapist put her hand on Jeannette's back to remind her that she was not alone in the room since she had lost visual contact with the group.

Group members offered Jeanette support and validation for her anger. Two group members called her during the week to see how she was feeling. The next session, she returned reporting that she had not binged once during the week. She also offered the following observation: "I didn't realize I was so mad at my family. I don't understand how such a stupid, sorry, little thing you had me do last week would make me realize I was so mad. But I feel better." Jeannette decided to tell the group about her rape to see if they thought it might be related to her bulimia.

Jeannette's breakthrough was that she stepped out of the caretaker role and was able to be taken care of in the group. Sober from alcohol, she was able to be in the scenario and feel her feelings more than in the past. She expressed her anger as well as her sadness. The therapist asked the group why they thought Jeannette had not resorted to bulimia for the week. Several people felt that Jeannette was able to express anger and vulnerability without her "I-can-handle-it-by-myself" posture. Subsequently, it was easier for the group to give her support. The group felt she did not have to suppress these feelings through bingeing or release them through purging. Someone suggested that crying was a way of purging one's self of feelings.

Ann

Ann, a 28-year-old lawyer, was the youngest of three children and the first one in her family to graduate from college. She lived at home with her parents, an arrangement that she planned to change in the next few months. However, something had always seemed to come up in the previous 2 years which delayed her moving out. The discrepancy between her living arrangement and her profession and age suggested that Ann was from an Overprotective Family.

Ann had been raped by a son of a close family friend 9 months previous to seeking therapy. She had kept her experience a secret from everyone but her best friend. Ann reported that her parents had noticed, and were concerned, that she appeared despondent and run-down in the last 8 months. Ann explained her behavior to her parents as work stress.

Ann had had an eating disorder for 10 years which she had also kept secret from her parents. Her laxative abuse, which started when she was 18 and beginning college, had significantly decreased once she started working as a lawyer. However, after being raped, Ann relapsed into her worst bulimia ever. She was bingeing and purging several times a day, taking as many as 60–80 laxatives at a time. She felt her bulimia was contributing to her tiredness and interfering with her ability to concentrate on her work.

Ann participated in an 8-week group in which all the women had been physically victimized. She felt a need to talk about being raped with people she felt would understand and not judge her. She wanted to tell her parents because they were her best support but felt that they would be devastated. Several group members urged her to tell her parents. As one woman said, "You are not to blame for being raped. You need comfort; you need to be loved. Your parents have always protected you. They'll believe you and they'll protect you." Ann agreed.

The therapist felt that a family sculpture might help Ann challenge the rules of secrecy and protectiveness that were currently undermining her emotional and physical health. The goal of the sculpture was to make it easier for Ann to approach her parents so that she could get support from them.

The therapist then moved Ann into enacting a scene. "Ann, pick someone in the group to be your mother and someone to be your father.

Okay. How might your mother and father comfort each other when they feel sad and devastated to hear that you were raped?" Ann replied with tears, "Dad would hold Mom to comfort her." The therapist asked, "Ann, what are you doing while they are looking and feeling so sad?" Ann asked a group member to be her sister who lived across the country. She had her hold an imaginary telephone in her hand talking to Ann's parents. Her brother sat with his back to her. Ann placed herself in a doorway observing the scene. She expressed feeling lonely, guilty, and scared.

The therapist then directed Ann toward a corrective sculpture: "Make the scene like you want it to happen." Ann put herself between her mother and father and had them encircle her with their arms without touching her. Ann said that, in this position, she was safe and protected and little again, a time when her parents would not let anything or anyone hurt her. She cried for 20 minutes. After a couple of minutes some group members asked if they could hold her, to which Ann nodded yes.

This was the first time Ann had cried in front of anyone since she had been raped. She revealed that she had been afraid that, if she told her parents, she would not be able to stop crying. The group asked her how she thought her parents would react to her now. Ann thought that while they would be sad they would offer her comfort.

Ann told her parents about being raped that same evening after her group therapy. She reported that all three of them cried. Her mom held her for an hour that evening. Both parents, although they had difficulty talking to her about their feelings or asking how she was feeling, spent a lot of time with her that week. Her symptoms were significantly reduced to one binge episode in the following week with less than 20 laxatives.

While the Overprotective Family impedes growing up, in Ann's case her parents' protectiveness was exactly what she needed to start working through her rape. She needed to feel safe and loved. The relief of crying in the group enabled her to have less fear about losing total control with her parents, and she was able to start cleansing herself from the rape experience.

Jessica

Jessica was 15 years old when she started an 8-week group treatment program. She lived with her mother and stepfather and their two biological children who were much younger than her. At the time of this intervention, Jessica had been bingeing and purging five times a week for 9 months. Her mother had suspected she was bulimic and confronted her 2 weeks before the group started.

Whenever Jessica would mention her family, she would start talking very rapidly. On one occasion she started describing her family:

My family is so screwy—or maybe it's me. Gee, I feel so guilty saying this. Okay, this is my perspective and maybe I'm off. It all changed 6 years ago when I was nine and my mom divorced my dad and 6 months later married this guy who I can't stand. He thinks he knows everything. What's worse is that he's an alcohol and drug counselor so he's always telling me what my problem is and saying it's just an alcohol or drug problem . . . I could go on and on about him. Let's see . . . my mom and stepdad, Jerry, have two children, my little brother, Pip, who's 5—they got married because she was pregnant but she denies it, but I can count—and Rachel who's 3. They are just the loves of my life; they are just like my kids; I would die if anything happened to them. But lately, Pip has started to boss me around like my stepfather, Jerry. I can understand child abuse. Sometimes he makes me so mad I want to hurt him, but I know it's not him I want to hurt, but Jerry. Don't get all worried here. I know I won't hurt Pip. My mom doesn't do anything, she just bosses me around. She doesn't disagree with what Jerry says to me so I'm mad at her too. I don't know what she does all day because when I get home from school, I have to clean the house and take care of the kids. I hate it. I can't wait 'til summer when I go to stay with my dad. I miss the kids, but not them.

The therapist thought that a family sculpture might help Jessica slow down and feel what she was experiencing in the family. The goal of the intervention was to help her to clarify what she needed from her parents. Her rapid speech seemed to be a way of covering up how upset she was in her family. Jessica was asked, "Could you show us just what you were telling us? Use people in the group to be your family members. You can put them in any position." Jessica smiled and asked, "Any position?" Jessica did the sculpture quickly, talking rapidly and nervously. She stopped smiling as she directed group members into position. She proceeded to ask the group member representing her stepfather to stand on a chair with his arms crossed against his chest; she indicated this was his superior position looking down at her over his round stomach. She put her mom beside and beneath him. She instructed her mom to smile but to struggle with her smile. Pip and Rachel were asked to kneel so that they would be little. They were next to Jessica instead of their parents. Jessica affectionately had her arms around each of them. In order to help Jessica identify her feelings, the therapist asked her to remain silent. Several times she started to talk but was motioned to stop. The third time she started crying frustratedly, "It seems hopeless!" She was given room to cry.

The therapist then directed Jessica to place her father and stepmother in her sculpture. As she started to do this she stopped and rolled up into a ball, saying that she felt sick. She sat on the ground with her knees pulled up and her arms hugging them. She began crying and then sobbing, "I miss him so much. I don't know why he left and didn't take me. I'm so miserable. No one takes care of me anymore. . . . I wish I was

Rachel and had a sister to take care of me. No one takes cares of me."
The therapist directed group members to sit around Jessica on the floor
to create a protective circle for her. Many group members were also crying
and were in similar postures as Jessica. Group members shared feelings
of loneliness, isolation, and ambivalence about wanting to be nurtured.

Because of Jessica's age and feelings of hopelessness and abandonment, her biological mother and father were invited in for separate consultations with Jessica. This intervention put Jessica back in a clear position of being a child instead of a surrogate parent to her younger siblings.
It also required that her mother find a baby-sitter for her siblings for the
consultation. This was the first time they had used a sitter besides Jessica
in 4 years.

The results of the consultations were that her father and stepmother
expressed a sincere desire to have Jessica live with them. Jessica's biological mother agreed to this change on a trial basis. Whether Jessica did or
did not go to live with her father was not as important as her hearing that
he wanted her. Family therapy with her mother and stepfather continued.
Her caretaking responsibilities were reduced to age-appropriate levels. Her
bulimia was reduced to once every 2 or 3 weeks by the end of four sessions with her mother and stepfather and two sessions with her father
and stepmother.

FAMILY SCULPTING IN THE FAMILY-OF-ORIGIN

Clearly, verbal intervention is advocated for education, history taking, and
at least the initial exploration of family communication and relationships.
Traditional verbal intervention such as re-enactments used in structural
family therapy, confrontation, paraphrasing, and verbal contracts have
value in working with bulimic families. Family sculpting is introduced when
verbal change and insight occur without an accompanying change in affect or behavior. An example of how this intervention can be used is illustrated with a Perfect Family, the Cowarts, described below.

The Cowarts

The Cowart family consisted of both biological parents, Ward and June,
their oldest son Josh (age 19), and their bulimic daughter, Amy (17). In
ten family sessions, the family had been able to make some changes in
their communication skills, such as allowing family members to finish their
own sentences, decreasing the frequency of tension-relieving jokes, and
listening better. However, it remained a difficult task to get the family
members to interact with one another with affect. As a family they had a

rigid politeness, which traditional verbal interventions so far had only amplified. Encouragement by the therapist to look hurt, angry, or disappointed when such feelings were described, or appropriate, was protested by rationalizing, minimizing, or intellectualizing the feelings or situations. Confrontation or interpretation of this typical interaction was politely accepted but did not result in significant change in these interactional patterns.

One day in session, Amy told her family that she had recently been arrested for shoplifting food from the neighborhood grocery. The family approached this problem very intellectually, asking her when it happened, from what store, and what did she take. They asked her why the police had not notified them, and so forth. All their questions were reasonable, but there was no visible emotional response. The more questions they asked her, the angrier Amy answered them. They still showed no visible emotional reaction.

Given how other attempts to elicit affect from this family had been difficult, the therapist attempted a family sculpting intervention. The therapist felt Amy's anger was a response to the lack of emotional response from her parents; the goal of the intervention was to elicit an emotional reaction from Amy's parents to her shoplifting.

The therapist turned to Amy and observed that she was sounding angry. Amy shrugged her shoulders. Then the therapist said, "Perhaps you have imagined this scene, Amy. Instruct your father, mother, and brother to assume the positions and facial expressions you thought they would have in response to what you have done. Start with your father." Amy instructed her father to look both disappointed and worried because she had been dishonest, her mother to look hurt and worried because she had not asked for help, and her brother to look concerned. As she proceeded to instruct and position each family member (with arms crossed against their chests to suggest judgment and anger), she fought back tears. She started crying as she started to cross her brother's arms, and instead he hugged her. Her mother's eyes started to water. After a while, the therapist asked Amy's mother to hug Amy. Josh stepped back. The therapist asked the father if he knew what he wanted to do. He replied that he wanted to join in but was not sure how. The therapist directed him to put his arms around Amy and his wife. Josh was also motioned toward the group and asked to put his arms around anyone in the family. Everyone looked emotional for the first time in therapy.

Subsequently, Amy was able to talk about how isolated and inferior she felt in the family and how much she needed their acceptance, particularly her brother's. She felt that he was the perfect child, and she could not follow in his footsteps; she felt that Josh and her parents looked down on her. She also expressed missing the hugs she used to get as a child.

The Cowarts experienced a dramatic breakthrough, which had not occurred during traditional verbal and structural interventions. The sculpture provided them a corrective emotional experience so they would feel how to give physical comfort to one another. In subsequent processing of this experience, it was ironic that Ward and June had tried so hard to not be judgmental and that their blank response had been interpreted to Amy as judgment. The therapist also explored Amy's reasons for shoplifting. It appeared that Amy was asking for a different kind of help from her parents. She wanted her parents to set limits. She also wanted to be free from having to try to be a perfect daughter for her parents.

The Hendersons

The Hendersons, Carol and Roger, had separated four times in the previous 4 years of their 17-year marriage. While they made a concerted effort to keep their three children out of their conflict, they did sometimes argue in front of Megan (age 16), Patrice (13), and Roger, Jr. (12). The children would become upset. Megan would often try to calm her parents down by telling them that they might feel differently about a separation in the morning. After such a fight, Carol would arrange for her parents, Bob and Edna, to take the children for the weekend. After each of these weekends, Roger and Carol would pick the children up and be very affectionate with each other. No further mention or overt exhibition of distress would be apparent until the next angry announcement of impending separation and another weekend with the grandparents. Such a pattern suggested a Chaotic Family environment and the strong possibility that alcohol was involved in the fighting.

Megan's bulimia started just after her 15th birthday. Her parents had a fight on Thursday; she broke up with her boyfriend on Friday; and she was diagnosed with mononucleosis the next week. Subsequently, she had to give up a starring role in her school play. During the 2-month recovery period from her mononucleosis, she lost 5 pounds.

Just after her Christmas vacation, Megan realized that she had gained 5 pounds. A pair of pants that she wore loosely during autumn now fit snugly. Megan and her mother went on a diet to lose 5 pounds each. However, after the diet, Megan gained back the 5 pounds within 3 weeks. She felt panicked and attempted to diet again. In a short period of time she started bingeing routinely, gained more weight, and resorted to vomiting in an attempt to "undo" her binge episodes.

Megan's grandparents discovered she was vomiting in their bathroom and informed her parents, Carol and Roger. Carol sought help immediately. Megan was vomiting at least once a day.

During the time frame of five family sessions, the therapist had received two telephone calls from Carol's mother, Edna. Edna was concerned that Carol and Roger's marital problems were at the root of Megan's distress. The therapist suggested that Edna lacked confidence in Carol and Roger's ability to sort out their marital problems, which somehow included Carol's parents, Edna and Bob. Carol's parents were invited to join the Hendersons in consultation.

Carol and Roger embodied a Perfect–Chaotic Family. They demonstrated an ability to control themselves from outbursts in sessions and were organized in giving a family history. They were cooperative with the therapist's suggestions. However, Megan's attempts to calm her parents during their fights suggested that at times she was functioning in a caretaker role. Family history around drinking was vague, and Megan and her siblings squirmed a lot during this topic.

In the first three-generation session, Edna indirectly accused Carol of inadequate parenting. Roger was silent, while Megan was protective of her mother. The therapist had seen such a pattern within alcoholic families and observed this to the family. Roger, Jr., said, "Dad drinks. Does that mean he's an alcoholic?" Carol's father, Bob, quickly interjected, "A man's entitled to a drink after a hard day of work."

The therapist decided to try a family sculpture to get around the denial and defensiveness that was likely to escalate during a talk about the role of alcohol in the family. Because Megan seemed so protective of her parents and Roger, Jr., seemed much less protective, the therapist asked Roger, Jr., to create the family sculpture. The therapist said, "Roger, can you make me a picture that looks like what happens when your parents fight? Put everyone in the picture including your grandparents. Let's start with deciding if you're at home or somewhere else." Roger created a simple sculpture. He put his parents in diagonal corners of an imaginary living room. He asked Megan to stand between them trying to connect her father's hand to her mother's hand. Patrice was trying to watch television. Roger, Jr., sat with Patrice but watched the scene between his parents and Megan. When the therapist prompted him to place his grandparents in the picture, he paused. He then put them across the therapy room in a space that represented their separate house. He gave his grandfather a book to read and had his grandmother on the phone calling Carol, his mom. The therapist asked him to assume his position again. Everyone held their position for a minute. The therapist went into the closet and came out with some bottles for props. She asked of the family, "Who should get these?" Bob and Roger simultaneously stepped out of position protesting that the exercise was silly and that the therapist was overreacting. Carol started crying.

As the therapist encouraged her to talk about her feelings of distress, Carol shared how desperate and distressed she had been as a teenager worrying about her own father's drinking. Now, she worried about Roger's drinking. The therapist asked Megan if she worried about her dad's drinking. She sheepishly looked at her father, then at the floor, nodding yes. The therapist asked Megan and her siblings to sit together. She asked Carol and Roger to sit together and Bob and Edna to sit together. With this structural intervention, the therapist stated that these groups needed to stay separate. Megan was not to be part of her parent's marriage; Edna was not to be part of Carol's marriage. The therapist also stated that she could not continue to conduct family therapy or help Megan in any significant ways until Roger and Carol went to an alcohol counselor. Roger was willing to stop drinking, and the children went to Alateen. Megan was referred to a treatment group for bulimia.

It is my experience that family therapy is not very effective while a parent is a practicing alcoholic (Root et al., 1986). Very direct, confrontative interventions are necessary to cut through the strong denial that exists in alcoholic families (Elkin, 1984). While it is very likely that this family would not come back to this particular therapist, the intervention was still probably therapeutic. The secret in the family was exposed. Megan's distress, and her siblings', was further clarified and defined. The therapist supported the family by giving them direction for more appropriate places to seek help in order to address their multiple problems.

DISCUSSION

Bulimia represents a developmental impasse in the transition from adolescence to young adulthood—whether the disorder is being addressed at 16 or 40 years of age. Therefore, family-of-origin work needs to take place at some point during recovery. While at the core of the work is the establishment of a balance between autonomy and closeness (Root et al., 1986), the content and origin of these issues may vary as demonstrated by the three different family types.

Patience is not only a virtue; it is absolutely necessary in doing work with bulimics and their families. While growing up opens new frontiers for a client and her family, it reflects movement into a new stage of family and individual development that is uncharted territory. Therefore, change may be slow; many bulimics have several years of growing up to accomplish.

Such a dramatic technique requires careful planning and intervention, particularly with clients who have been physically and/or sexually abused. The therapist needs to have sensitivity as to how physical proximity and postures may trigger affect and flashbacks to traumatic events—even after the therapy session is over (Root & Fallon, 1988). Clients need to be given overt permission to decline to participate in sculpting and to regulate whether and how they are physically touched. When a client has an individual therapist in addition to a group therapist, I recommend that the two therapists coordinate treatment planning to maximize the benefit of this technique to the client.

There are few situations in which strong recommendations are made against the use of family sculpting. However, I would discourage its use with clients who are psychologically very fragile. The emotions this technique may elicit with a fragile client may precipitate decompensation, which is perhaps the ultimate fear of some bulimic clients. Even in the inpatient setting, therapists need to evaluate the appropriateness of this technique for each client carefully. As mentioned earlier in this chapter, the use of this technique is not recommended for family-of-origin members when sexual abuse is actively ongoing or unresolved in the past.

Clients who are especially comfortable with physical movement or expression, such as athletes, dancers, actresses, joggers, and aerobic exercisers, appear to be most receptive to family sculpting. Clients of family and cultural backgrounds that are more expressive are also very receptive to family sculpting.

As in any form of family therapy, it is ultimately important that the therapist has resolved significant issues in her or his own family-of-origin, particularly around loss, anger, dependency, and intimacy. Otherwise, the therapist will be limited as to how far she or he can take the client with this intervention. Additionally, the therapist must have comfort with her or his own body, or the discomfort will be apparent to clients and limit the direction of the family sculpture. I recommend that, before a therapist uses family sculpting with clients, he or she try it out personally to understand its impact.

While a co-therapist team is not necessary for family sculpting, such a team provides some advantages in facilitating and processing sculptures. As in any co-therapy situation, it is helpful to have more than one perspective. Additionally, one therapist can focus on directing the sculpture, and the other can watch the reactions of all the clients or family members. Lastly, a co-therapist team allows both compensation of each other's limitations due to therapists' family-of-origin issues and feedback about these unresolved issues.

Family sculpting provides an adjunctive technique to verbal therapies. It can be useful in circumventing the defenses of rationalization, minimization, and intellectualization that block affect. While the results of family sculpting are sometimes dramatic, it is neither magic nor a better form of family therapy intervention than others. It is an alternative technique to facilitate movement through a developmental impasse.

REFERENCES

Duhl, F. J., Kantor, D., & Duhl, B. S. (1973). Learning, space, and action in family therapy: A primer of sculpture. In D. A. Block (Ed.), *Techniques of family psychotherapy: A primer.* New York: Grune & Stratton.

Elkin, M. (1984). *Families under the influence.* New York: Norton Books.

Fallon, P., & Root, M. P. P. (1986). Family typology as a guide to the treatment of bulimia. *American Mental Health Counselors Association Journal, 8*, 221–228.

Garfinkel, P. E., & Garner, D. M. (1982). *Anorexia nervosa: A multidimensional perspective.* New York: Brunner/Mazel.

Johnson, C., & Flach, R. A. (1985). Family characteristics of 105 patients with bulimia. *American Journal of Psychiatry, 142*, 1321–1324.

Kog, E., Vandereycken, W., & Vertommen, H. (1985). Towards a verification of the psychosomatic family model: A pilot study of ten families with an anorexia/bulimia nervosa patient. *International Journal of Eating Disorders, 4*, 525–538.

McGoldrick, M., & Gerson, R. (1985). *Genogram in family assessment.* New York: Norton Books.

Minuchin, S., Rosman, B. L., & Baker, L. (1978). *Psychosomatic families.* Cambridge: Harvard University Press.

Moreno, J. L. (1946). *Psychodrama.* Beacon, NY: Beacon House.

Perls, F. S. (1969). *Gestalt therapy verbatim.* Moab, UT: Real People Press.

Perls, F. S. (1976). *The gestalt approach and eye witness to therapy.* New York: Bantam Books.

Root, M. P. P., & Fallon, P. (1988). Victimization experiences as contributing factors to the development of bulimia in women. *Journal of Interpersonal Violence, 3*(2), 161–173.

Root, M. P. P., Fallon, P., & Friedrich, W. N. (1986). *Bulimia: A systems approach to treatment.* New York: Norton Books.

Satir, V. (1964). *Conjoint family therapy.* Palo Alto, CA: Science and Behavior Books.

Satir, V. (1972). *Peoplemaking.* Palo Alto, CA: Science and Behavior Books.

Schwartz, R. C., Barrett, M. J., & Saba, G. (1984). Family therapy for bulimia. In D. M. Garner & P. E. Garfinkel (Eds.), *Handbook of psychotherapy for anorexia and bulimia* (pp. 280–307). New York: Guilford Press.

Stanton, M. D., & Todd, T. C. (Eds.). (1982). *The family therapy of drug abuse and addiction.* New York: Guilford Press.

Strober, M. (1981). The significance of bulimia in anorexia nervosa: An exploration of possible etiological factors. *International Journal of Eating Disorders, 1*, 28–43.

Strober, M., & Humphrey, L. (1987). Familial contributions to the etiology and course of anorexia nervosa and bulimia. *Journal of Consulting and Clinical Psychology, 55*(5), 654–659.

Watzlawick, P., Beavin, J. H., & Jackson, D. D. (1967). *Pragmatics of human communication.* New York: Norton Books.

Yalom, I. (1975). *The theory and practice of group psychotherapy* (2nd ed.). New York: Basic Books.

6

Psychodrama and the Treatment of Bulimia

Monica Leonie Callahan

Since 1981, I have been exploring ways of using psychodrama as part of individual and group psychotherapy with bulimics in an outpatient setting. Almost all of my clients are women; their ages range from the late teens to the early 50s. Psychotherapy is only one part of the treatment. I encourage clients, as needed, to consult with a physician, meet with a nutritionist and attend meetings of support groups such as Overeaters Anonymous (OA). I do not require a commitment to specific changes in eating behavior in order to begin treatment; indeed, the ambivalence about such a commitment is often the issue that must be dealt with first.

This chapter introduces the reader to psychodrama in the treatment of bulimics. "Bulimia" here refers to the DSM-III (American Psychiatric Association, 1980) definition of the disorder, which is less restrictive than the definition of bulimia nervosa in the DSM-III-R (American Psychiatric Association, 1987). In particular, the women I describe may or may not meet the DSM-III-R criterion of regularly engaging "in either self-induced vomiting, use of laxatives or diuretics, strict dieting or fasting, or vigorous exercise in order to prevent weight gain."

Others have written extensive reviews of the literature focusing on psychodrama (Bischof, 1970; Buchanan, 1984; Haskell, 1975; Kipper, 1986; Z. T. Moreno, 1959; Starr, 1977; Yablonsky, 1976) and on the treatment of bulimia (Emmett, 1985; Garner & Garfinkel, 1985; Neuman & Halvorson, 1983). A number of authors (Boskind-White & White, 1983; Browning, 1985; Neuman & Halvorson, 1983; Roy-Bryne, Lee-Benner, & Yager, 1984; Shisslak, Schnaps, & Swain, 1986; White & Boskind-White, 1984) refer to action methods such as role playing, gestalt techniques, and assertiveness training used to treat eating disorders, but none of these applications utilize psychodrama as a primary methodology.

The chapter begins with an overview of the basic principles, objectives, and techniques of therapeutic psychodrama. I discuss how psychodrama is best applied to the treatment of people with bulimia and then demonstrate the use of these techniques to address four central clinical issues. For each issue, I present a psychodramatic group exercise and a reconstruction of a full-blown psychodrama pertaining to that theme. A general discussion follows.

PSYCHODRAMA

Psychodrama is a form of therapy and education that uses a wide range of action methods to examine subjective experience and to promote constructive change through the development of new perceptions, behaviors, and connections with others. Participants enact past situations, present dilemmas, future expectations, dreams, fantasies, emotions, and ideas— all occurring in the "here and now" of a special sort of heightened reality. It is the job of the "director"/therapist to help create an atmosphere conducive to such experiences and to develop therapeutic action structures jointly with the "protagonist," or central character, and with the members of the group. Psychodrama is usually conducted in groups, but it has been adapted for use with individuals as well (Stein & Callahan, 1982).

Psychodrama was formulated by Jacob L. Moreno (1946, 1953, 1973; Moreno & Moreno, 1959, 1969) during the years 1908–1925 in Vienna and was brought by him to this country in 1925. Over the next half century, Moreno further developed and published his ideas for psychodrama, sociometry, role theory, social systems theory, and group psychotherapy. He also founded a residential center for the practice and training of psychodrama in Beacon, NY.

Moreno was an idealist. Drawing from a background in philosophy and theology, he viewed people as possessing a transcendent ability to create through the workings of an inexhaustible inner energy that he termed "spontaneity." Spontaneity is defined as the ability to generate novel, appropriate responses to old situations and effective responses to new ones. Spontaneity is also the ability to infuse the familiar with new life and to live in general with vitality and authenticity. The goal of psychodrama therapy is to remove existing blocks to spontaneity so that the natural creativity fundamental to psychological health and growth can flourish. This goal is best accomplished by creating a context that approximates real life and by treating spontaneity as it emerges in observable behavior.

Along with spontaneity and creativity, Moreno emphasized the basic interconnectedness of people; in particular, he stressed their need for one another in order to establish an identity and to lead a meaningful life. He postulated a natural flow of feeling perceptions between people that, when left unencumbered, can greatly enhance spontaneity. This occurs, for example, in the ideal situation of role reversal, when one person is able accurately to grasp on many levels the subjective experiences of the other by putting herself in the other person's place.

Moreno studied spontaneity in its moment-to-moment behavioral manifestations. He believed there is a continuous process of "warming up" or preparing for a particular act or feeling state. People use "starters" to warm themselves up, such as mental images, anticipatory physical movements, or the external aspects of an unfamiliar role. Some starters enhance spontaneity, while others, including addictive substances, only appear to do so; instead, they have destructive effects and prevent the healthy development of "self-starters." An example of the use of such dysfunctional starters is the way some people rely on food to coax themselves through anxiety-producing tasks or to produce desired emotional states. The therapeutic goal would be to help them develop alternative starters for achieving the same outcomes.

Another major component of Moreno's thinking was his conception of roles. Moreno viewed people as natural role players. According to him, the self emerges from a constellation of roles, and the status of an individual's role repertoire—for example, the variety of roles available and whether these roles are congruent with inner experience—is an important indication of psychological health. Roles are formed in an interpersonal context and develop differently depending on how they are reciprocated and influenced by the roles of others. Spontaneity is curtailed when people are locked in a rigid system of roles that won't permit growth or change. Thus, for example, some bulimics become quite adept at role playing in the process of adapting their behavior to accommodate others. But beneath an outer expressiveness and flair for the dramatic, these women are often cut off from their inner experience, and they feel empty and confused.

Learning new roles occurs in three stages: (1) "role taking," trying on the externals of a role; (2) "role playing," gaining comfort and spontaneity in a role, and (3) "role creating," changing a role by infusing it with unique, personal elements. The power and effectiveness of psychodrama stems from the fact that roles can be assumed, at least initially, without being experienced as part of the self. In this way, role taking and role playing provide a kind of psychological protection that helps an individual explore unfamiliar, threatening, or otherwise unacceptable areas of concern.

Moreno believed that the goal of psychodrama is to achieve a "catharsis of integration" through action experiences in the here and now. This form of catharsis produces change not only through releasing pent-up anxieties and emotions, but also by bringing about new perceptions and, at least potentially, a reorganization of the self. In the words of

Z. T. Moreno (1971), "The greatest depth of catharsis comes . . . from embodying those dimensions, roles, and interactions which life has not, cannot, and probably never will permit."

In J. L. Moreno's view, catharsis does not attain its full therapeutic impact unless it occurs in an interpersonal context. The importance of connectedness with others underlies the three-part structure of a traditional psychodrama session in which the enactment is sandwiched between the "warm-up" and "sharing" phases. During the initial warm-up, central themes emerge and the group develops the underpinnings of trust and mutual involvement needed to support the "action" phase. Following the action, in the sharing phase, the protagonist is reintegrated into the group as members speak in turn of their identification with the psychodrama. This phase may also be a time for "de-roling" (helping people relinquish particularly compelling roles), for giving feedback to the protagonist, for making interpretations, and/or for contracting for further work.

Along with producing catharsis, psychodrama may heighten the effects of more general curative factors in group psychotherapy. For example, participating together in the enactment of an individual's drama can be an experience of considerable intimacy, especially when the therapist, role players, and group members are able to accurately sense and portray the protagonist's inner world, follow her lead, and facilitate a spontaneous release of emotion. In this way, psychodrama can enhance the group's function as a "self-object" by providing a special sort of mirroring, as Kohut (1977) described it.

Psychodrama can also be a means of highlighting and working through transferences occurring in the group process. For example, the choice of someone to play a significant role may reveal transferential feelings toward that person and may provide an opportunity to work through those feelings. Transferences and projections that emerge in the group's overall interaction can also be dealt with psychodramatically. For instance, a particular member may dominate a number of sessions with one emotional crisis after another, drawing forth repeated attempts to help from some members while alienating others. Psychodrama techniques can be used to help the other group members discover the function this person is serving for them, both individually and as a group.

Psychodrama's curative effects depend on how it is used. If the goal is behavioral learning or role training, action can be structured to emphasize the use of modeling, anxiety reduction, behavior rehearsal, feedback, and positive reinforcement. A client might enact a stressful situation known to trigger bingeing and purging and then try out alternative ways to cope with the situation. Alternately, if the goal is bringing into awareness and counteracting destructive internal objects, action can be structured to help the protagonist personify her inner voices, release repressed emotions, and affirm the weakened parts of her self. In bulimia, such self-destructive internal dynamics are often played out in the relationship with food, as in the emotional responses during an episode of bingeing and purging.

Detailed descriptions of the wide array of psychodrama techniques and action structures have been provided elsewhere (Blatner, 1973; Hale, 1981; J. L. Moreno, 1946; Z. T. Moreno, 1965). The following are five basic techniques that appear in the clinical examples. These are simplified definitions, as each technique has many nuances and variations.

The "soliloquy" is a monologue in which the protagonist expresses inner thoughts and feelings as if she is talking to herself, but out loud. This technique may be used to help the protagonist warm up to a situation or to help break through resistances and emotional blocking (see case 1 and 3 later in the chapter).

In "doubling," a group member physically joins the protagonist and attempts to give voice to unexpressed feelings and thoughts as the drama proceeds. The protagonist is given the option of rejecting or accepting and incorporating any expression and action by the double. Doubling may be used to provide support, to elicit emotions, to stimulate thinking, or to offer a gentle sort of confrontation (see case 3 and 4).

In "role reversal," the protagonist exchanges parts with the person with whom she is interacting in order to perceive the world—and, more importantly, to perceive herself—from the other's point of view (see cases 1, 3, and 4).

In the "mirror" technique, another group member portrays the protagonist and duplicates as accurately as possible her actions in the previous enactment. This gives the protagonist an opportunity to observe her own verbal and nonverbal behavior and to consider how it affects others (see case 1).

In the "aside," the action is stopped in midstream, and the protagonist is asked to express her feelings and thoughts at that moment. This technique may be used to stimulate insight and the awareness of emotions or to help break through unproductive patterns in the drama (see case 3).

PSYCHODRAMA AND BULIMIA

When I invite someone in my group for bulimics to act as the protagonist in a psychodrama, the response may be great enthusiasm or thinly veiled terror, but it is invariably intense. Reactions often stem from fears of being forced to reveal a vulnerable inner self that is felt to be unworthy or to express intense emotions that are experienced as unmanageable.

Psychodrama may seem like an improbable treatment of choice for the bulimic, who isolates herself from others, maintains a tight hold on her emotional life, and, above all, fears a loss of control. The idea of enacting in front of others a behavior that produces so much shame and self-doubt is almost unthinkable. Furthermore, people with so many negative feelings toward their bodies would be expected to resist something involving so much movement in proximity to others.

Nevertheless, I have found psychodrama techniques to be highly effective for many bulimic clients, in particular, helping people in their efforts to overcome blocks to emotional experience and to gain access to hidden parts of the self. This is facilitated by the use of multiple nonverbal and imaginal cues that engage participants on many levels simultaneously. Psychodrama also provides opportunities to experience, practice, and strengthen the healthier aspects of the self, and sharing such intense experiences with others can help counteract the isolation so characteristic of people with bulimia.

There are ways of adapting psychodrama techniques to the special needs of the bulimic. Some individuals in the group may only be able to work on their own issues indirectly by playing roles in other people's dramas or by doubling other members. The therapist can make good use of the playfulness of some psychodrama techniques, as in the personification of favorite binge foods. For example, someone could take the role of "ice cream" and interact with various group members as a way of exploring the function ice cream serves for them. With respect to the bulimic's sensitivity about her body, techniques may be altered so that they are less threatening. For example, bulimics can be given the option of sitting rather than standing in a particular exercise, or methods can be used that require only limited movement, such as speaking to an empty chair that represents a person or a part of the self.

CASE STUDIES

The following clinical examples were selected to demonstrate the use of psychodrama to address four major areas in the treatment of bulimia: (1) eating behavior and the relationship to food; (2) body weight and body image; (3) intimacy issues; and (4) self-experience and self-structure. The examples consist of group exercises and reconstructions of psychodramas based on actual sessions.

Eating Behavior and the Relationship to Food

The Clock Exercise

Group members are asked to imagine the face of a clock with specific positions for 12, 3, 6, and 9 o'clock spread out on the floor of the room.

They walk silently in a circle, mentally passing through the hours of the day, and then stop at a time when food typically becomes a problem for them. When everyone has stopped, each person is asked in turn to talk in the present tense about what she is doing, thinking, and feeling. This procedure is repeated several times. Finally, people are asked to focus instead on a time of day when they feel particularly strong emotionally and untroubled about food. Everyone then sits down and discusses the exercise.

The clock exercise can also have a more specific focus, for example, how group members feel about their bodies at different times of day. Along with talking at each stopping place, each person could assume a physical position to express her feeling. The clock exercise often produces material for further exploration during the same or later sessions.

Case 1: Laura's Psychodrama

Laura was a 44-year-old woman, about 80 pounds overweight, who had been through a long series of weight-loss programs; however, she was unable to complete any of them. She was never able to stay slim for very long and attributed this difficulty to problems in her marriage and to feelings about her abusive, alcoholic father. She talked of her fear that if she lost weight she would have to face her husband's lack of physical responsiveness and the overall emptiness in their marriage of 18 years. She also blamed her inability to lose weight on her father, who had called her "fat and ugly" throughout her childhood. He had often accused her of being just like his overweight mother, a mentally ill woman who had neglected and abused him. Laura was in reality a talented and appealing woman, but she suffered from deep feelings of shame, self-doubt, and loneliness. She felt best when she took part in performances at a community theatre, for which she had won some local acclaim.

At the time of her psychodrama, Laura had attended individual therapy for a year and a half and she had been in the group for 9 months. Her initial depression had subsided, and she had begun to deal with feelings about her family and about her past. She still felt isolated, however, and had not yet made any real changes in her use of food. She had participated in psychodramas focused on others and had herself worked as protagonist on career and family issues, but she had never before worked directly on her eating behavior. This session was a turning point for Laura, as she herself spoke of it later. Subsequently, she began attending OA and a women's support group at her church. More significantly, soon after, on her own initiative, she began to experiment with changing her eating habits by eliminating sugar from her diet. She was able to sustain this for several months before a family crisis necessitated the interruption of therapy.

During the warm-up, Laura said she felt hopeless about her bingeing, a behavior that usually occurred late at night when her family had gone to sleep and she was finally alone. I suggested that she use this session to take a look at her experience of that vulnerable time and to try to come up with alternatives to bingeing. The action began with Laura using furniture and other objects to set up her living room and kitchen. As a warm-up to the situation, I asked her to imagine that it was a typical night and soliloquize about her day.

LAURA: My body feels tired, but my mind is still awake. I spent the whole day chauffeuring my daughter around and talking to people on the phone about the flea market for the church. Everybody wants me to do things. I should never have volunteered, even though it's once a year. Now it's nice and quiet, and I just want to forget about everything. I feel kind of antsy—I think I'll see what's in the refrigerator.

Laura continued to speak as she went through the motions of searching the refrigerator, sitting down in front of the television with her favorite binge foods, and eating. She performed this scene with less spontaneity than she had shown up to that point, and she seemed embarrassed. With the idea of helping Laura learn to anticipate and interrupt her compulsive behavior, I asked her to select someone to represent herself and replay the whole scene as a kind of mirror. Laura would observe in the role of a wise and compassionate counselor to herself. The woman she chose to portray herself played the scene of bingeing in front of the television very effectively. Using small boxes piled high in her lap to represent the food, she eagerly stuffed cookies, cupcakes, and chocolate into her mouth. I stopped the action and asked Laura as counselor to reflect out loud.

COUNSELOR/LAURA: That's disgusting! You're a fat, lazy pig. Is that all you can do with your time? No wonder you're all by yourself!

Laura had not been able to warm up to the assigned role, scolding and abusing herself instead as she habitually did internally. As a way of providing more guidance, I aligned myself with the counselor and asked her to try to see through Laura's outward behavior to the sensitive person inside and to help her find another way to deal with her feelings. The counselor/Laura then suggested that Laura take a walk in her flower garden, listen to the birds, and write in her journal.

Laura returned to her original role and followed this advice. As she took a walk in her garden, which she described in vivid detail, she spotted a family of birds. She chose someone to play the mother bird, then reversed roles with her and sent a message to Laura, the gist of which was as follows:

BIRD: I am part of nature and I am beautiful, and so are you!

Finally, Laura returned to her own role and listened to the bird repeat her words so that she could feel the full impact of her own message and, it is hoped, begin to internalize it.

Body Weight and Body Image

The Mirror Exercise

Group members stand facing an area of the wall that serves as their imaginary mirror. They are given the option of closing their eyes and are asked to visualize themselves in the mirror. One by one, they describe what they "see" and then address their image. Responses are typically negative descriptions and distortions of their bodies, followed by harsh criticisms and demands for change. Each person then takes one step back and speaks from the role of someone significant in her life who might say or think similar negative things about her. Following this, each person takes another step back and speaks from the role of someone significant in her life who appreciates and supports her struggle. Finally, everyone takes two steps forward and speaks again as herself to her image in the mirror. What is said this last time usually reflects what was said in the second, more supportive role. Everyone then sits down and talks about the experience.

One variation of this exercise is to ask people to reverse roles with their image after they speak from each assigned role and respond to what was said. This method requires that people face outward; a darkened room or private corner may help them feel less self-conscious.

Case 2: Bonnie's Psychodrama

Bonnie was a 35-year-old woman, about 60 pounds overweight, who had a history of alternate bingeing and restricting, with wide fluctuations in her weight. Her periods of thinness had been achieved through extreme dieting and compulsive exercise. The last such period had occurred during the early years of her brief marriage to an up-and-coming, status-conscious businessman to whom her appearance was very important. After the first year of marriage, Bonnie began to suspect that her husband was having affairs during business trips, though he repeatedly denied her accusations. When the affairs started to become known around town, she initiated divorce proceedings. A bitter battle ensued over the division of property, and her husband used Bonnie's occasional bouts of compulsive spending to claim that she had squandered their money. The day after the divorce became final, her husband married an 18-year-old model.

Bonnie spoke of feeling humiliated, but she showed little emotion aside from a disdainful tone of voice. She talked wistfully about having been thin and attractive but seemed ambivalent about losing weight. She had been divorced for 2 years but hadn't dated at all, though several men had shown interest in her. Bonnie talked very little about her large family, but she did mention how afraid she and her siblings were of her minister father, who had been very strict and protective of the girls.

At the time of this session, Bonnie had been in group therapy for about 4 months; it was close to the end of the time-limited group. My hope was to help her move closer to resolving her ambivalence about changing her eating behavior by focusing on her weight and its defensive function. The psychodrama could also provide opportunities for her to express her accumulated anger.

I asked Bonnie to choose group members to represent her extra weight and to physically surround herself with them. She chose six people and had them form a tight ring around her. I asked how she felt. She said, "Very comfortable," and everyone laughed. When asked what or who was outside the circle, she said, "People, especially men who are interested in me, and some people in my family." I asked her to choose someone to represent a hypothetical "interested" man. She took this role first while the person she had chosen stood in her place temporarily. As the man, Bonnie was quite seductive.

MAN: I've been watching you ever since you started working here, and I can't take my eyes off you. Are you busy Saturday night? Or what about the weekend—why don't we go down to the shore? My friend has a beach house, and he's not using it.

Bonnie resumed the role of herself, and the person chosen to play the man repeated these words, adding to them in the spirit of the role. When asked how she was feeling, Bonnie said she felt safe where she was and did not even acknowledge what had just been said. As the man came closer and became more aggressive, she responded more directly: "Forget it! Leave me alone! Find someone else to take advantage of."

I then asked Bonnie to think of a family member she would place outside the circle, and she chose her sister, who had been her running partner in her latest thin phase. She selected someone to play her sister, but began by portraying the role herself.

SISTER: Look at all that weight you've put on! Honey, just trust me. I'll get you back on a diet, and you'll be skinny in no time. We can run around the track like we used to. And look at your hair—you've really let it go. You've got to stop feeling sorry for yourself!

When Bonnie resumed the role of herself, I had the person playing her sister speak these words and at the same time try to pull her out of the "weight" circle. As Bonnie resisted and moved away from her sister, she asked the circle to come with her, at which the group laughed sympathetically.

This seemed like a good point to turn the focus of the drama to the function of the weight encircling Bonnie. I asked her to reverse roles with someone in the circle and tell "Bonnie" inside the circle what she, as the weight, was doing for her. The other members of the circle would follow her lead. At first Bonnie and the others told the inside "Bonnie" how they protected her from disappointment, from abusive relationships, from sexual exploitation, from her family's high expectations, and from painful emotions in general. Bonnie then returned to the center of the circle and people repeated what had just been said. At this point one member of the circle began to speak of the positive things Bonnie was missing in life by hiding behind her weight.

CIRCLE MEMBER: We keep you from experiencing all of what it is to be alive. We keep you from knowing the joys of sexuality and a loving relationship. We keep you from letting people know all the good things you have to offer as a person. We keep you numb and preoccupied so that you don't feel the ups and downs, the sorrows and joys that give meaning to life.

Bonnie was moved to tears and later referred to this message as having been very meaningful and encouraging.

As a form of closure, I asked Bonnie to do something with her circle of weight to signify where she stood at that moment. She pushed against the circle (people had locked arms) with some force but without enough to break through. I encouraged the members of the circle not to let her easily push her way through, as it seemed important to leave Bonnie with a true sense of her remaining ambivalence.

Intimacy Issues

A Self-Presentation Exercise

In this exercise, group members think of a significant person in their life, past or present, who has had something to do with their relationship to food. One by one, each takes the role of that person and "visits" the group in that role. People are given two options: either they can stand outside the group, warm up to the role, and then enter as the visitor, or they can sit in a chair facing away from the group while preparing for the role and then turn their chair back when they are ready to begin. In the role of the visitor, each person is asked to tell the group about himself or herself and then to talk about the group member he or she is introducing (her actual self). During this time, the therapist may ask questions and may invite group members to do the same. The visitor is then thanked for coming and walks away (or turns the chair back around). The group member becomes herself again and is invited to talk about the experience, including feelings toward the person whose role she played.

This exercise can be altered to define the visiting person more specifically or to include more than one role. For example, each member could choose someone she believes has been part of her problem with food and then someone who has been helpful with respect to that problem.

Case 3: Donna's Psychodrama

Donna was a 38-year-old low-weight bulimic and the unemployed mother of two teenage children. Her first marriage had ended in divorce after 3 years and she was now "happily" remarried. She had never developed job skills or pursued her career interests as she had married and become pregnant soon after high school and had been supported financially ever since.

Donna had been secretly bingeing and purging since high school, when she had been a beauty queen and quite popular. While suffering inwardly during that time, she had maintained a pleasing and confident manner, especially in social situations with her parents, who were active in politics and highly visible in the community.

Donna spent her days chauffeuring her children, following an intensive regimen of exercise, fixing up her house, cooking elaborate meals, and attending work-related social functions with her husband, a prominent lawyer. Her life felt empty to her and she had no close friends in her area. Donna had been in therapy intermittently for the previous 10 years, but she had been open about her bulimia only during the last 3. She had attended a number of groups for eating disorders but, by her own admission, she had dropped out too soon for them to be of any help to her.

At the time of her psychodrama, Donna had been attending group therapy for 6 months. At the beginning of this session, she expressed feelings of hopelessness about ever being able to stop bingeing and purging. Her husband's attempts to be supportive left her feeling confused and frustrated. I invited her to explore her feelings toward her husband with the idea that these might somehow be connected to her bulimia.

Donna began by portraying a typical scenario preceding a bulimic episode. She had spent hours that day planning and cooking dinner. Now everyone had eaten, and she was in the kitchen cleaning up and picking at the leftover food on the plates. I asked her to soliloquize.

DONNA: Another boring day. I hate this life. Why do I even try to cook something special for him? He takes it for granted. He asks me how things are going with my "problem," but does he really understand? Then again, at least he asks me; he really does make an effort. I shouldn't be so critical. Why am I so worried about what he thinks of me? Why am I so insecure about his feelings toward me—like at those awful parties?

"Those awful parties" were cocktail parties connected with Donna's husband's work. I invited her to show us what happened at a typical party. She chose people to play the roles of her husband, his male colleagues, their wives, and some female colleagues. I also asked her to choose someone to be her double.

The scene began with her husband, played by Donna, talking confidently, while drinking, about his successes at work. He began flirting with one of the women, complimenting her and acting intensely interested in what she was saying. Donna then resumed her own role while the scene was replayed with a group member representing her husband. I stopped the action and asked her for an aside. Donna spoke of feeling older and less attractive than the other women. Her double was much more able than she to express anger about her husband's flirtatious behavior, accusing him of needing to prove that he could still attract women. I asked Donna what it would be like to tell her husband how she felt, and she said she didn't know how to do that without jeopardizing their relationship.

I then invited Donna to use the psychodrama as a chance to try talking with her husband in a new way. In the previous scene she had acted in a subservient manner toward her husband, so I had her place him standing on a chair looking down at her in the hope that such exaggeration would help stimulate the expression of her feelings. Donna was better able to express her anger toward her husband with him so obviously "above" her, and she did so with a chorus of other group members who had all been invited to double her.

DONNA: I hate your flirting! I don't know why you need to do that. And I hate always being the one to compromise, to make things comfortable for you, to support your career. I have needs too, and I need to take the time to do some things for myself. I am thinking about going to OA meetings and I may not be at home as much at night. You're going to have to understand. You ask me about my bulimia as if you're expecting a quick solution—like it's just a matter of self-control and why do I keep doing it if I'm happy with you. Well, there's a lot more involved in my problem, and maybe you don't want to hear about it because you wonder if you have an addiction yourself.

Donna reversed roles with her husband, and the group member playing her husband repeated what she had said. She then returned to her own role and considered out loud how she had sounded and which things she might actually say to her husband. Donna was surprised to hear herself be so confident and expressed relief at having vented her feelings. She decided to talk to her husband about going to meetings and about her bulimia, though she was still unsure about showing her anger.

Donna reported some positive changes in her marriage that she related to this session. With more time, it might have been helpful to explore whether Donna's difficulties with her husband harkened back to problems in earlier relationships; my suspicion was that unresolved issues with her parents, now emerging in her marriage, were somehow connected to her eating disorder.

Self-Experience and Self-Structure

A Self-Projection Exercise

A chair is put in a central location and group members are asked to use their imagination and place in the chair the part of themselves that is afraid of change and doesn't want to give up the bulimia. One by one, each person is given a chance to enact an inner dialogue with that part of herself, either alone or with the help of another group member. Each member begins by sitting in the empty chair and taking the role of the part of herself that she projected—assuming its body position, thoughts, and feelings—and then soliloquizing. Following that, the therapist guides each person in a series of role reversals between the part in the empty chair and the part of herself that emerges in the original chair. There is some advantage to performing the exercise in dyads, as this gives each person a chance to view and hear the different parts of herself.

This exercise can be used to highlight other inner conflicts as well, depending on how the initially projected part of the self is defined. For example, group members could be asked to begin with the part of themselves that is afraid of close relationships. Another variation is to have each person choose two group members to role play the two sides of the conflict so that she herself can stand back, observe her own struggle, and find a way to intervene.

Case 4: Individual Psychodrama with Fran

Fran was a 26-year-old single woman who had been bulimic for 11 years. She had also had periods of cocaine and alcohol abuse and some stealing to support her addictions. She was close to finishing her master's degree in a helping profession but was not sure whether she wanted to work in that field.

Fran had always occupied a special position in her family. Even after her family knew she was bulimic, she continued to be held up to her sisters as the strong, successful, and thin one. In her early teens, she had served as confidante to her mother, who was depressed and very unhappy with her marriage. Fran had always desired a better relationship with her father, who was a workaholic, critical toward himself and others, and emotionally distant.

Fran's family, though living far away, continued to be involved in her life through frequent phone calls, packages, and visits. Their style of closeness left little room for individuality, and, as a result, Fran had become an expert at assuming roles to accommodate others. She felt that her family and friends didn't know the "real" Fran, and she herself was unsure of who she was or what she wanted.

Beneath her cheerful and confident exterior, Fran was quite fearful and periodically would be overcome by intense surges of emotion. She had a repetitive history of self-destructive relationships with men, in which she would feel overpowered and demeaned and at the same time extremely dependent. It was the turmoil of one such relationship, along with the worsening of her bulimia, that led her to seek treatment.

Fran's psychodrama occurred after 5 months of individual therapy. She had begun to attend OA and to keep a journal, but she had yet to establish control over her bingeing and purging. I had introduced the possibility of using psychodrama techniques at the start of therapy, and we had used them in two previous sessions.

In this session Fran talked about how she walked around most of the time feeling like the devil was perched on her shoulder, watching and commenting upon her every move. She acknowledged that this figure probably represented a part of herself and that sometimes she felt like two people. I invited her to explore this duality by acting it out. My hope was to strengthen her ability to counteract what seemed to be a highly rejecting and self-destructive inner voice. I asked Fran to stand behind her chair in the role of the devil and talk to "herself" in the empty chair.

DEVIL: You never do anything right! Sit up straight! All you do is talk, talk, talk, and then you go home and eat, eat, eat. You're disgusting! Serves you right if you gain weight—your stomach looks bigger already. No wonder: you haven't been exercising enough! You're lazy, and I caught you cheating again with those reports. They're skimpy, and you know you should be much more thorough. And that journal of yours—you should be embarrassed reading that to Dr. Callahan. You don't even write in complete sentences.

Fran then sat in the chair and became the other part of herself, a part that sounded and acted like a lively and rebellious child. To help Fran make the transition, I suggested that she first move around in the role, at which point she got up and paced nervously back and forth. The words soon followed, encouraged by an occasional doubling statement from me.

FRAN: I can't stand this anymore! I can't live up to your standards. Leave me alone! I'm tired of everything I do and say being wrong—why can't I just live my life? I don't care anymore. I'm so tired of everything. Why shouldn't I eat if I want to? [Fran was getting more and more agitated at this point.] I want some ice cream right now, and I hope you're satisfied! I'm going to get two gallons and turn on the television and eat. I'm so mad! I don't know what to do.

Fran reversed roles a few more times, alternating between herself and the devil.

At this point, sensing that it would be acceptable to her, I joined in the role playing. I wanted to help Fran develop a more accepting and nurturing attitude toward herself. The belief that her own needs were legitimate would be a first step toward finding constructive ways to meet them. I took the role of the part of herself she had just played and gave her the task of trying to calm "me" down, to reassure me, to help me feel better about myself, and to help me consider the possibility of giving up bingeing and purging.

At first it was difficult for Fran to respond to the role I was playing with anything other than her accustomed self-criticism and punitiveness. I used my role to help her warm up to her assignment by asking for help in various ways and by responding warmly to her positive efforts. Fran eventually became quite confident and calming in this new role, and her remarks suggested the beginnings of a new perspective on herself.

FRAN/NEW ROLE: You have a right to be angry—the way you never give yourself a break. You don't have to be perfect! You're doing the best you can, especially when you consider all those years you depended on bingeing and vomiting to deal with things. But it's time to stop hurting yourself and to start using the resources you have. It'll be hard but you can do it! Try to do what they're telling you in OA—take 1 day, even 1 minute, at a time and call someone when you you're upset—maybe even find yourself a sponsor. You're important! You're worth it!

The action ended with me reversing roles with Fran and repeating what she had said so she could experience the effect of her words.

It was not long after this session that Fran became much more involved in OA and began to be "abstinent" for several days at a time—the first major step on her road to successful recovery. She often referred back to this psychodrama, in particular when she tried to understand what had precipitated a loss of abstinence.

DISCUSSION

These case studies present a somewhat idealized and oversimplified picture of psychodrama and its application. The sessions from which the examples were drawn evidenced a good match between the client's readiness, the group's receptivity, and the methodology. An effective psychodrama is often the culmination of a series of preparatory individual and/or group sessions, and a number of sessions following the psychodrama may be needed to integrate its effects with the rest of the protagonist's experience. Closure is particularly important with bulimics, who are prone to dissociation. The intense experience of an emotional psychodrama may be temporarily "forgotten." But if the emotions generated by a psychodrama are not worked through sufficiently during the sharing phase, the resulting emotional tensions may be acted out subsequently in an episode of bingeing and purging.

The portion of the session following a psychodrama is important for other reasons as well. For example, transferences among the group members may be heightened by the enactment and, with the help of some discussion, brought to a new level of awareness. Psychodrama can also have a powerful impact on transference toward the therapist, especially as the therapist moves in and out of the active role required to direct the drama. The greater involvement of the therapist in psychodrama, relative to other therapies, may be jarring to some and reassuring to others—in any case, it can provide meaningful data for therapeutic work.

Psychodrama at its best requires more than the skillful use of techniques. Its effectiveness depends on the clinical sensitivity and maturity of the therapist, on the relationship between the therapist and client, and, in the case of group therapy, on the evolution of the group. Such factors can determine whether, for example, a particular psychodrama is experienced by the protagonist as an invasion of privacy or as a freely chosen opportunity to share and explore private experiences. A sense of control is particularly important for bulimics who are beginning to risk the letting go of long-established defenses. The factors mentioned above can also determine whether the protagonist experiences the psychodrama as the product of the therapist and/or the group, or whether she feels it to be her own personal creation. A sense of ownership is crucial for bulimics, who are experts at accommodating others at the cost of failing to develop a secure sense of self. In my experience directing bulimics, it is a good idea to check frequently with the protagonist concerning her experience of the psychodrama at that moment and to offer the protagonist as many choices as possible regarding the structure and progress of the action.

Psychodrama is not intended for everyone, and certain techniques should be used with discretion. Not all people, for example, have the capacity to tolerate the features of psychodrama that require a well-developed ability to separate fantasy from reality and to differentiate the self from others. For example, clients with a borderline personality organization may have difficulty distinguishing between a psychodrama experience and reality or maintaining a secure sense of themselves while taking on the role of others. It may be difficult for them to relinquish roles and role perceptions of others following an enactment. Techniques that involve rapidly switching roles, enacting parts of the self, or personifying objects can be confusing and frightening for more disturbed clients. Also, the emotional intensity of techniques such as doubling demands a tolerance for a certain degree of intimacy that some people find overwhelming.

A final note of caution: Psychodrama is a powerful method not only for the client but for the clinician and may heighten the effects of countertransference. For example, the therapist may become narcissistically identified with a particular psychodrama as a production, especially if the protagonist is accommodating and the therapist has unmet needs for creative expression, recognition, or control. Also, in working with bulimics, the therapist directing a psychodrama may experience the client's own perfectionism and performance anxiety.

There are a number of applications of psychodrama other than those described here that are relevant to the treatment of bulimics. For example, psychodrama can be employed effectively in an inpatient setting, where the immediate availability of other staff and other groups may permit more intensive, confrontational psychodramas. Furthermore, psychodrama need not focus solely on the concerns of individuals but can also be used to examine and work through key moments in group development. For example, in a case of frequent absences by an ambivalent group member, other members might be asked in turn to reverse roles with her and then consider how they identify with her and what function she serves for the group. Such absences can stimulate fears of the group disintegrating, and the group might explore this in a dramatized future scenario or "future projection" (Z. T. Moreno, 1959). Another possibility is the use of sociodrama, which employs psychodrama techniques to examine issues more generally rather than focusing on the specific experiences of individuals. One sociodrama, for example, might explore societal expectations concerning thinness and their ramifications for bulimics. Group members could take the roles of people, institutions, or other sources of expectations and direct messages to several people representing "all bulimics." The group could then explore in action the effects of these messages and attempt to generate constructive ways of coping with them. Empirical studies of the clinical effectiveness of psychodrama are limited (Kipper, 1978), and I am not aware of studies focusing specifically on the use of psychodrama with bulimics. Research is needed in particular to address the questions of which bulimic clients benefit most from psychodrama, when psychodrama is contraindicated, and which psychodrama techniques are effective at particular phases of treatment.

In summary, psychodrama techniques, in the hands of a skilled and clinically sensitive therapist, appear to have a great deal to offer the treatment of people with bulimia. Psychodrama works on many levels simultaneously and is able to accommodate diverse theoretical orientations. Thus, as shown in the case studies, psychodrama techniques can be directed toward the goals of both cognitive–behavioral and psychoanalytic approaches—a frequent combination in working with bulimics. Psychodrama may be particularly useful in helping clients overcome blocks to emotional experience and in helping them work through internal conflicts that help sustain their eating disorders.

REFERENCES

American Psychiatric Association. (1980). *Diagnostic and statistical manual of mental disorders* (3rd ed.). Washington, DC: Author.

American Psychiatric Association (1987). *Diagnostic and statistical manual of mental disorders* (3rd ed., revised). Washington, DC: Author.

Bischof, L. J. (1970). *Interpreting personality theories* New York: Harper & Row.

Blatner, H. A. (1973). *Acting-in.* New York: Springer.

Boskind-White, M., & White, W. C. (1983). *Bulimarexia: The binge/purge cycle.* New York: W. W. Norton.

Browning, W. N. (1985). Long-term dynamic group therapy with bulimic patients: A clinical discussion. In S. W. Emmett (Ed.), *Theory and treatment of anorexia nervosa and bulimia* (pp. 141–153). New York: Brunner/Mazel.

Buchanan, D. R. (1984). Psychodrama. In T. B. Karasu (Ed.), *The psychosocial therapies: Part II of the psychiatric therapies* (pp. 783–798). Washington, DC: American Psychiatric Association.

Emmett, S. W. (Ed.). (1985). *Theory and treatment of anorexia nervosa and bulimia.* New York: Brunner/Mazel.

Garner, D. M., & Garfinkel, P. E. (Eds.). (1985). *Handbook of psychotherapy for anorexia nervosa and bulimia.* New York: Guilford Press.

Hale, A. E. (1981). *Conducting clinical sociometric explorations: A manual for psychodramatists and sociometrists.* Roanoke, VA: Author.

Haskell, M. R. (1975). *Socioanalysis: Self direction via sociometry and psychodrama.* Long Beach, CA: Role Training Associates of California.

Kipper, D. A. (1978). Trends in the research on the effectiveness of psychodrama: Retrospect and prospect. *Group Psychotherapy, Psychodrama and Sociometry, 31,* 5–17.

Kipper, D. A. (1986). *Psychotherapy through clinical role playing.* New York: Brunner/Mazel.

Kohut, H. (1977). *The restoration of the self.* New York: International Universities Press.

Moreno, J. L. (1946). *Psychodrama* (Vol. 1). New York: Beacon House.

Moreno, J. L. (1953). *Who shall survive?* New York: Beacon House.

Moreno, J. L. (1973). *Theatre of spontaneity.* New York: Beacon House.

Moreno, J. L., & Moreno, Z. T. (1959). *Psychodrama* (Vol. 2). New York: Beacon House.

Moreno, J. L., & Moreno, Z. T. (1969). *Psychodrama* (Vol. 3). New York: Beacon House.

Moreno, Z. T. (1959). A survey of psychodramatic techniques. *Group Psychotherapy, 12,* 5–14.

Moreno, Z. T. (1965). Psychodramatic rules, techniques and adjunctive methods. *Group Psychotherapy, 18,* 73–86.

Moreno, Z. T. (1971). Beyond Aristotle, Breuer and Freud: Moreno's contribution to the concept of catharsis. *Group Psychotherapy and Psychodrama, 24,* 34–43.

Neuman, P. A., & Halvorson, P. A. (1983). *Anorexia nervosa and bulimia: A handbook for counselors and therapists.* New York: Van Nostrand Reinhold.

Roy-Bryne, P., Lee-Benner, K., & Yager, J. (1984). Group therapy for bulimia: A year's experience. *International Journal of Eating Disorders, 3,* 97–116.

Shisslak, C. M., Schnaps, L., & Swain, B. (1986). Interactional group therapy for anorexic and bulimic women. *Psychotherapy, 23,* 598–606.

Starr, A. (1977). *Rehearsal for living: Psychodrama.* Chicago: Nelson Hall.

Stein, M. B., & Callahan, M. L. (1982). The use of psychodrama in individual psychotherapy. *Journal of Group Psychotherapy, Psychodrama and Sociometry, 35,* 118–129.

White, W. C., & Boskind-White, M. (1984). Experiential-behavioral treatment program for bulimarexic women. In R. C. Hawkins, W. G. Fremouw, & P. F. Clement (Eds.), *The binge-purge syndrome: Diagnosis, treatment, and research* (pp. 77–103). New York: Springer.

Yablonsky, L. (1976). *Psychodrama: Resolving emotional problems through role playing.* New York: Basic Books.

7

Dance/Movement Therapy with Bulimic Patients

Arlynne Stark
Simona Aronow
Theresa McGeehan

Dance, the most basic of all art forms, involves the direct expression of self through the body (Hanna, 1979; Sorell, 1967). As such, it is a powerful modality for therapy. Based on the assumption that body and mind are interrelated, dance/movement therapy works directly with the body, using movement and dance to establish a more realistic body image and to effect changes in feelings, cognition, and behavior. Patients are helped to develop self-awareness, to work through emotional blocks, to gain a clear perception of themselves and others, and to effect behavioral changes (American Dance Therapy Association [ADTA], 1985). Dance/movement therapy, as a result, is often an effective treatment modality for bulimic patients.

Patients with bulimia suffer a distortion of body image, low self-esteem, and poor self-concept, often resulting in problems in interpersonal relationships. In addition, they often have difficulty identifying feeling because of their dissociation from bodily sensations. Through the use of dance/movement therapy, bulimic patients are encouraged to recognize tension in their bodies as a sign of feeling. This recognition allows healthier controls and choices to replace self-destructive binge and purge cycles; it also assists bulimics in eventually allowing feelings to be expressed symbolically in movement. Focus on interpersonal relationships in the dance/movement therapy sessions provides patients with alternative ways of relating to other people; thus, they are able to decrease their sense of isolation (ADTA, 1985).

The first section of this chapter summarizes the history and development of dance/movement therapy, its theoretical basis, its goals, and the therapeutic process. Next, the chapter focuses on the use of dance/movement therapy with bulimic patients. Specific methods and techniques are introduced and illustrated by brief case studies. Throughout the chapter, suggestions are offered (primarily from our inpatient work with groups and individuals) for possible applications of techniques and methods that may be of interest to other mental health professionals.

While we have provided techniques and examples of ways in which dance/movement therapy methods may be used in the treatment of bulimic patients in particular, we also wish to convey the potential value of dance/movement therapy as an effective therapeutic modality in general. It is important, however, for other professionals to use sound clinical judgment in deciding when and how to incorporate these techniques into existing treatment modalities.

HISTORICAL DEVELOPMENT OF THE PROFESSION

Dance/movement therapy has its roots in ancient times, when dance was an integral part of life. It is likely that people danced and used body movement to communicate long before language developed. Dance expressed and reinforced the most important aspects of cultures. Societal values and norms were passed down from one generation to another through dance, reinforcing the survival mechanism of the culture (Bartenieff & Lewis, 1980). In many societies today, dance still functions as part of celebrations, rites of passage, and other important events.

The direct experience of shared emotions on a preverbal and physical level in dance is one of the key influences in the development of dance/movement therapy (Chaiklin, 1975). The feelings of unity and harmony that emerge in group dance rituals provide the basis for empathetic understanding between people. For the individual, dance may safely disclose deeply buried fantasies and allow symbolic expression of personal potential and conflict. Dance, in making use of natural joy, energy, and rhythm, fosters a consciousness of self. As movement occurs, body sensations are often felt more clearly and sharply (Schmais, 1985). Physical sensations provide the basis from which feelings emerge and become expressed. Through movement and dance, preverbal and unconscious material often crystallizes into direct feeling states or personal imagery. It was the recognition of these elements, inherent in dance, that led to their eventual use in dance/movement therapy (Bernstein, 1979).

Pioneers

The development of dance into a therapeutic modality is most often credited to Marian Chace, a former dance teacher and performer. Over the years, she refocused her work from teaching dance technique to assisting individuals in developing and expressing their personal needs through movement (Chace, 1975). She began to work with children and adolescents in special schools and clinics as well as in her own studio, taking referrals from psychiatrists, psychologists, and other members of the health professions. In 1942, she was invited to work at St. Elizabeth's Hospital in Washington, DC. There, she put to work her understanding of the importance of the body's relationship to emotional expression. Over the years, the success of her work with extremely regressed nonverbal and psychotic patients at St. Elizabeth's Hospital gained national recognition. Patients who had been considered hopeless were able to engage in group interaction and to express feelings in the dance/movement therapy sessions. For many patients, establishing a movement dialogue, and supporting it with verbalizations related to feelings, images, thoughts, and memories, was often their first step toward recovery.

In the 1950s and 1960s, other modern dancers also began to explore the use of dance as a therapeutic agent in the treatment of emotional disturbances. Trudy Shoop and Mary Whitehouse on the West Coast and Franziska Boas and Liljan Espenak on the East Coast furthered the development of dance as therapy. Although these pioneers developed different approaches, each used dance as the context for her work. Their shared therapeutic goals were to foster integration in the body, leading to a feeling of wholeness and aliveness; to utilize movement and dance as a means of experiencing and expressing the full range of feelings; to share group and individual expression of feelings; and to externalize and express emotional material, including conflicts, memories, and fantasies, through symbolic action (Bartenieff, 1975).

General Goals and the Therapeutic Process

There are three primary arenas in which dance/movement therapy works: (1) the body and its action; (2) interpersonal relationships; and (3) self-awareness (Stark, 1982). Some specific goals related to body action are to foster a healthier body unconstricted by tensions, conflicts, and feelings; to help patients activate the body, thus permitting cathartic release of tension and feelings; and to develop a more realistic body image so that individuals may experience a sense of bodily integration and coordination.

In the second arena, dance/movement therapy establishes a basic level of communication through its direct use of rhythm and physical interaction. Group experience allows increased self-awareness through the visual feedback that occurs from observing how other people move. By noticing feelings expressed in the bodies of others, the patient may begin to identify and recognize her own feelings. In the microcosm of the world presented by the group, patients receive and give direct feedback about themselves and learn to develop a broader range of behavioral options.

Goals in the third arena are based on the assumption that being aware of one's bodily experience fosters and deepens self-understanding. The individual must have a body sense, essentially a preverbal experience, before a verbal or conceptual pattern can develop. The most direct expression available to the individual is through the body. That is, the physical experience of one's muscular actions provides an immediate way of knowing and experiencing one's self. When the importance of words is reduced, a more direct observation of nonverbal behavior results. For individuals with strong verbal defenses, movement may provide a more reliable identification of feelings than words. For bulimic patients, who often feel isolated, have difficulty identifying and expressing their feelings, and have poor interpersonal relationships, participation in group dance/movement therapy may be particularly valuable.

Group Sessions

The flow of a group dance/movement therapy session is established as the therapist facilitates the patients' spontaneous movements and connects them to the movements of others with such methods as mirroring the action, extending it, changing it, or moving in opposition to it. This linking of material is based on the therapist's assessment of the process as it unfolds. A typical group session consists of three parts: warm-up, theme development, and closure. The warm-up serves to heighten the patients' awareness of their physical and emotional state. The therapist looks for group movement themes to develop in the session. A typical warm-up flows through the body in a sequential manner to establish movement connections and to center and ground the patients. For example, peripheral movement in the hands may be sequenced through the arms into the torso and down through the legs. The quality of movement is developed in the same way. Light, tentative movement of the arms away from the body may become stronger and more direct and may include pushing or punching. As the emotional content expressed by the group is developed more fully on a bodily level, an integration of feelings, thoughts, and actions occurs. As a result of a thorough warm-up, patients usually feel more relaxed, coordinated, and ready to activate and use their bodies expressively. The warm-up also provides a beginning awareness of feelings and thoughts and their link with body action. For example, a stretching movement of the arms and hands might develop into a pushing movement. Patients may become aware of their desires to "push something away." As the body action becomes stronger, specific feelings and accompanying thoughts (e.g., "I'd like to push my mother away") often occur.

The therapist structures the group's movement through his or her kinesthetic response to the patients' movement or according to the common movement theme of the group to capture the essence of the feeling observed. By mirroring and exaggerating expressive behavior, the therapist encourages each patient's awareness of feelings through visual feedback. The movement behavior is then expanded in a symbolic dance reflecting conflicts, wishes, or dreams; the therapist may initiate movement and encourage associations, imagery, or content.

The therapist must be alert and responsive to the the group's ability to tolerate these expressions. If the affect is developed too quickly, or if the movement becomes too large or too emotionally loaded, patients may experience overwhelming emotion and loss of control. Emotional overload will lead to resistance, which can be more successfully approached by backing up to a safe level of movement (affect) and progressing to full expression from another angle. Sometimes resistance itself becomes the theme. Thus, the movement session develops in waves of expression, recuperation, expression, recuperation. Movement flow changes and develops from the evolving therapeutic process as well as from group and individual needs.

Once the affect is fully developed, expressed, and worked through in movement, the therapist leads the group to resolution and closure nonverbally with movement and verbally with a discussion of the session. Closure provides an integration of the physical, emotional, and intellectual aspects of the patients.

It is the therapist's ongoing observation, assessment, and modification of movement flow that separates dance/movement therapy from movement tasks or exercises.

USE OF DANCE/MOVEMENT THERAPY TREATMENT WITH BULIMIC PATIENTS

Bulimics often have difficulty in identifying and expressing feelings. Dance/movement therapy addresses many of the elements thought to be involved in recovery from bulimia: "improving body awareness and body image, developing a sense of self and identity, recognizing conflicts, developing positive coping skills and personal strengths, and overcoming isolation" (Raskin, 1983, p. 62). Stempler (1983) also supported this view by noting that "movement therapy can facilitate changes in the bulimic's self-deprecating attitude" (p. 6). Moreover, Krueger and Schofield (1986) suggested that "for eating-disordered patients there is no authentic movement" (p. 327), resulting from a lack of awareness of internally directed feelings early in life. Although early parent-child interactions may have formed the basis for it, the lack of internally generated feelings and authenticity probably still exists for most bulimics. As such, many bulimics have difficulty allowing their true feelings to be expressed nonverbally.

In order to understand how dance/movement therapy can address some of the therapeutic goals previously mentioned, it is important first to review the more common movement behaviors characteristic of bulimics.

Characteristics of Bulimic Patients

In the absence of formal research studies regarding movement characteristics of bulimic patients, we have observed from our clinical work that most bulimics portray several of the following movement characteristics. We also offer possible interpretations of each movement behavior.

Peripheral movement. It is common for bulimic patients to use the distal and peripheral parts of the body for gesturing. That is, movement rarely flows into the trunk or core of the body. This seems to reflect the bulimic's pattern of keeping feelings at a distance and being out of touch with sensations and bodily needs.

Purge posture. Bulimics often sit or stand with sunken chests, shoulders curved forward, and chins sticking out in a posture characteristic of depressed patients. The jutting chin and hunched shoulders are similar to the position of the chin and head when purging. The authors have labeled this position the "vomit/purge posture."

Inactive trunk. Often bulimics do not engage in movement that flows through and utilizes the trunk area. Thus, there is very little adjusting, adapting, molding, and responding with this part of the body. Movement in the trunk area often appears flat. Unlike anorexics, who are often quite rigid in the torso, bulimics may be very passive and appear to merge with others or objects in the environment; for example, they may fold themselves around or conform to the contours of a chair as though it were a container for them.

Little use of space in the environment. This characteristic may indicate difficulty in reaching out and effectively interacting with the environment.

Exaggerated quickness and time urgency or no sense of time. Bulimics often stop and go abruptly between movements, rather than making a more natural transition. This is thought to be associated with impulsivity.

Superficial affect. Bulimics often present a false smile or are overly animated. Those who tend to use a lot of body movement may project what seems like a false or performing image to others.

Loss of integrated body connections. An integrated connection between upper and lower body parts is lacking. Often, movement that occurs in the upper part of the body does not flow freely through and into the lower part of the body; similarly, movement that begins in the lower part of the body appears disconnected from the upper body (i.e., like a marionette).

Active/passive mode. The bulimic patient often operates in either a very active or very passive mode. Going from one extreme to the other appears to be the norm, rather than balancing and modulating between the two extremes.

Most bulimics are out of touch with body sensations and feelings. Movement observed in bulimics conveys the impression that they attempt to deaden their bodies or to be overly active to prevent awareness of deeper feeling. In some cases, these individuals have been physically or sexually abused. Regardless of their history, most bulimics dislike their bodies and have poor self-images and self-concepts. Dance/movement therapy fosters awareness of body sensations and feelings. Bulimic patients can become aware of how they abuse their bodies (by bingeing) to ward off uncomfortable sensations and feelings.

The dance/movement therapist will often use movement for the purpose of modifying or changing the dysfunctional movement characteristics mentioned above. Through movement interventions, new learning and feelings can occur. Many of these movement characteristics are directly or indirectly addressed in the following section on treatment issues and techniques.

TREATMENT ISSUES AND TECHNIQUES

Dance/movement therapy addresses the problems underlying bulimic behavior using a multidimensional approach. The goals established for therapy are to develop trust; develop body awareness and a more realistic body image; develop a clearer sense of self and body boundaries; encourage autonomy and enhance self-esteem; encourage more appropriate interpersonal relations, thereby overcoming loneliness, isolation, and depression; and facilitate identification, tolerance, and expression of emotion in appropriate, constructive ways.

In the following section, each goal is discussed in terms of Mahler's object relations theory (Mahler *et al.*, 1975) and related therapeutic interventions. Case studies are offered for illustration. Although the goals and techniques were developed primarily from our clinical experience with hospitalized patients (primarily in group work), many can be used as part of outpatient treatment for both individuals and groups. Also, while the discussion of treatment goals, interventions, and techniques artificially separates underlying developmental and emotional issues, many interventions suggested address more than one goal simultaneously. Moreover, because developmental tasks are continually refined, they resurface and are readdressed throughout the course of treatment.

In order to assist patients toward self-understanding, we believe that verbal processing is important. This may occur following an intervention that the patients perceive as difficult or toward the end of a session as part of the closure process. A verbal discussion is useful to help clarify and integrate feelings, thoughts, and behaviors and to foster trust and intimacy among group members.

Trust

The first goal, developing trust, recapitulates the primary symbiotic relationship between the child/patient and primary caretaker/therapist. Movement interventions addressing this goal focus on developing rapport and giving nurturance within the safety and acceptance of the therapeutic relationship. To facilitate this, the therapist and patient may need to work on body awareness and body trust before moving into relationship trust.

1. The therapist uses his or her own body to empathize with and mirror patients' nonverbal behaviors kinesthetically. The therapist can synchronize with, or reciprocate, the patients' posture, gesture, breathing, eye contact, body rhythms, and/or movement qualities (e.g., passive, quick, tense, strong). Since self-consciousness is an issue with bulimics, it is important to mirror them in a manner that does not mock them but rather creates a feeling of "being with." The nonverbal exchange simulates symbiosis, provides the therapist with information about the patients' feelings, and gives patients the experience of being understood and accepted on an unconscious body level.

2. Some additional interventions toward the development of trust and nurturance include the use of touch and massage. It is important to respect any resistance or aversion to receiving nurturance evidenced by the bulimic patient due to fear of intrusion. The level of resistance may be related to the high incidence of physical and/or sexual abuse in this population. Thus, it is important for clinicians to be sensitive to patients' readiness to engage in self-touch. However, the use of touch can provide a corrective experience for patients who are ready to explore physical contact that is different from the kind they have learned to fear; it can also help with self-acceptance.

Self-massage can be used to encourage body awareness. It can be presented in an educational way to reduce anxiety about intimacy and sexuality. Feet, hands, and shoulders are most comfortable to work with initially for self-massage. In group situations, if patients begin to trust one another, exchanging back rubs or foot massages can be a way to develop a sense of mutually reciprocal caring and nurturing.

Other nurturing forms of contact between group members involving touch include sitting back to back and rocking in a mutually satisfying rhythm, standing and rocking with the group in rhythm, standing and leaning back to back while holding each other up, or one patient holding another patient and gently rocking her.

While being held and rocked, D. began to cry. She talked about how the experience reminded her of her mother who died several years earlier. She acknowledged her need and desire to be nurtured and how she missed the relationship where this need was first met.

3. Fabrics can be used to support the development of nurturance. For example, patients can wrap themselves in blankets, parachutes, or sheets to elicit an experience of being warm, safe, and protected. Sometimes, however, this can stimulate sensations and feelings of being trapped and overprotected. In such instances, scarves and other soft materials can be used to foster nurturance by having the patients gently run the fabrics over parts of their bodies.

4. "Hiding Behind Walls" is a technique that uses pillows and blankets to represent barriers to intimacy and the need for protection and safety. As individuals within the group sit isolated from each other, the therapist may choose to accentuate the common feeling of isolation and insecurity by suggesting that group members wrap themselves in blankets. Rhythmic soothing music can be used to support this process. The group is eventually encouraged to risk leaving the safe place to make contact with others by reaching out. Eventually, patients can free themselves from the false security of the hiding place and replace it with human contact. Often, patients must confront awkwardness, insecurities, and fear of rejection.

The group began with patients hiding behind blankets and holding on to their pillows. The therapist questioned them about the comfort they felt: "Where else in your lives do you experience this kind of safe but lonely feeling?" she asked. She then asked the group to begin to make contact with the other patients in the room. Eye contact began, and the child-like game of peek-a-boo unfolded. The theme became "now you see me, now you don't." The therapist stated the theme. Patients were encouraged to expose more of themselves by coming out of the blankets [womb]. They were reassured of the safety of the group. Patients verbalized feeling vulnerable, scared, and resistant to trust. The group was encouraged to assist one another in coming out of the blankets. Reaching, lifting, and holding movements evolved and were supported and encouraged by the therapist. Several patients began to cry. The group got physically closer. Patients started actively holding and hugging each other. Gradually the strong affect of needing to be held passed. The group was brought to closure with each person hugging herself.

When patients are unable to give up their defense of "hiding," the therapist encourages them to remain in hiding and to become aware of the choice they are making. Giving permission to do this in a group transcends isolation and acknowledges the patients' need for obtaining nurturance and security the only way they can allow themselves, however dysfunctional.

5. The "Trust Falls" exercise is another technique with which to address the issue of trust. Group members form dyads and decide who will be passive and who will be active. The passive patient is instructed to stand as stiff as a board with arms folded across her chest and to fall toward her partner while maintaining stiffness. The role of the active patient is to catch and rebalance the partner. The roles are then reversed. The dyads can then be brought into a group circle. Each patient is given the opportunity to stand in the circle's center. Here, the falling is repeated but the passive patient can fall in any direction. The surrounding people do not rebalance the patient but gently push her to fall in another direction. The result is often a feeling of being rocked like a baby.

6. A variation of the Trust Falls exercise uses a stretch band, an elastic cloth large enough to accommodate the group. The band enhances safety and a sense of being held up through tactile stimulation around the body and by providing a literal container for the dyad or group. Patients stand inside the stretch band in dyads or as a group and lean away from each other.

7. Another useful technique employs a parachute or sheet. The group stands in a circle holding its outer edges. Each person is then lifted in the parachute or sheet and rocked by the other patients.

Body Awareness and Body Image

Body awareness helps individuals focus on sensations and feelings within the body as well as the movement potential of the various body parts. Through body awareness, patients can begin to discriminate their own body cues. Awareness helps to facilitate a sense of control over the body and eventually over the external world.

Bulimics tend to cut off body sensations as evidenced by bingeing or depersonalization. Rather than relying on their own body cues and signals, bulimics often try to determine what responses and behaviors please other people. The dance/movement therapist may address body awareness in many different ways. The most basic awareness of the self comes from breathing (Siegel, 1984). A baby adapts its own breathing to its mother's and develops synchronous respiration, thus setting patterns for future intimacy. In addition, this adaptation assists with the formation of body ego and body image. Rhythmic steady breathing can recapitulate this early experience with the mother. Breathing exercises can also reestablish these primary connections to one's body as they foster an awareness of sensations and tension areas. As body connections return, it is not uncommon for feeling to return, thus allowing both positive and negative feelings to crystallize. Feelings of frustration and anxiety may also appear and intensify as some patients experience how out of touch they are with their emotions. The anxiety beneath blocked feelings can be overwhelming for some patients. It is, therefore, important for the dance/movement therapist to channel the sensations into a positive and meaningful experience.

1. Full breathing is a technique that charges the body and enhances feelings of aliveness. At the same time, it fosters the release of tension and encourages relaxation. In the full-breathing process, the individual breathes deeply, expanding the chest cavity equally in several directions. The torso expands front and back, widens into the ribs and lengthens along the spine. It is helpful to have patients see the technique demonstrated and even touch the therapist's torso in order to feel the breath changes. Patients then feel their own torsos to experience where breath comes in fully and where it is being held. This is best done seated. As breathing deepens, sound will often emerge.

2. Another breathing technique has patients sound the vowels while lying down. Each sound resonates in a different part of the torso (Bartenieff & Lewis, 1980). This technique is particularly effective in drawing awareness to different body parts. Moreover, the resonating sound helps to stimulate and unblock tension areas. Another method of enhancing breathing uses the sound of "sss" or sighing to let oxygen out and increase exhalation. It is important to rest and pause in between cycles to prevent hyperventilation.

3. For some patients, this kind of breathing work is difficult and frustrating because of the urge to keep feelings repressed. Therefore, it is often helpful to use props to facilitate the process, for instance, blowing a balloon or feather across the room, blowing up a balloon, or blowing on one's own hand.

Further development of body awareness can be achieved through a series of closed-eye processes in which images are introduced verbally by the therapist. This method allows patients to notice feelings as the imagery links feelings, the unconscious, and consciousness.

1. Patients are asked to lie down in a comfortable position on their backs with arms at their sides. The therapist asks them to start with deep breathing to promote relaxation and to enter a state of inner concentration and body-level attention. After a few minutes of breathing, patients are asked to scan a variety of memories or sensations. First, they scan the bodies from head to toe, one body part at a time, for places where there is tension and holding. Next, they scan their bodies part by part for both

pleasant and unpleasant memories associated with each body part. Last, they scan their minds for memories related to their bodies from birth forward to the present. The patients may note outstanding memories, especially early traumas.

Whenever possible, images are later brought to consciousness through verbalization or movement enactment. They may form the basis for later expressions of rage, grief, joy, and fear related to past hurtful or pleasant experiences. The reader may want to refer to Kearne-Cooke's chapter on imagery (Chapter 2) and to *Transforming Body Image* (Hutchinson, 1985); both include many suggestions for imagery work with the body.

2. It is also helpful for some patients to use drawing in conjunction with this exercise as a way to capture inner sensations and to provide an object that recalls their experience. The reader may want to refer to Morenoff and Sobol (Chapter 8) and Fleming (Chapter 14) on art therapy for some specific suggestions and techniques.

3. Another major area of body awareness involves sensing body parts, their connectedness to each other, and their potential range of motion. In this process, patients can become more realistic about both their abilities and limits. Developing awareness must be approached in a noncompetitive and nonjudgmental manner to minimize stress and foster self-acceptance and acceptance of others.

Sometimes an educational, structured model reduces anxiety and provides containment for affect. Patients are taught basic anatomy and body structure by using anatomy books, a model skeleton, direct palpation, and body experience. Especially important are helping patients to locate the anatomical bony landmarks (e.g., shoulder joints) and to learn to differentiate between essential muscle (which has volume) and body fat. Patients can develop a sense of what "normal" is structurally and identify features that are consistent from person to person. These realizations help patients to regard their own bodies more realistically.

4. A warm-up of stretching and using each body part, first in isolation from other body parts and then in relationship to them, allows patients to gain awareness of the use and function of body parts.

5. The Bartenieff Fundamentals ™ (Bartenieff & Lewis, 1980) are a series of simple exercises for developing an awareness of bodily integration and for fostering efficient, effective use of the body. There are six basic exercises and many variations that support the basic connections in the body. Other systems of body work useful in recognizing body awareness are those of Moshe Feldenkrais (1972) and of Matthias Alexander (1969).

Body awareness creates a solid foundation for body image development. Fisher (1986) defines body image as the way in which people assign meaning to their body experience and to various body parts. The following examples illustrate ways to work with body images in relationship to one's self.

1. To begin to loosen up images and associations, the group leader calls out a body part, starting with less threatening areas such as the face, elbow, and eyes. Patients respond quickly with associations to body parts, saying as many words as come to them and talking simultaneously. As the group becomes more comfortable, body parts that are more threatening and contain more affect may be identified, such as hands, breasts, and genitals. Anyone in the group may call out the body parts. For this process to work successfully and to be authentic, patients must feel safe with each other.

2. Images, drawings, or collages can be translated into movement; small gestures, whole-body actions, or short movement phrases can be constructed to symbolize both current body perceptions and body ideals. For example, one hand might gesture in ways to suggest pleasing and accommodating others, while the other hand may express what the patient would really like to do (e.g., a punching movement). Patients can conduct a movement dialogue between the two images. This facilitates resolution of the conflict between the two perceptions of the self, the real and the ideal.

3. "Bigger than Life" is another technique that works with people with distorted body images. The technique employs music and exaggerated freestyle dance movements. Patients select a body part they are obsessed with and exaggerate its size; they pretend that the body part continues to grow in size and weight until they can barely move. The therapist supports the process by encouraging imagery to enhance the quality of the movement. For example, some patients pretend to carry a boulder or to "drag the weight of the world." When all the patients can barely move, the are instructed to peel the images off their bodies and pile them into the middle of the group circle, thereby symbolically liberating themselves from their distortions.

Sense of Self and Body Boundaries

Developing a clear sense of self and of body boundaries requires self-differentiation. Developing body boundaries is important for bulimics, who need to strengthen their capacity to hold and tolerate the intense feelings they have previously controlled through bingeing and purging. Some patients fear they will split apart or go out of control as feelings deepen, emerge, and demand expression. Defining body boundaries thus helps patients develop a clear sense of limits as well as a sense of being able to depend on their bodies.

1. Lying on the floor with their eyes closed, patients are guided through relaxation exercises and are asked to explore the shape of their body edges and surfaces as well as the volume of their body parts both visually and through self-touch.

2. Patients are instructed to roll forward, backward, and sideways on floor mats. If they can allow the soft surfaces of their bodies to roll and not just the bony landmarks, they can develop an awareness of their body boundaries and definitions.

3. Pushing against a wall with hands, back, or sides can help define the edges of the body. Likewise, patients can push outward with their hands or feet by increasing the tension in them and stiffening themselves, as if sensing an imaginary wall or bubble around their bodies. Pushing can also be done with another individual, shoulder to shoulder, back to back, or hand to hand.

4. Next, the patient is asked to move in a spontaneous way and to freeze her movement when asked to. The frozen movement usually gives a specific feeling and bodily sensation. This exercise can also be done when the individual decides when to freeze. Some patients will require instruction from the therapist as to when to freeze, while others will make choices on their own. These differences may be related to the ability to be self-directed.

5. An additional way of defining one's self in space and clarifying boundaries is through exploring personal space. This is explored up and down, out to either side, and in front and in back. It is also explored at high (above one's head), middle, and low (near the floor) levels. Imagery can be used with this process to help patients describe their personal-space sphere. For example, one person may perceive her space as a protective bubble or as though it had walls. Sometimes patients are asked to imagine the space as a house, which they can design out of any material they wish. It is their house and no one may enter unless invited. This imaging process defines and protects the boundaries of the self. Often, images used by patients take on personal symbolic meaning.

S.'s house was made of glass because she trusted that no one would break in. C.'s had to have two doors so she would not feel trapped. P.'s was made from shells and was set on the ocean. The shells were there so she could tell if someone was coming close by the sounds of the shells.

The process of beginning to define body boundaries may trigger the process of realizing individual needs and questioning how these needs can be met. For example, a personal space that evokes images of solid walls might be indicative of a need to protect one's self from other people and/ or harm. Patients can be encouraged to see how these personal images may influence their feelings and behaviors. Body sensations can then begin to be repeatable, recognizable feeling states that can eventually be identified, and the patient can have some control as a result.

Autonomy and Self-Esteem

The fourth goal, encouraging autonomy and self-esteem, recapitulates the practicing subphase of Mahler's separation–individuation process (Mahler *et al.*, 1975). The dynamics of this stage of development culminate in the psychological birth of "I," the rudiments of a unique and separate identity. Exploration and experimentation in therapy can result in a clearer sense of self, which can then generalize to life outside the therapy setting.

Movement dynamics characteristic of this stage of development begin with pushing and pulling and later evolve into more self-directed movements. The individual's focus shifts from need gratification to assertion and exploration. There is a heightened awareness of muscles and attainment of sensation and motor action. Muscles are used aggressively. It is a time of activating one's sense of self and having some impact on the environment.

To develop a sense of autonomy, it is important for patients to experience their real body center and the two weight centers. This includes a clear sense of balance and awareness of stability and mobility in both the upper and lower parts of the body. Balancing helps to develop body and ego definition.

1. Shifting from one foot to the other and then centering the body, and finding the two weight centers (strength in the pelvis and levity in the chest), promotes a sense of bodily integration. This is essential learning for individuals who need to learn to mobilize their bodies in order to feel and express assertion.

2. Patients shift their weight from one foot to the other, moving side to side or forward and back with knees slightly bent, balancing the lower body in a stationary position while moving the upper body in different directions and positions. They balance on one foot or they walk with attention focused on when their weight shifts from one foot to the other.

3. Two people hold each other wrist to wrist (facing each other) and create a mutual balance. As one person shifts position by bending her knees and dropping her pelvis toward the floor, both the upper and lower body of the partner must adjust to keep the countertension within the body and between the two people. The mutual balance and accommodation must be maintained as the partners switch position, and the other bends knees and lowers to the floor. This seesaw-like activity helps to activate the weight center in the pelvis and requires stability for both participants. Much accommodation and continual shifting of body center will naturally occur. If done successfully, both partners will experience an ability

to accommodate without losing their sense of bodily integration and connection.

4. Patients' ambivalence about taking a stand can be given expression through pushing-and-pulling movements. Allowing the ambivalence to be expressed in movement can clarify the patients' feelings by making the struggle conscious. The therapist can suggest that patients push against walls, floors, doorways, or each other. Pulling movements can be activated using sheets, blankets, or stretch bands in a tug-of-war. Patients are asked to monitor whether they can maintain balance and a sense of self without being pushed or pulled over. This technique helps to stabilize their bodies and provides a sense of control and mastery that is needed for working with deeper aggressive feelings.

5. Frequently, a person expresses autonomy in relation to others through the use of assertion, anger, and/or aggression. Through physically using the large muscles of the body and matching the movement quality with the voice, patients can observe their impact in the world. For example, patients may be encouraged to stamp their feet and shout "no." Using objects can sometimes provide a safer release of feeling. For example, the group can be encouraged to throw and kick beach balls or rip up newspapers. The therapist asks the group to label an object and to imagine that it represents issues, memories, or conflicts the patients are trying to resolve. Beanbag chairs and sponge balls are also effective props. The therapist begins the process of picking them up, throwing them, mushing them, molding them, and kicking them. The group is encouraged to follow suit. Similarly, bataca bats can be used to hit the wall, chairs, or pillows. This exercise can be expanded to pillow fighting, bataca fighting with another patient, or playfully grabbing something away from another patient such as a ball or sheet.

6. If the group members are amenable, they can be encouraged to imitate the body movements and sounds of aggressive animals, especially lions, bears, and tigers. However, especially if affect is strong, it is important to handle closure by having the patients join together in calmer, less aggressive movements. This will help to make them feel safe and less vulnerable.

7. Fostering leadership within the session is another method of supporting autonomy while building self-esteem in the context of the group. "Changing leadership" is a technique that begins with all patients standing in a line. The patient at one end begins leading the group in a large line around the room. The patients in line imitate the leader's movements. When another patient wants to take over the leadership, she begins a new movement or direction in space. She needs to make her movement very obvious and clear so the rest of the group will refocus their attention on the new leader. Leadership may shift at any time.

8. Another technique, called "flocking," can also be used. The group

stands together in an amorphous shape, and one patient volunteers to lead. The group imitates the movement of that person as long as the group's movement flows in the leader's direction. When the group spontaneously changes direction, the person now in front leads, and the group imitates the new leader's movement. Anyone can break away from the original group formation and start their own subgroup. The effect is a chorus of people either moving together or subgroups moving simultaneously. In the process of relating to the movement of others, the patient can learn to be empathetic with another person without merging and losing her sense of self. This technique helps to promote a clear sense of self versus separateness.

Interpersonal Relationships

The fifth goal of treatment is socialization and developing appropriate interpersonal relationships. Another intent is to provide an experience of pleasure in the body in the context of a group and to overcome loneliness, isolation, and depression. Developmentally, this stage recapitulates Mahler's rapprochement subphase of the separation–individuation process.

Bulimics have great difficulty being themselves with others (Mahler, et al., 1975). The real self in touch with spontaneous impulses, feelings, and desires is split off and repressed. As a result, bulimics often attempt to validate themselves through others. Characteristics of perfectionism and overachievement stem from the need for constant recognition. Boskind-Londahl (1976) wrote that the self-image of bulimics is constructed around societal expectations of the ideal. This unrealistically high standard contributes to self-deprecating thoughts and feelings and the desire to hide their real selves from others.

Movement interventions can focus on self-expression in relation to others and the outside world by developing the creativity and spontaneity of the hidden self and encouraging the experience of pleasure from social interaction. However, it is important to begin on a body level. The therapist strives to help bulimics integrate movement in and through their entire torsos, providing a feeling that all body parts are connected and the body self is whole. This kind of movement fosters integration in the body and serves as a basis for self-expression.

1. Patients can sculpt in empty space or use other group members to create shapes. Other patients can be instructed either to touch or not touch. The reader may want to refer to Root on family sculpting for more ideas (Chapter 5).

2. Spatial distancing is another technique useful in exploring interpersonal relationships. Patients are instructed to alternately distance themselves and move closer to other patients until they locate a place that

is comfortable in relation to the other group members. When this exercise is complete, patients are asked to think about the distance they maintain in their personal relationships and their feelings about intimacy.

3. Mirroring with a partner can clarify the subtle shifts in awareness of self-initiated versus other-initiated behavior while encouraging spontaneity. Patients choose a partner and agree about who will lead and who will follow. The process starts using only the hands or one body part; it gradually involves more of the body until full body movement is employed. All communication between participants is nonverbal. Patients switch roles after the therapist believes that the leader has experienced moving with spontaneity and creativity. When both patients have had an opportunity to lead, the therapist asks them to continue without designating a leader. This part of the session is less structured and encourages free exchange and movement dialogues through nonverbal communication. Mirroring indirectly addresses the issues of isolation and fear of intimacy.

4. In another process, patients are asked to come together as though a picture will be taken of the group. The patients hold their position for a few moments, noticing where they have located themselves in relation to other group members. The photographic session can take on a movement action and/or dialogue.

5. As patients develop more realistic body images and senses of self, they can be more available to feedback from others about the images they project to the world. This is a crucial turning point in therapy. It is essential that bulimic patients receive realistic feedback about what impression they actually make on others and that they realize that they are accepted for who they are and not for how their bodies appear. The following technique utilizes projection and observation as means of noticing commonly held attitudes and beliefs.

Each patient is asked to walk back and forth across the room. The other patients are asked to focus on their own kinesthetic experience (body sensations and feelings) while observing the patient's walk. The therapist then asks the group to give written feedback about what the individual's posture conveys. What is this person's body saying? What is missing? The group's observations are read aloud and the walking patient confirms or refutes the feedback. The therapist then asks the patient and the group what they feel is preventing fulfillment of the walker's needs.

R. executed her walk across the room with sagging shoulders, downcast eyes, and tension through her arms and fists. Feedback from the group described feelings of loneliness, discomfort, anger, shame, hurt, sensitivity, and longing for acceptance. The group felt R. needed reassurance, confidence, and self-acceptance. R. confirmed the group's perceptions but was surprised that she projected this image to others. When asked what prevented her from fulfilling her needs, she replied "Guilt."

6. Another useful technique at this stage of therapy is imitative walking. The therapist suggests that patients adopt other people's walks, not only exhibiting the walk but becoming it. Each patient does this by taking on the rhythm, energy, posture, and speed of the other person's walk. Patients can also be asked to imitate the walk of family members. By miming the walks of people who have been close to them, patients can learn how they have incorporated other people's attitudes and characteristics in their own movements—or how their movement styles differ.

7. In another technique, similar to the one above, a patient is asked to begin a movement that is repeated over and over. Another patient joins in, executing a different movement that is related and attached to the first person. Other group members join, and eventually a moving machine is created. People can add sounds to their movements. The task here is to be related to the movement of others, yet maintain individual, separate movements and a sense of self.

Self-Expression

The last goal in our work with clients is authentic self-expression. Self-expression is risking being one's self regardless of other people's responses. Self-expression is being truthful with what one feels and finding a way to communicate that externally. Developmentally, self-expression is related to Mahler's stage of object constancy, in which one's own individuality begins to consolidate and one's contradictions find some resolution (Mahler et al., 1975). This also coincides with development of gender identity.

Using more authentic self-expression provides a channel for previously denied intolerable feelings. These often include inner rage, sexuality, and the need for nurturance. It is an empowering experience to reclaim and express one's feelings, and self-expression offers bulimics a feeling of being adult and effective in the world.

1. To help encourage authenticity, small authentic gestures are used. These movements may have meanings that large active external movements may mask. Examples of authentic gestures include the small pushing-and-pulling or opening-and-closing gestures of the hands that emerge during times of ambivalence. Other meaningful gestures can be making eye contact after feeling ashamed, a spontaneous punch while talking about one's father, or two hands interlocking and folding together while talking of feeling more connected to others.

2. As clients develop more authentic reactions, they often must learn how to modulate feelings so that they are expressed appropriately. The acquisition of this skill is important for bulimics as they rarely modulate their feelings or behaviors. In movement, modulation is learned through

exploring opposite movement qualities. Patients are helped to experience extremes as well as gradual transitions from one extreme to another. For example, patients may be asked to find a body posture that is very small and closed and one that is very large and open. As they move from one to the other, they pay attention to the feelings in each posture as well as how sensations and feelings change throughout the continuum. According to Laban (1960), affect and modulation of affect can be observed in movement qualities. Although specifics are beyond the scope of this text, all therapists can observe differences in the qualities and usage of weight, time, space, and flow in order to understand differences in personality and expression of affect.

3. Emotions such as anger are usually threatening. Expression may be enhanced by the use of props (beanbag chairs, punching bags, balls, stretch bands, parachutes, masks, etc.). Props are introduced when the therapist believes that the affect that is surfacing needs a focus or container to reach full expression. The prop selected depends on the quality of the movements in need of support. It serves as a support and is removed when it is no longer needed. Props are not used when patients are able to directly confront their feelings and express themselves to others.

4. Imagery is also used to address issues too threatening to face directly. Imagery provides a metaphor that can later be related to the real problem. For example, the image of taffy can act as a metaphor for conflict between two people where boundaries are diffused and responsibility is unclear. The movement qualities are parallel to, and thus clarify, the qualities of the conflict: in this example, both are sticky, difficult to manage, and hard to separate from.

Anger can be expressed with punching, kicking, and throwing. Beanbag chairs, pillow fighting, and punching bags work well as they are not as threatening as direct contact. Newspapers and phone books can be slashed, torn, and shredded. Slashing can also be done with foam swords or other safe objects that cut through space.

Parachutes work well in regulating expansive, overwhelming tension or anxiety. Group members form a circle around the edges of the parachute and shake it as if removing crumbs from a table cloth. The intensity of the tension or anxiety is mirrored in the billowing of the parachute. The therapist may use this as a lesson in setting limits by instructing the patients to shout "no" when the billowing reaches the threshold of tolerance. Patients can learn what their limits are and how to modulate anxiety levels.

Frustration can be manifested by wringing, twisting, struggling movements. Patients are asked to imagine wringing out a wet towel, or they can actually wring a dry towel, stretch band, or parachute. Having a tug-of-war imitates the frustration and struggle for control over food, family members, and/or staff. The tension builds to its maximum and is suddenly released when one side collapses.

Guilt can be crystallized using images of heavy burdens, such as carrying the weight of the world on the shoulders. Shame can be reflected in images of a building collapsing in on itself or looking down at the floor. Images that help to crystallize fear are being in an arctic outpost where it is extremely cold, lonely, and desolate or gripping something and not letting go. An image for loss of control is that of a skier going downhill and not being able to stop or a car without brakes.

DISCUSSION

Before attempting to implement dance/movement techniques, it is important for therapists to take into account each patient's level of functioning, motivation for change, and readiness to utilize her body as a vehicle for self-learning and self-expression. Some patients will be extremely fearful of using their bodies as vehicles for therapeutic change. While the techniques described are particularly useful in working with inpatient groups, many of them can be adjusted for individual work and/or outpatient treatment. Careful attention must be given to patients' resistance, however; often the movement is experienced as too direct and immediate. In such instances, verbal preparation before and discussion afterward will help to ease any anxiety or discomfort.

In our experience, groups of bulimic patients tend to display extremes in the dynamics of the movement session and to act out their ambivalence. Initially, the group may express a desire to just relax and experience acceptance of where they are at that time without striving to do anything but focus on themselves. Later in the session, the group may insist on structure, requesting specific exercises such as the Bartenieff Fundamentals ™, body drawings, or work with posture. Still later, the group may request a return to a more unstructured approach. The group can only tolerate the lack of structure until frustration and anxiety build to an intolerable level; then they will ask for structure. Conversely, when in a structured situation, they will begin to feel too restricted. It is recommended that therapists adjust and modify the sessions and interventions based on patients' needs and appropriate treatment goals as well as what the therapists are experiencing with the patients in the session.

It is important to mention the shifts in the patient–therapist relationship that may occur as a direct result of moving together. Often, issues related to intimacy surface since moving together serves to augment the experience of "being with" another. Because the therapist is often serving as a role model, he or she will need to pay particular attention to how his or her presence and participation in movement affects the therapeutic process. In our experience, participation in group sessions serves to enhance the therapeutic process. Moving together in a one-on-one interaction may stimulate both positive and negative outcomes. Obviously, these are dependent on each patient's issues and transference responses.

Because movement provides such direct access to emotional content, it is important for therapists who are not trained in dance/movement therapy to be particularly cautious and sensitive to the power of movement. Otherwise, patients may feel that they are going to lose control or express uncontrollable rage. An educational versus a more psychodynamic approach to the techniques and methods offered is recommended for untrained therapists using dance/movement.

Collaboration with other therapies can be extremely effective. Dance/movement therapy sessions can be part of verbal group therapy; dance/movement therapy can be combined with another creative/expressive therapy, such as art or drama therapy; and individual verbal psychotherapy sessions can be scheduled immediately following dance/movement therapy sessions. The collaboration of approaches allows for a further enrichment and enhancement of the material. For example, feelings, issues, and conflicts that emerge in a dance/movement therapy session can be further explored and enacted in drama therapy or psychodrama. Likewise, the visual representation available in art therapy can be augmented and further clarified by incorporating movement as part of the treatment process. Dance/movement therapy either before, after, or as part of verbal group therapy may help to elicit feelings and to release affect in a safe and structured manner, or it may assist with the development and working through of group issues and themes.

While dance/movement therapy has gained recognition as a valuable therapeutic modality, there is a need for clinical research studies to lend additional support to its validity. Two potential areas for further research are developing assessment tools for diagnostic formulation and determining which clinical interventions are the most successful for which particular individuals. It is our belief that the set of movement characteristics discussed in this chapter could form the basis for clinical research.

Finally, it is important to again mention that, while the techniques offered in this chapter may seem relatively simple, they do require a level of sophistication in movement observation and understanding of body movement (preferably including a dance background). Training of dance/movement therapists is done on the master's level. The clinical programs, which are 2 years full-time, include extensive coursework in dance/movement therapy theory and skills; movement observation; nonverbal behavior; group dynamics; human growth and development; and psychotherapy and research. Clinical practica and a full-time internship are also required. The American Dance Therapy Association sets the educational standards, monitors the approval process for institutions, and provides professional registration and certification for its members.

In conclusion, mental health professionals in many areas may find the goals, techniques, and methods of dance/movement therapy useful in their work with bulimic patients. These techniques include fostering body awareness, developing a more realistic body image, developing affect and themes into action, transforming movement into expression, stimulating social interaction, and providing relaxation. The professional's desire to develop a sensitivity to nonverbal communication as a vehicle of personal expression in therapeutic work can offer a new and valuable dimension in work with bulimics.

REFERENCES

Alexander, M. (1969). *The resurrection of the body*. New York: Dell.

American Dance Therapy Association. (1985). Untitled brochure. Columbia, MD: Author.

Bartenieff, I. (1975). Dance therapy: A new profession or a rediscovery of an ancient role of the dance. In H. Chaiklin (Ed.), *Marian Chace: Her papers*. Columbia, MD: American Dance Therapy Association.

Bartenieff, I., & Lewis, D. (1980). *Body movement: Coping with the environment*. New York: Gordon & Breach.

Bernstein, P. (Ed.). (1979). *Theoretical approaches in dance-movement therapy* (Vol. 1). Dubuque, IA: Kendall/Hunt.

Boskind-Londahl, M. (1976). Cinderella's step-sisters: A feminist perspective on anorexia nervosa and bulimia. *Signs: Journal of Women in Culture and Society, 2*, 342–356.

Chace, M. (1975). Untitled article on professional history. In H. Chaiklin (Ed.), *Marian Chace: Her papers*. Columbia, MD: American Dance Therapy Association.

Chaiklin, S. (1975). Dance therapy. In S. Arieti (Ed.), *American handbook of psychiatry: Vol. 5: Treatment*. New York: Basic Books.

Feldenkrais, M. (1972). *Awareness through movement*. New York: Harper & Row.

Fischer, S. (1986). *Development and structure of body image*. Hillsdale, NJ: Lawrence Erlbaum Associates.

Hanna, J. L. (1979). *To dance is human*. Austin, TX: University of Texas Press.

Hutchinson, M. (1985). *Transforming body image: Learning to love the body you have*. Freedom, CA: Crossing Press.

Krueger, D., & Schofield, E. (1986). Dance/movement therapy of eating disordered patients. *The Arts in Psychotherapy, 13*, 323–331.

Laban, R. (1960). *The mastery of movement*. London: MacDonald & Evans.

Mahler, M., Pine, F., & Bergman, A. (1975). *The psychological birth of the human infant*. New York: Basic Books.

Raskin, C. (1983). *The effects of dance therapy on body image in bulimic women*. Unpublished master's thesis, Goucher College, Baltimore, MD.

Schmais, C. (1985). Healing processes in group dance therapy. *American Journal of Dance Therapy, 8*, 17–36.

Siegel, E. (1984). *Dance-movement therapy: Mirror of ourselves*. New York: Human Sciences Press.

Sorell, W. (1967). *The dance through the ages*. New York: Grosset & Dunlap.

Stark, A. (1982). Dance/movement therapy. In L. Abt & I. Stuart (Eds.), *The newer therapies*. New York: Reinholt.

Stempler, M. (1983). *The use of movement therapy as an effective treatment modality with bulimic females: A pilot study*. Unpublished master's thesis, Loyola Marymount University, Los Angeles, CA.

8

Art Therapy in the Long-Term Psychodynamic Treatment of Bulimic Women

Andrea Morenoff
Barbara Sobol

Bulimia is a chronic, habitual behavior that may be associated with a wide range of pathology. This chapter addresses this symptom as it exists in a population of older, characterologically impaired women who were treated in our clinic over a period of several years. This is an exhausting and demanding population to treat, in many cases requiring long-term therapy and an arsenal of techniques to address symptomatology that is highly resistant to cure or improvement. Alan Goodsitt's statement (1985), written of anorexics, applies to this population as well:

> Their difficulty in relating inner experiences is yet another manifestation of defects in the self-organization. These patients fail to relate inner experiences because they have an impaired capacity to live within the body-self. They are out of touch with their core experiences. There is a failure to integrate bodily, cognitive, and affective experiences into an organized core self. (p. 60)

In a long-term group for bulimic women with borderline characteristics, we developed a treatment approach that involved a combination of individual and group therapy. This combination has been tried by several eating-disorders programs (Yager & Edelstein, 1985). In fact, Yager and Edelstein (1985) wrote that patients with borderline character features *require* concurrent group and individual psychotherapy.

Within such a framework, we used a pattern of treatment in which we moved deliberately, as needed, from art therapy to verbal therapy, from past to present focus, and from behavioral to cognitive to psychodynamic issues. We called this pattern of deliberate change in therapeutic modalities "tacking." We chose this approach to address the complexity of a population who demonstrated strong resistance to traditional therapeutic interventions and had maintained their symptoms over a period of years.

What remained consistent in the therapy were the issues of self-esteem, the integration of the fragmented aspects of the self, and the function of the bulimic symptom. Long-term treatment goals included the development of greater self-esteem and of a capacity for higher levels of self-regulation. These goals addressed the symptom as well as the clients' entire level of functioning. It was our determination that a significant reduction in the frequency of the bulimic symptom would be a more reasonable goal than symptom extinction.

Verbal therapy was always the primary mode of treatment. This allowed us to respect the need of the clients to maintain their intellectual defenses. This chapter addresses in depth the incorporation of art therapy techniques, which allowed us to challenge the clients' defenses without assaulting them.

THEORY

Two of the earliest practitioners and teachers of the discipline of art therapy in the Untied States were Margaret Naumburg (1966) and Edith Kramer (1971), each of whom wrote books linking psychoanalytic theory to the use of art in therapy. As the field has developed, other art therapists have expanded on the writings of Kramer and Naumburg or have contributed works on the use of art therapy in conjunction with various other theoretical models, including gestalt therapy, cognitive therapy, and family therapy. Particularly relevant to our work are the writings on art therapy and self-psychology by Mildred Lachman-Chapin (1979) and Ruth Obernbreit (1985).

Elinor Ulman (1961, 1974), founder of *The American Journal of Art Therapy*, offered succinct definitions of the discipline:

> Essential to art therapy is that it partake of both art and therapy. For this purpose these terms may be briefly defined as follows: "Art" is the meeting ground of the inner and outer worlds as experienced by human individuals. "Therapy" aims at favorable change in personality or in living that endures beyond the therapeutic session itself. (1974, p. 14)

> [The motive power of art] comes from within the personality; it is a way of bringing order out of chaos—chaotic feelings and impulses within, the bewil-

dering mass of impressions from without. It is a means to discover both the self and the world, and to establish a relation between the two. In the complete creative process, inner and outer realities are fused into a new entity. (1961, p. 20)

A client sitting down to paint or draw—whether spontaneously or guided by suggestions of the therapist (through the giving of a specific task)—faces an unknown territory that may be experienced as challenging or frightening. As Ulman wrote, it is impossible for either the therapist or the client to "chart in advance [the] voyage of discovery" (Ulman, 1974, p. 14).

We invited our eating-disordered clients to express artistically their deepest internal imagery—representations of self and object and of the world as each client uniquely experienced it. The theoretical assumption here is that images a person makes emanate from their correlates in her inner (mental) representational world (Hammer, 1958). For characterologically impaired clients, the inner representational world has been highly distorted from earliest childhood, and the distortions continue, in adulthood, to affect the clients' perception of their environment and their ability to function within it. It is postulated that distortions, impairments, or fragmentation will be seen in the images on paper. After careful consideration, the therapist can then choose to reflect gently with the client on the meaning of the images, to make interpretations, or to hold that information for later reflection, depending on the receptivity of the client and the stage of treatment.

In offering art therapy tasks to our clients, we were seeking, either implicitly or explicitly, to elicit the truest and most honest expressions of "self" possible at that moment; to do so within a nurturant, nonjudgmental atmosphere; to stimulate the expression of affect; and to make available, for reflection, distortions in perception or other observable evidence of dysfunction.

It is important to emphasize that bulimic clients are acutely sensitive and perceive a wide range of external stimuli as threatening to their fragile sense of self. In a world often perceived as hostile, they do not believe they have the strength to tolerate their sense of despair, anxiety, or rage. Thus, they protect their internal representational world from scrutiny behind a defensive wall constructed in part from their bulimic behavior. The bulimia, therefore, not only allows for a discharge of tension and fulfills a habitual component, but it also enables the client to anesthetize herself against and dissociate herself from her underlying pain. Behind the defensive wall, the disallowed feelings are a part of an intricate system with elements of grandiosity, magical thinking, primitive and idiosyncratic mood-regulating mechanisms, distorted perceptions of reality, and inappropriate affect. The use of art therapy, as we have constructed it, gives us a peek behind this wall and an additional avenue of access to the interior life of the client.

By means of the graphic images, not only do we become acquainted with the world behind the bulimic symptom, but we also learn to take it seriously. We interpret it as an accurate reading of the clients' mental state and thereby open a dialogue with the pathology. We work with this pathology both in group and in individual therapy. However, when the symptom demands attention, for example, if bingeing or fasting become exacerbated, we move in whatever direction seems appropriate (tacking) in order gently to persuade the symptom to recede. Often this involves behavioral and structural work and sometimes includes family intervention.

In working with our population, we believe that the goals of treatment as described above are most effectively met when the use of art takes place in a group setting. This setting affects the pace of the work by inhibiting process that may become too threatening and move too quickly. The group setting also enhances and supports the clients as they observe each other's process and give each other feedback.

In using art in group therapy, one should be mindful that the act of creation is essentially "a solitary act. . . . The first audience is an audience of one—the artist [herself]" (Ulman, 1974, p. 14). Making art in a group allows clients to include others in their private, creative experience. Such sharing can generalize to other experiences of social interaction.

Lachman-Chapin (1974) called attention to the interplay between the solitary creative act and group dynamics. She distinguished two different approaches to the use of art in a group. In one, the art is secondary to the group process and is used for the purpose of fostering group interaction and observation. In this mode, the art may often take the form of pictographs or quick sketches with relatively little emotional or artistic investment. The other alternative is having art as the primary focus, with clients creating the best product they can. In this approach, the therapist encourages the formal development, over time, of "something highly meaningful and personal . . . and the experience is [then] shared" (Lachman-Chapin, 1974, p. 16). Lachman-Chapin also presented a third alternative, a balance between these two approaches. This third approach comes closer to our group model, in which the intent is to access unconscious material *and* to create a shared personal work. However, this process is controlled by giving the art tasks at specific intervals and thereby modulating the extent of the intrusion into the unconscious.

THE THERAPY STRUCTURE

The women who were seen at this clinic using this modality ranged in age from 25 to 50 years. They were in lower-middle to upper income brackets and, with few exceptions, had some formal education beyond high school. They were single, divorced, married, or cohabiting. They were referred to the clinic initially by other therapists, weight management centers, and physicians. Later referrals came through advertising and word-of-mouth; that is, they were self-referred. All clients had had some previous therapy, although not necessarily for an eating disorder.

The groups were open-ended, contained from four to seven women, and ran a natural course from approximately 2 to $2\frac{1}{2}$ years. All clients were seen first in individual therapy for at least 6 weeks before they were allowed to enter a group. In situations where all clients were new, we recommended a 6–10-week minimum individual evaluation. This made it possible for a relationship to form with the primary therapist and to determine if the client was able or willing to make a commitment to long-term work. The format of the group work was clearly explained before the client began. Each client entering a group was asked to make a 6-month minimum commitment.

Two female therapists (the authors—a social worker and an art therapist) were the group leaders. Each group met for $1\frac{1}{2}$ hours once a week; art therapy tasks were given approximately once every 6 weeks. All clients were in individual therapy (usually, although not always, with one of the group leaders) for 1 hour on a day other than the group day. Clients were invited to contact their individual therapists between sessions for reassurance and other concerns. Specific contracts around such contacts were usually made. Contact between group members outside of therapy was not allowed. Extra individual sessions were offered to clients as needed for crisis intervention; such intervention was done using traditional psychotherapy or art therapy, depending on the issue. All clients were referred for physical examinations before treatment began. Where appropriate, psychiatric evaluations were required.

As previously noted, this was a population with marked borderline characteristics, though bulimia was always the primary presenting issue. Clients reported bingeing–vomiting patterns varying from several times a day to several times a week. A smaller number were laxative abusers. In addition to the eating disorder, clients' histories included alcohol and drug abuse (prescription and street drugs), prostitution, forgery, theft, compulsive spending, gender confusion, and family histories of suicide and psychosis.

The general design called for the group to proceed in phases toward insight, maturity, and self-regulation. Understanding the dynamics of bulimia, awareness of affect, acquiring relationship skills, ability to confront others appropriately, and achieving greater capacity for honest self-scrutiny were among the developmental tasks to be learned.

The attention of the therapists and the focus of the art were directed at the general developmental level of the group. However, members who were new to the group were supported and assisted in functioning at whatever level they were able. The art assignments, although designed to elicit certain specific responses, were general enough to apply to almost any phase of the therapy.

CASE STUDIES

To illustrate this technique, we have selected three clients and have chosen examples of their artwork done in group during the course of their treatment. The three clients are referred to as Marcia, Susan, and Candy.

Marcia was a married woman in her early 40s. She had been bulimic (a laxative abuser) for more than 15 years. She reported a history of serious depression, several extramarital affairs, a suicide attempt, and the abuse of prescription pharmaceuticals.

Susan, at 31, had been sustaining a very high frequency of bingeing and vomiting for 12 years. During the course of treatment she maintained a low normal weight. She was socially isolated, a compulsive debtor, and had a family history that included active psychoses, suicides, and anorexia. She was single and lived alone through most of her therapy.

Candy began treatment at the age of 29. She had been bingeing and vomiting for 10 years and, at the time of treatment, was a recovering alcoholic. She had a recent history of prostitution and of drug abuse. Throughout most of her treatment she was living with her fiancé.

The art examples presented here were in response to several assignments: (A) a self-portrait; (B) an alternative self-portrait; (C) an early memory; and (D) a positive childhood experience with mother.

All the tasks presented here were given to the clients in a large room adjacent to the regular group room. In this space, a large table and several smaller tables were arranged; the floor was also an option as a work space. The following materials were made available: blocks of tempera paint, liquid tempera paint, pencils and erasers, pastels, and crayons. The choice of materials, the availability of a wide array of colors, and the comfortable, inviting space were all seen as conducive to self-expression. For some tasks the clients were asked to close their eyes for a few minutes while the therapists played music or led an exercise in guided imagery. Tapes were chosen by the therapists from among commercially available tapes and were selected for their appropriateness to the task. Scripts for the guided imagery were written by the therapists, again with their appropriateness for a specific art task in mind.

Either therapist would give the instructions for the tasks. Clients' questions would then be answered, after which they were given approximately 45 minutes in which to paint or draw. Only a minimum of interaction was encouraged. Discussion took place in the regular group room. Clients who had finished carried their paintings back inside and hung them up; they could contemplate them while waiting for the other group members to finish.

Self-Portrait and Alternative Self-Portrait

The use of the assigned self-portrait laid a foundation for differentiating among clients in terms of body image and availability of affect. The physical experience of self in these clients reflected a range of internal distortions, some of which were rooted in very early mother–child interactions. By keeping the instructions simple and open to interpretation, we offered little to the client around which to structure a cognitive response. It was our expectation that this would stimulate an expression of affect that would be free from the cognitive censoring processes usually present in verbal recollections and descriptions.

Figures 8-1 and 8-3 were made in response to assignment A, the non-directive self-portrait, for which the instructions were, "Paint a picture of yourself; paint the whole person and not a stick figure." A title was requested.

Figures 8-2 and 8-4, painted several weeks later during the next art therapy session, were responses to assignment B, the alternative self-portrait, designed to counteract the negative self-images that had appeared in assignment A. Clients were invited to do a relaxation exercise in which they were to visualize a place where they had felt "a sense of happiness or peace." When ready, the clients were asked to open their eyes and then paint portraits "within a real recent or past situation in which you felt similar feelings of happiness or serenity." Additionally, each client was given more individualized directions that referred to the imagery of the original self-portrait from assignment A.

Marcia: "The Real Me"

Marcia painted a figure whose head and face are prepared as if for public view (Figure 8-1). The face is carefully made up, with a bright, fixed smile and a meticulously arranged, fashionable hairdo. The body below the neck is startlingly different. First of all, it is a frontal view compared with the three-quarter view of the head. Moreover, the body is nude and is cut away to reveal an accurate and detailed depiction of the digestive organs. Within this anatomical representation of Marcia, there is one small symbolic element: a cartoon-like drawing of her heart.

When invited to describe her painting, Marcia became very bitter. She said she felt that she had become her digestive system. She called

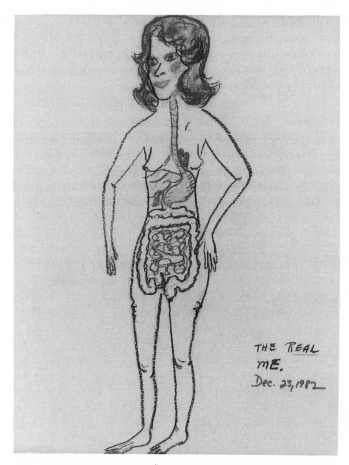

THE REAL
mE.
Dec. 23, 1982

Figure 8-1. Marcia's first self-portrait, "The Real Me."

attention to and expressed displeasure with her small breasts and her "pretty" face. When asked how she might make the picture more pleasing to herself, she said, "I would take a little off the thighs." (Note the wrinkled flesh on the outline of the thighs.) This painting contains marked depersonalization both in the mannequin-like head and the mutilated body. It was apparent from group members' facial expressions that they reacted to this graphic and cruel self-as-specimen depiction.

The therapists chose to acknowledge the eating-disorder component in a matter-of-fact manner but avoided further comment on the bitterness of Marcia's remarks or the distortion in self-concept evident in the graphics. As group leaders, we had indeed invited the expression of distortions through the purposeful vagueness of the assignment and had anticipated using the information for both diagnosis and treatment. However, in order to create some balance in perception, we directed Marcia's focus to the presence of the heart. We suggested that the heart was different from other aspects of the painting and that it represented, perhaps, a small yet hopeful element of self-love.

Marcia: "I Dug It!"

Figure 8-2 is Marcia's alternative self-portrait, made during the following art session. Marcia was reminded that the heart in her earlier painting represented the affective focus, the hopeful part. We asked her to draw a new image of herself that would be governed by this hopeful, positive heart, this time with the heart as the center of focus. In this painting,

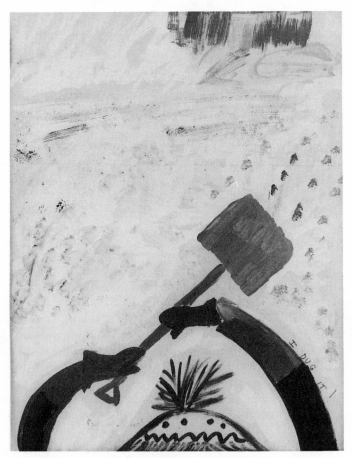

Figure 8-2. Marcia's second self-portrait, "I Dug It!"

Marcia barely enters the picture; she is heavily clothed and is visible only from behind. She depicts herself with a naive, childlike, joyful quality and appearance. Her body is energetic, with arms upraised, unlike the distorted and distressed frozen image of "The Real Me." There was a visible softening and sense of delight as Marcia recalled for the group her experience of being outdoors, alone, shoveling snow after a heavy winter storm. The therapists intervened very actively to counter Marcia's imbalance in self-perception. We suggested to her (and to the group) that there was another aspect of her self available to her—the capacity for delight and vitality that was often eclipsed by her identification with the eating disorder and her attendant self-loathing. In addition to providing feedback to Marcia, we encouraged group members to focus on their capacity to find and give a positive response. The group leaders modeled appropriate nurturant responses and shut down or limited other kinds of responses at this stage of therapy.

Susan: "Meditation"

Susan is a slender and curvaceous woman with a small waist and large breasts. In her pastel drawing (Figure 8-3), she depicted herself as a heavy,

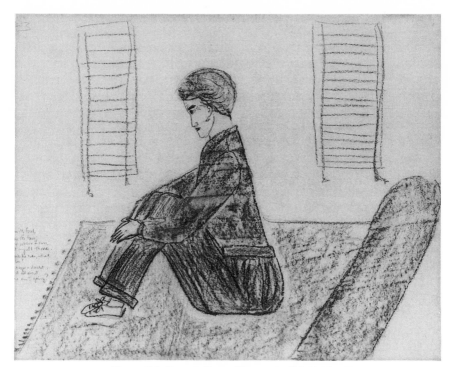

Figure 8-3. Susan's first self-portrait, "Meditation."

rigid, masculine figure. Her body proportions are distorted. In the drawing, she is sitting on a mat in an austere, bare room between two closed blinds. Her body pose is self-contained, hands clasped around her knees, her head down. Her expression is introspective, serious, and frowning. The colors are dull and are blended with black. The figure may be interpreted as withdrawn and tense. The group members expressed surprise that Susan would draw herself as so masculine. The therapists, however, focused on acceptance of the image. Rather than confront Susan with the rigidity, we asked her to identify within the picture elements that might be read as "soft." Susan pointed out the rather dainty hands and feet, drawn proportionately much smaller than the rest of the body.

As with Marcia, during the next art session, we asked Susan to focus again on the softer aspects of her picture, the hands and feet. She was

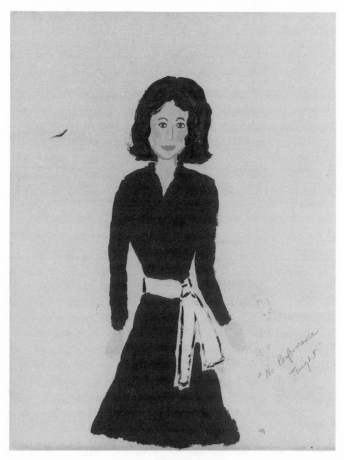

Figure 8-4. Susan's second self-portrait, "No Performance Tonight."

asked to draw herself again with this image as the inspiration in order to arrive at a self-representation that was different but equally true for her.

Susan: "No Performance Tonight"

In the subsequent picture (Figure 8-4), Susan painted herself as a thin young woman in a purple dress with a yellow sash. Her body is still rigid, but there is a clear attempt to show herself as pretty. The rendering of Susan's characteristic tentative and worried look is sensitive and accurate. Unlike the previous picture, body proportions appear quite accurate. However, where there were disproportionately large and heavy legs in the first picture, here there are no legs. In this early set of pictures, Susan graphically presented the gender and identity confusion with which she entered therapy and which were subsequently linked to her bulimia. Because these issues were so clearly expressed in the art early in therapy, the therapists were alert to other, verbal evidence of distortions. As therapy progressed, Susan made many more pictures that expressed ambivalence about being an adult woman. These pictures were used as points of reference throughout the work. In contrast to Marcia's work, Susan's "mutilation" of her self-image takes the form of denial of her body and diverts concern from the self toward thinness and asceticism.

An Early Memory

Figures 8-5 and 8-6 were responses to assignment C, which invited the clients to depict themselves in their early developmental systems in order to give the therapists information on how the clients perceived their early relationships. It was our intent to elicit an expression of feelings that are frequently out of intellectual recall. This provided an historical context for the client and gave us a working hypothesis for diagnostic and treatment purposes. The content of the drawing was the focus for the clients in creating the pictures; the expression of affect was the primary focus for the therapists in examining them. The task was given with the simple instruction, "Draw an early memory," with no further elaboration.

Susan: "Let Go of Me!"

Figure 8-5 is a dramatic painting of a mother and child done mainly in vivid blue (mother's dress) and yellow (child's shirt) with slashes of magenta paint for the mother's fingernails and mouth. It shows a grasping mother with clawed hands holding Susan while averting her head. Susan's consciously stated intent was to depict herself as the victim of a demanding, overbearing mother. However, the therapists perceived much more ambivalence in the picture than the client was able to recognize. Graphi-

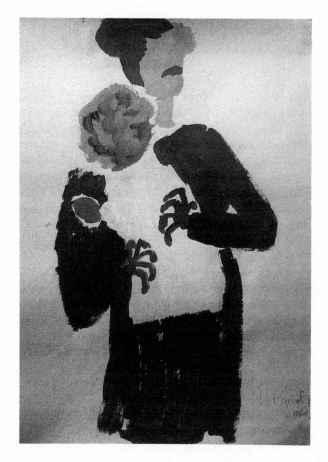

Figure 8-5. Susan's painting of an early memory, "Let Go of Me!"

cally, the baby is without depth and is incorporated into the mother's form. It is unclear who is asking to be let go of—who rejects whom. In both the graphics and the content, there appears to be a symbiotic but conflicted relationship in which mother and daughter both have difficulty with separation. As Susan gradually gained the ability to verbally acknowledge this ambivalence and her rejection of her mother as inadequate, the therapists were able to use this painting as a reference in making interpretations. The feedback given to Susan at the time of the task was affirmative and reinforced her ability to express powerful emotions. It left the door open for future attention to identifying these emotions and acknowledging their complexity.

Candy: "Wicked Witch of the South"

Figure 8-6 is a colorful painting that looks somewhat like a storybook illustration of a child's room. To the left of center, Candy used a lot of white and bright, flat, primary colors. However, the figure in the upper right-hand corner—a witch's face surrounded by clouds and bats—is done in uneven strokes of brown, black, burnt sienna, and a muddy magenta. The picture is meant to show the room Candy and her younger sister shared as children. Candy, in the upper bunk, is shown only as a bumpy shape huddled under the covers. She is cowering in fear from a dream image of the "Wicked Witch of the South" and wishing she could leave the room to go to her mother. The figure of the witch hovers just above the door to mother's room.

This was one of many paintings in which Candy was unable to depict herself within the frame of the painting. In talking about her picture, Candy was able to describe her sense of fright and aloneness with her protection (mother) out of reach. Candy stated that she could not move from her bed to get comforted because of the spectre of the witch over the door.

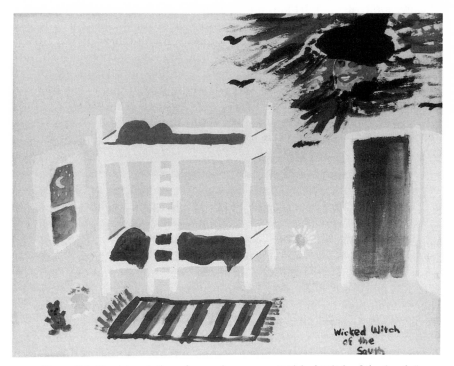

Figure 8-6. Candy's painting of an early memory, "Wicked Witch of the South."

Although she strongly implied that the Wicked Witch of the South and her mother, who is a Southerner, were one, Candy did not verbalize this. That she could neither explicitly state what her picture implied nor place herself within the frame was interpreted by the therapists as avoidance and evidence of a need for emotional distancing. However, this interpretation was not shared in group. Instead, we affirmed Candy's resourcefulness in her ability to use color and the cheerful presentation in her depiction of the scene, as well as noting the absence of depression. Working from this and other early paintings, we formulated a view of a disengaged family with a powerful but emotionally absent mother. Candy's continuing inability to place herself in her drawings was an indicator that deep intrusion into her unconscious process would be inadvisable at this point in treatment. Rather, a cognitive and behavioral approach continued to be more appropriate.

A Positive Childhood Experience with Mother

Figures 8-7 through 8-10, responses to assignment D, came at a much later stage of therapy. This assignment addressed a healing process (specifically, some of the hurt and anger with clients' mothers that was elicited in assignment C). This was a deeper probe beneath the negativity to discover if, where, or in what way, the capacity for nurturance was buried. The assignment was therefore more specific in its instructions, which were given in two stages: (1) to paint an early and positive experience with mother; and (2) to produce a second painting (without much time for reflection) that represents the "heart" or essence of the artwork produced for the first stage. This combination of tasks was designed to reach toward the source of the client's capacity for pleasure, joy, and, ultimately, self-love.

Candy: Untitled

Figure 8-7 is an outdoor scene painted in soft shades of green and representing the front yard of Candy's childhood home. At the center of the picture, framed by the landscape, a small child-like figure in a bright red dress, reading a book, sits on a swing that hangs from a large, leafy tree branch. Candy said that this was meant to be her mother. As in Figure 8-6, Candy herself is not visible in the picture but rather is implied somewhere just outside the frame, approaching her mother. According to Candy, she is about 8 years old and has just left school after a humiliating encounter with a teacher. She is running down the road, seeking the comfort and protection of home. The mood of anticipation described by Candy seems more important than the actual shared moment of pleasure with

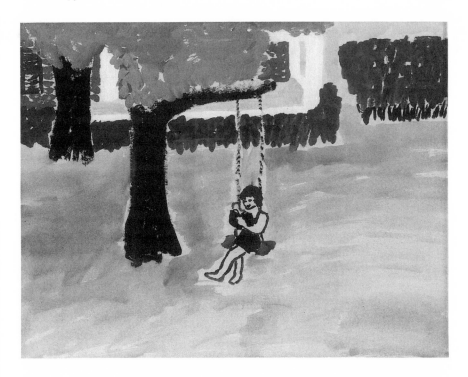

Figure 8-7. Candy's untitled painting of a positive childhood experience with her mother.

her mother. Physical and emotional distance seems to be expressed both explicitly (landscape setting) and implicitly (Candy's physical absence from the picture) in Candy's presentation of this early scene.

Candy's second painting (Figure 8-8), the "heart" of the primary art work, shows only a pale blue sky and the ropes of the swing reaching up to a tree branch. The ropes are foreshortened, as if seen from below. Candy reported that this is the view from her mother's lap as her mother holds her on the swing. The image conveys Candy's delight in the sunny sky simultaneous with her longed-for contact with the love-object, mother.

Candy was able to depict both the anticipation of pleasure (Figure 8-7) and the sensation of release from anxiety (Figure 8-8). However, she seemed unable to depict the facilitating link between these two events—the moment when mother and child were together on the swing. The missing link of interpersonal engagement was seen by the therapists as central to Candy's behavior as an adult. In her adult life, she had established a pattern of turning away from healthy relationships and toward the dysfunctional experiences of prostitution and substance abuse. Candy's therapy had revealed a long history of overstimulation and lack of

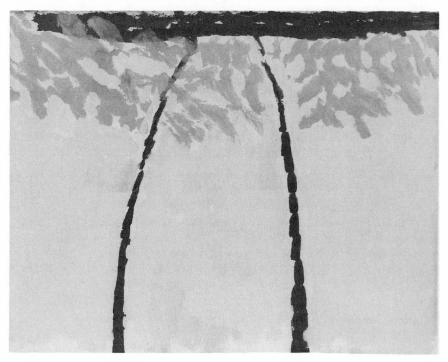

Figure 8-8. Candy's untitled painting of the heart of her childhood experience with her mother.

resolution in her relationship with her mother. Over time, Candy was able to recall numerous incidents in which her mother shared stimulating stories from her own experience yet was unable to offer guidance or comfort to her daughter. Thus, Candy's dysfunction was seen by the therapists as a pathological defense against her experience of a narcissistic and emotionally disengaged parent.

The feedback the therapists gave to Candy emphasized that her ability to experience pleasure and relief came from within herself. Her confident use of color and line, as well as her verbal explanation of the positive experience shown in her painting, were used to support this view of the self. We stressed that she was able to create from her environment a legitimate sense of joy and well-being despite her reluctance to depend on other people. In subsequent work, that belief in herself was expanded into a tentative but growing sense of trust in others and a relinquishing of her dependence on antisocial behavior.

Marcia: Untitled

In response to the instructions, Marcia painted, with great care (Figure 8-9), a detailed picture of herself at about age 8, dancing with her mother in the kitchen. A poorly defined object to the right, identified by Marcia as a record player, is painted in murky colors; Marcia, her mother, and the curtained window are painted with delicate strokes and in light, clean colors. The smiling mother is dressed in a feminine blouse and has a rose in her hair, red lips, and a locket around her neck. Marcia is clearly a child here, in a frilly and delicate light-blue frock and pigtailed hair. Mother and daughter are dancing together. Marcia's back is to the viewer. Marcia described this as a scene in which she is teaching her mother the dance steps she had just learned in school that day. In her narrative about her painting, Marcia characterized the dancing as a task or requirement, the goal of which was to please her mother. In contrast to Candy's paintings, in which she experienced pleasure in the absence of an awareness of mother, Marcia's painting suggests that her mother is experiencing pleasure outside any awareness of Marcia.

Marcia depicts an enmeshed parent–child relationship. Mother's delight is at the center of Figure 8-9. Although Marcia is present, we know nothing about the quality of her affect in that moment. Marcia's role is to

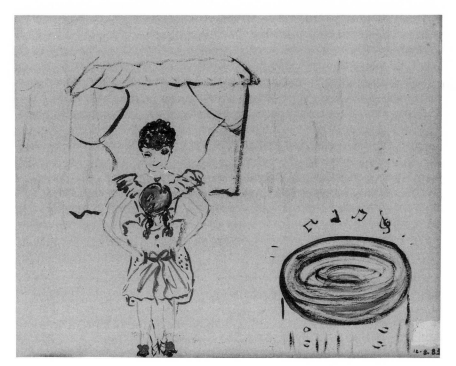

Figure 8-9. Marcia's untitled painting of a positive childhood experience with her mother.

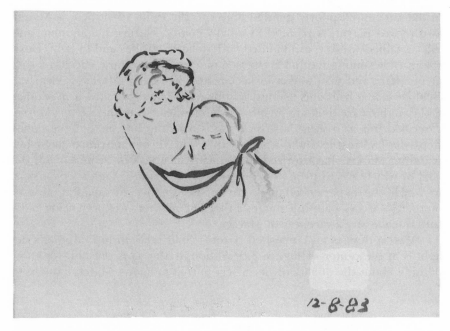

Figure 8-10. Marcia's untitled painting of the heart of her childhood experience with her mother.

be her mother's facilitator. It seems that providing pleasure for a narcissistic parent had become her *raison d'etre.*

In the second artwork (Figure 8-10), the essence of the painting was a startling revelation to Marcia of her fusion with her mother and their failure at achieving the desired separation–individuation. The painting is of two faces distinct at the top but joined at the jaw, sharing a disproportionately large, wide, smiling, red mouth. This symbiotic attachment had led Marcia away from any awareness of her own innate capacity for pleasure. In its stead was a series of "significant others" from whom she had attempted to derive her sense of self-worth. The dependency on others, who had, by her report, consistently disappointed her, created in her an enormous amount of anger that was gradually attended to in therapy. The information about Marcia's symbiotic attachment that became available in these paintings allowed the therapists to direct her attention to the need to make her pleasure in life more clearly her own. The authenticity of her half of the smiling face was explored over time. She was challenged by the therapists and the group to work toward the achievement of an internalized sense of self that would eliminate the pathologic fusion and dependency.

Termination

Subsequent art tasks (and the related group and individual therapy) continued to seek out, to discover, and to label the building blocks with which these clients could construct new and more appropriate defensive structures. These new defenses (or options) were necessary to respond to the genuine early deprivation and wounds experienced by all of these clients as well as to the new stressors they encountered as adults. The restructuring took place in many arenas: the behavioral, the cognitive, the emotional, the affective, and the interactive. Each client's artwork, collected during the course of treatment, served to document the change and growth process.

As group therapy entered the final stages, we felt it was important for each client to review her unique collection of art. Because this particular group was ending for everyone at the same time, one extended session was devoted to this review. In other groups, when only one group member is leaving, a review of only that person's artwork may be the subject of all or part of a group session.

In the group meeting, slides of each woman's pictures, arranged chronologically, were presented to the clients in the quiet, darkened room. This event promoted and allowed clients to share a view of themselves as multilevel, complex human beings, who were changing, yet who had consistent cores. This view of themselves was an antidote to the all-or-nothing, dichotomous self-concept that is characteristic of so many bulimic clients. Because the final group was part of a termination and self-reflective process for each client, we chose only to show the slides and affirm each person's identity; we then continued the work of reflection and termination in individual therapy.

DISCUSSION

In the cases discussed above, and with most of our clients, the bulimic symptom was perceived to be the primary source of pain. However, the evidence gained from our clinical experience confirms that the bulimia protects and ensures the maintenance of the underlying pathology and thereby prevents significant long-term improvement. Thus, to treat this population exclusively for the eating disorder is shortsighted. The client's plea to achieve a "cure" through the annihilation of the symptom should not seduce the therapist into mistaking the symptom for the illness. Premature symptom reduction may in fact exacerbate the underlying pathology. Clients are likely to become even less trusting of themselves and their capacity to make lasting changes; also, there is a serious risk that they will learn to distrust the therapeutic process completely. Although it is essential to address the bulimic symptom throughout the course of therapy, one must not allow the client to believe that this is the total work. Rather than treating the symptom in isolation, we engage the client in a process that aims toward making profound changes in the structure of the self.

To accomplish this restructuring, it is necessary to discover the nature of the essential breakdown in the client's development. By using art therapy techniques, we are able to gain access to deeply held issues that are often outside conscious recall or verbal recounting. Additionally, art therapy allows us to identify, describe, and monitor the specific structural defects that are unique to each individual client.

To elicit authentic self-expression, therapists should create a setting and an expectation that invite the client to engage and invest freely in the artwork. This means providing ample space and time, minimizing distractions, and offering appropriate reassurance that any effort will be respected and accepted.

Initially, there will be a limited amount of information available to the therapists beyond the specifics of the eating disorder (or other behavioral manifestations of dysfunction). Therefore, it is recommended that instructions given early in therapy be purposefully vague and open-ended, yet able to be personalized; for example, "Draw an early memory," "Draw a place you'd like to be," or "Draw a picture of yourself." It was our experience that some structure or instructions were helpful in reducing anxiety and allowing clients to trust the process of doing art.

Subsequent art tasks may be drawn from more specific knowledge of the clients. It is suggested that therapist(s) draw hypotheses concerning underlying pathology from evidence accumulated earlier from both verbal expression and earlier art works. These hypotheses can generate the direction therapy should take as the work proceeds. For example, Susan's drawings (Figures 8-3 and 8-4) showed dramatic contrasts in her image of herself. This generated the hypothesis that she had a fragmented self-concept. Later in therapy, another assignment was designed to give more information that would explore the validity of this hypothesis. The following task was given: "draw a secret part of yourself that others don't know." This assignment required the client's increased trust in the therapists and the therapy process. It encouraged the client to reveal more closely held self-concept material. Thus, in the later stages of therapy, assignments may be more challenging, less didactic, more interpretive, more supportive of increased interaction with other group members, and, if necessary, more confrontational.

Throughout this process, art tasks should be presented in a way that supports the individual's developmental needs. Some examples of assignments requiring greater ego strength might include the following: "Draw a picture of yourself in relation to this group," or "Draw a picture that approximates the feeling you get when you are bingeing." Such assignments focus on what is most currently painful to the clients, such as their isolation or their sense of shame in their relationship to food.

In all stages of therapy, it is suggested that the therapists be nurturant and nonjudgmental. The artworks should be described rather than critiqued. It is up to the therapists to model this behavior for the group. For example, rather than saying, "What a beautiful tree," one should say, "You made a large, leafy tree in bright colors." In making interpretations, the therapists must be careful to refer to what is actually visible in the graphics or to what the client has already reported that she perceives in the graphics. Oftentimes, images that may be disturbing are not described or acknowledged (or even recognized) by the client. In our treatment model, the therapist is advised to respect that avoidance. When unduly disturbing or provocative images are presented, it is the responsibility of the therapist to respond with caution and to pay attention to the client's expressed or implied need to keep what is still unmanageable (even though graphically expressed) at a preconscious level. This can be done by actively focusing on a positive aspect of the image, thereby creating a more balanced internal perception. Clients overly stimulated by their own disturbing imagery may be invited individually to produce art works that are soothing and supportive of the self. It is critical to remember that art tasks can elicit primary process material that must be handled with sensitivity and care.

Finally, it should be noted that there are clients for whom this complex, multidisciplined approach is contraindicated. This approach, although gentle, is essentially a challenge to long-held and often malfunctioning defensive structures. It requires that clients maintain their ability to function while moving in and out of their pathology. Extremely fragile clients, such as those with a suspected thought disorder or active suicidal ideation, should not engage in this process and should be supported in keeping their defensive structures intact. In such instances, a less threatening cognitive and behavioral approach may be more effective. Our therapy model is also not recommended when clients have easy verbal access to their issues and are able clearly to articulate their affective experiences. If a client indicates that she has a functional capacity for integration, a simpler and less dismantling therapy should be the therapy of choice. Our therapeutic model is designed to be an effective, broad-based, multidimensional approach to be used in cases where the eating disorder is chronic, unyielding, and long-term.

CONCLUSION

This chapter has described a program of therapy that involves the following: (1) individual psychotherapy in which the client–therapist relationship is established; (2) concurrent group therapy in which interpersonal relationships are examined and practiced; (3) art therapy techniques used in group to gain access to deeper issues; and (4) a tacking approach to allow maximum flexibility in addressing the bulimic symptom and the underlying pathology.

This is a clinical therapy model and, as such, provides no long-term follow-up data. Clients for whom this model was successful were in therapy from 3 to 5 years. Success in treatment was determined by a significant reduction in the bulimic symptom as well as by lifestyle changes that reflected improved self-integration and higher ego functioning. For about 70% of our clients, the bulimic symptom was significantly reduced. Moreover, improvement in emotional well-being was observed in therapy, reported by the clients, and dramatically recorded in their artworks. These artworks reflected an increasingly realistic self-concept, an improved capacity for healthy interpersonal relationships, and a greater ability to be effective in meeting their own emotional needs. Finally, for all of our clients, the eating disorder was no longer perceived by them to be the source of their dysfunction. It ceased to be the central focus of their lives.

REFERENCES

Goodsitt, A. (1985). Self psychology and the treatment of anorexia nervosa. In D. M. Garner & P. E. Garfinkel (Eds.), *Handbook of psychotherapy for anorexia nervosa and bulimia* (pp. 55–82). New York: Guilford Press.

Hammer, E. F. (1958). *The clinical application of projective drawings*. Springfield, IL: Charles C. Thomas.

Kramer, E. (1971). *Art as therapy with children*. New York: Schocken Books.

Lachman-Chapin, M. (1974). A partnership with other expressive arts. In B. I. Levy (Ed.), Symposium: Integration of divergent points of view in art therapy. *The American Journal of Art Therapy, 14,* 16–17.

Lachman-Chapin, M. (1979). Kohut's theories on narcissism: Implications for art therapy. *The American Journal of Art Therapy, 19,* 3.

Naumburg, M. (1966). *Dynamically oriented art therapy: Its principles and practice*. New York: Grune & Stratton.

Obernbreit, R. (1985). Object relations theory and the language of art: Tools for treatment of the borderline patient. *Art Therapy Journal of the American Art Therapy Association, 2,* 11–18.

Ulman, E. (1961). Art therapy: Problems of definition. *Bulletin of Art Therapy, 1*(2), 10–20.

Ulman, E. (1974). Innovation and aberration. In B. I. Levy (Ed.), Symposium: Integration of divergent points of view in art therapy. *The American Journal of Art Therapy, 14,* 14.

Yager, J., & Edelstein, C. (1985). The outpatient management of bulimia. In W. H. Kaye & H. E. Gwirtsman (Eds.), *A comprehensive approach to the treatment of normal weight bulimia* (pp. 47–75). Washington, DC: American Psychiatric Press.

9

Music Therapy Improvisation Techniques with Bulimic Patients

Paul Nolan

Music therapy improvisation is useful in facilitating psychotherapy because it stimulates the awareness and expression of emotions and ideas on an immediate level. The nonverbal, structured medium allows individuals to maintain variable levels of distance from intrapsychic and interpersonal processes. The abstract nature of the sonic qualities of music provides flexibility in how people relate to, or take responsibility for, their own musical expressions. The nonverbal expression may be a purely musical idea, or it may be part of a personal expression to the self or to others; the flexibility afforded the individual within music therapy improvisation can accommodate both levels of expression simultaneously. When a person interacts musically with others, she may experience, separately or simultaneously, the overall group musical gestalt, the act of relating to and interacting with others, and her own feelings and thoughts about herself, her music, and/or the interactions.

Group musical experiences seem to stimulate verbal processing, possibly due to the various levels of interaction available to the group members. When facilitated by the therapist, musical experiences and subsequent verbal processing provide excellent opportunities for patients to experience and integrate areas of conflict, as well as areas of ego strength, that may not have been previously available to them.

This chapter addresses the role of music therapy improvisation techniques within group treatment of bulimic patients. Except for the work of Parente (Chapter 15), there are no known published references in the treatment literature that describe the use of music therapy with people with eating disorders. Thus, one purpose of this chapter is to introduce the reader to the potentials of using music therapy to address specific treatment issues of bulimia. A second purpose is to describe a specific model of music therapy improvisation that facilitates expression of affect in the here-and-now, provides a successful experience in the mastery of tension regulation, identifies intact areas of ego functioning that may not be apparent to the patient, challenges cognitive distortions, and provides a means for practicing alternative interpersonal behaviors.

The first part of this chapter describes theoretical concepts that apply to the process of group music therapy with bulimics and a rationale for the use of music therapy with this population. The second part focuses on the methods of group improvisation with case studies provided as illustrations. This particular model emphasizes the use of music therapy within a group format.

THEORETICAL CONCEPTS

Music therapy integrates easily with most current theoretical concepts and orientations of psychotherapeutic practice. I have been influenced particularly by psychodynamic and ego psychology authors, specifically D. W. Winnicott and Heinze Hartmann. The interpersonal theories of Harry Stack Sullivan and Karen Horney play a lesser, although significant, role in this model of music therapy group improvisation.

Key concepts from the work of these authors apply to certain dynamics of bulimia as well as to the matter in which music therapy improvisation is used. Winnicott's (1953) concept of transitional objects and transitional phenomena relates to bulimics' attempts to evoke the representation of symbiosis through bingeing (Goodsitt, 1985). The use of music is an attempt to replace the binge with a healthier transitional phenomenon so that the patient may reduce withdrawal responses to anxiety during therapy. Hartmann (1958) described those ego functions that can emerge in treatment that replace the bulimic's maladaptive defense mechanisms. This process can provide access to the inner self. Musical expression can provide access to the primitive level of ego functioning through fantasy production, which provides an alternate means for reaching conflictual material. Sullivan (see Mullahy, 1952) and Horney (1945) provide clinical understanding of the interpersonal conflicts of the bulimic.

The contributions of all the above-mentioned authors are described in this chapter in the order of their significance to this model of group music therapy. Due to the intrapsychic and interpersonal processes that are manifested in the process of music therapy improvisations, two or more theoretical concepts may be employed simultaneously in the case studies. I do not assume that all readers are familiar with the presented concepts of Winnicott and Hartmann as they apply to this approach to music therapy. Therefore, the concepts are described in detail.

Transitional Objects and Transitional Phenomena

Winnicott (1953) introduced the terms "transitional objects" and "transitional phenomena" in describing a developmental stage that usually begins for the infant between 4 and 12 months. A transitional object may be defined as the first possession created by the infant that is relied on to allow for the transition from the first oral relationship with the mother to the true object-relationship. The object may be a favorite piece of cloth, part of a blanket, a toy, or a teddy bear. Transitional phenomena are the personal patterns of object use, including gestures, various oral activities, and manipulations. Winnicott introduced the terms "transitional object" and "transitional phenomena" for "designation of the intermediate area of experience between the thumb and the teddy bear" (p. 89). The activities are still oral in character but the status of the object has changed. Within the earliest stages of oral activity, the infant creates the mother as part of herself. The mother's adaptation to this "primary creative activity" contributes to this illusion, which is not challenged until the task of weaning enters into development (Winnicott, 1953). The disillusionment inherent in the weaning process places more of a demand on the formation of transitional phenomena. It is during the disillusionment inherent in the weaning process that transitional objects are used to provide early forms of self-soothing during times of stress, particularly when going to sleep. Within the personal patterns of use or transitional phenomena, lies the discovery of objects that are not part of the infant's body. This process provides the early stages for the formation of object-relations and later reality testing.

Another function of the transitional object, as described by Goodsitt (1985), is to allow the infant to develop the ability to control her inner states of tension. During the symbiotic stage of development, the mother soothes the infant and protects her from stimulus overload. During weaning, this function is transferred to the transitional object, which the child totally controls, and which provides a sense of well-being and security. If adequate mothering occurs, these functions are internalized and become part of the child's mental structure. If this internalization fails, the individual cannot separate successfully because of the inability to provide her own sense of security. Other complications may include fusion of fantasy with reality when under stress, inability to regulate anxiety states, and seeking external sources for security.

Winnicott included the earliest stages of musical development as part of the transitional phenomena. In the mouthing of an object, the infant may use babbling or her first musical notes as accompaniment. In this early use of transitional objects, the infant's accompanying vocal sounds and anal noises may become more important than the actual mouthing of the object. The personal pattern of use, as part of the transitional phenomena, allows the infant to begin to link external reality (the object) with the subjective experience (accompanying vocal sounds). In this manner, the transitional phenomena functions as a resting place for the perpetual human task of keeping inner subjective reality, magical thinking, and symbiotic longing separate from, yet interrelated with, outer objective reality.

Transitional objects may change in childhood, but their function of use remains the same. The child may find her teddy, or other toy, to be absolutely necessary during times of stress or when a depressed mood threatens. Music as a transitional phenomena experience is demonstrated in the way "an older child goes over a repertory of songs and tunes while preparing for sleep" (Winnicott, 1953, p. 89).

As with the achievement of any developmental milestone, transitional objects and phenomena never go away; rather, they widen in their application throughout later stages in life. Over time, the use of transitional phenomena broadens to include areas of play, artistic creativity and appreciation, dreaming, and religious feelings.

Within the binge–purge cycle in bulimia, there exists a pathological use of transitional phenomena. Goodsitt (1985) reported that patients with eating disorders suffer from intense chronic or recurrent tension states. They are driven to reduce these tensions through "intense external self-stimulating activity" (p. 63). Bulimics tend to binge, vomit, or use strenuous physical exertion to regulate their tension states. This extreme external stimulation reflects the bulimics' inability to develop self-soothing capacities in controlling the states of tension described by Goodsitt. However, the binge is only temporarily successful in achieving control over tension; anger, guilt, and a sense of having lost control result when the realization of the binge fully enters consciousness. The consequent purge may serve the purpose of self-punishment, an expression of anger, and a means to return to a sense of self-control. Over time, the cycle may become a compulsive process to regain control over anxiety and unacceptable impulses, even though this process may be distressing to the individual. Thus, the attempted use of binge–purge behavior as a transitional phenomenon to reduce states of inner tension or negative feelings is not successful. Feelings of humiliation and shame following the purge often result in resignation and a sense of failure, which contribute to a reluctance to enter treatment, increased isolation, and secrecy (Browning, 1985).

Ego Psychology

In contrast to Freud's understanding of the ego as the arbitrator of conflicts between demands of the id and superego, Hartmann (1958) recognized the conflict-free portion of the ego in his construct of ego psychology. The functions of this portion develop as the result of an individual's adaptation to her environment and include motor development, speech, thought, perception, intention, and comprehension of objects (Cumming & Cumming, 1962). Hartmann separated these ego functions from those deriving from the conflict-born ego, which are usually referred to as defense mechanisms. Successful adaptation is generally the result of both defensive functions and conflict-free ego functions.

Hartmann attributed the capacity for fantasy (not grounded in the defense mechanism of denial) to the conflict-free ego. Fantasy may remove one from external reality in response to conflict; it may also allow the surfacing of needs and goals from one's inner reality. Hartmann referred to this process as "regressive adaptation," that is, adaptation that requires a detour through regression. This form of adaptation, although more primitive and archaic than the defense mechanisms, provides the genesis for acts of creativity and artistic endeavor. Hartmann acknowledged the role of instinctual drives (primary process) in the arts, but he distinguished conflict-free ego functioning as a separate phenomenon. Regressive adaptation allows a release from external reality with enhanced mobility of the ego. This mobility can access feelings on a primitive level through the detour of regressive adaptation, which bypasses the inhibiting defense mechanisms.

Within my clinical experience, and according to reports of other music therapists and our Hahnemann University graduate students, the emergence of conflict-free ego functioning is frequently observable in the musical behaviors of chronically psychotic state hospital patients. At times during music therapy sessions, a patient may suddenly break into a spontaneous song, synchronizing with the musical structure, and demonstrate a significant increase in his/her level of functioning. Following the music therapy session, the patient usually returns to a state of withdrawal characteristic of an infantile defensive functioning state.

In an acute hospital setting, I witnessed a similar outburst from a near-catatonic schizophrenic. Although unable to speak or move freely, the patient could play complicated chord progressions to remembered songs when handed a guitar. Barring his inability to maintain the tempo of the music with the rest of the group, his motoric control and musical ability demonstrated a higher level of contact with reality (the music) than his otherwise regressed ego could produce.

Hartmann's concept of regressive adaptation is helpful for the music therapist working with bulimic patients. For example, within group musical improvisations, tension levels may be increased in response to dissonant, loud musical expressions. Subjective extramusical associations may arouse a patient's inner state of tension, which in other situations would result in withdrawal or purge behavior. However, patients may later report that they sensed themselves "merging with the beat," and, instead of fearing a loss of control, they may actually report a feeling of safety. The therapist may understand this response as a result of the patient's ability to shift into an altered state of consciousness, allowing a release of conscious restrictions. This process actually enhances patients' involvement with outer reality, while maintaining contact with their inner selves through regressive adaptation.

Interpersonal Psychotherapy

The music therapy approach described in this chapter evolved within a group therapy setting. The benefits of group treatment with eating-disordered patients was described by Piazza and Steiner-Adair (1986) as follows:

> Group therapy provides eating-disordered patients with a social context in which they can develop a more healthy identity within the context of the network of group relationships, an arena to practice and develop interpersonal skills, and a shared experience in which the importance of relationships and communication is supported and reinforced. (p. 29)

Many bulimics present with problems in interpersonal relationships, and often this is a central issue in treatment (American Psychiatric Association, 1980; Barrett & Schwartz, 1987; Vandereycken & Meermann, 1984); therefore, influences from interpersonal psychotherapy approaches are helpful in understanding and dealing with these issues.

While the interpersonal relations approach of Harry Stack Sullivan and the interpersonal "basic attitudes" approach of Karen Horney are considered to be neo-Freudian (see Kutash, 1976), these approaches emphasize the importance of interpersonal relationships in personality. Both authors utilized classical psychoanalytic training in their work, but they significantly changed their perspective from intrapsychic to interpsychic.

Specific aspects of Sullivan's model that influence group music therapy improvisation with bulimics relate to their distorted interpersonal assumptions, as well as the concept of empathy as the "nonverbal communication of emotional states" (Cottrell & Foote, cited in Mullahy, 1952, p. 196). The use of music therapy improvisation within interpersonal psychotherapy models has been described by Broucek (1987, p. 111), who wrote that the very act of "music improvisation is, by its very nature, an interpersonal process."

Complaints of low self-esteem, feelings of inadequacy and inferiority, and reports of self-deprecating thoughts frequently relate to an interpersonal context that is often traceable to distorted interpersonal assumptions. In music therapy groups, distorted interpersonal assumptions will become apparent to the therapist during verbal processing, when participants report their perceptions of the musical interactions. For example, at the close of an initial music therapy group, one patient showed a distorted negative self-appraisal when asked how she viewed her role in the group. She stated, "When I first came into the room and saw all of these women, I said to myself, 'Everyone here has a wonderful, happy life but me.'"

Often, the feedback of group members, actual tape-recorded material, and the therapist's interventions can increase the resistance of the patient in accepting that she distorts. The anticipated negative response appears to be syntonic with feelings of inadequacy. However, by encouraging experimentation with new musical behaviors and an increased focus on external reality (the music of the group), regular patterns of anticipated responses are interrupted. Patients must then challenge their view of group events. This is particularly evident when patients begin to ask for and accept feedback about the role their sounds played in the entire musical production.

In her book, *Our Inner Conflicts* (1945), Horney established a theory based on interpersonal attitudes used by individuals as solutions to anxiety. Each part of the theory involves a mode of interpersonal relating that is also apparent in music therapy improvisations with bulimics. Horney identified these interpersonal attitudes as moving away, moving toward, or moving against others. These attitudes are adaptive in our development until they result in compulsive, rigid, or indiscriminate behavior or become mutually exclusive. Within music therapy improvisation, experimentation with new behaviors is encouraged to challenge distorted assumptions about how one comes across to others. For example, a patient may believe that she is not deserving of support or positive acknowledgement from others. Her musical choices may consistently place her in a passive, quiet role. Her sounds may consistently attempt to fit in with whatever music is presented. Ultimately, the patient may never create a sound or a rhythm that is not already played by another. Although this person may be moving toward the music or group, in a symbiotic manner, she is also moving against herself by interacting in a subservient pattern: "I'll do as you do, because you are better." Using Horney's model, this "moving toward" attitude may be interrupted if the patient is placed in a position where she is encouraged to make sounds in a leadership manner, receiving musical support from the other participants. Patients in music therapy groups have reported that, although it was initially difficult to allow themselves to accept musical support from the group, actually hearing their own music as its own entity was a new and rewarding experience. Within these experiences, patients can develop the insight that their musical expressions are not as bad as they anticipated and that they are capable of eliciting support from others in the group.

Rationale for Music Therapy

The emotional, or affective, response to music has been described by many psychodynamic theorists. Noy (1966, 1967), in his summary of these theories, wrote that affective responses stem from the arousal of libidinal drives, the transformation of unconscious content through sublimation, and the flexibility of the repression mechanism. Kohut (1957) described the pleasure experienced from music as resulting from the discharge of libidinal energy within the control of the ego.

Physiological components of the affective response are traced to the limbic areas of the brain where orientation, physiological changes, and primitive forms of emotion result from musical stimulus (Kreitler & Kreitler, 1972). Thus, the response to music is traced to physiological and psychological processes.

Both unconscious and primitive physiological responses to music can result in the formation of mental imagery and associations that may relate to the listener's past or to aspects of her present emotional and cognitive states. This is due to the capacity of music to bypass the censor without arousing the same defenses as does verbal language (Noy, 1966, 1967). Since music does not relate to the world of objects and is not explicit in its denotation, it is viewed as a relatively nonthreatening language (Meyer, 1956). The nonverbal and nonspecific characteristics of musical expression allow for the most subjective involvement possible without environmental and structural restrictions or limitations. The ability of music to elicit extramusical associations and images is one of the bridging processes between musical expression and the conscious awareness of feelings. This is perhaps the most significant contribution of music to therapy with bulimics. Meyer (1956) believed that "music arouses affect through the mediation of conscious connotation or unconscious image processes." (p. 256). The imagery or associational responses are from the realm of the individual's experience and are "the stimuli to which the affective response is really made" (p. 256). The process of eliciting associations and imagery during music therapy sessions gives rise to defensive functioning, as well as to deep primal areas not readily accessible through strictly verbal communication.

METHOD

It is assumed that the reader has had minimal or no experience in observing music therapy sessions; therefore, a detailed description of the materials and methods follows. Case material is cited to illustrate the techniques. Theoretical points raised earlier are reintroduced in an attempt to integrate theory with practice.

Definition of Improvisation

Apel and Daniel (1974) defined improvisation as "the art of spontaneously creating music . . . while playing, rather than performing a composition already written" (p. 140). Bruscia (1987) described music therapy
improvisation as "inventive, spontaneous, extemporaneous, resourceful,
and [involving] creating and playing simultaneously" (p. 5). He stated that
it does not always result in "music" *per se,* but that it is a process. Within
clinical improvisation, the therapist is a participant–observer focused primarily on the music in terms of the therapeutic relationship. Stephens
(1983) suggested that the therapist acquires three roles within group music therapy improvisation: (1) initiator of direction; (2) supporter, or ground,
to the music; and (3) guide toward the forward direction of the group.
The therapist must have the "ability and sensitivity to accept clients non-
judgmentally, and to respond musically in empathic and intuitive ways to
the person moment by moment" (Boxill, 1985, p. 96).

Improvisation provides the therapist the means to relate to the patient on actual and symbolic levels. Within the therapeutic relationship,
there is a directness of intention in the therapist's choice to support, confront, ignore, and/or move with the patient's musical gesture or expression. Within this actual component of therapeutic relating exists the symbolic realm of how the music and relationship relate to the patient's
extramusical world. The music therapist must possess the musical sensitivity and skills to create and respond to musical forms, or sound gestures,
with flexibility in the use of musical elements (melody, harmony, rhythm,
timbre, style, etc.).

Materials

For clinical improvisation, melodic and rhythmic musical instruments are
chosen that do not necessarily require formal music training for their use
in producing an organized musical sound. For example, xylophones with
movable tone bars may be arranged by the music therapist so that an
individual may play a sequence of tones with a musical result. Some tonal
scale arrangements, such as the pentatonic scale, allow even a random
sampling of tones to produce a musical "statement" identifiable within a
definite tonality, or key. This allows an individual without training to "make
sense" in her tonal and rhythmic expressions. In this model, two xylophones of different tonal ranges are placed opposite each other within
the group circle. Higher and lower pitched melodic instruments allow for
more variety in musical associations. Both sides of the circle include instruments of the hand percussion family, such as tambourines, claves,
maracas, triangles, hand-drums, deep-pitched drums on stands, a sus-

pended cymbal, and other percussion instruments. In this setting, a guitar is available for the therapist to provide harmonic and melodic feedback and support.

Instruments are carefully selected to allow some degree of success in the music improvisations. The creation of musical statements or compositions is not the goal within music therapy improvisation. Once the participants recognize that they are capable of producing sounds that convey some degree of meaning, they are capable of using their instruments intentionally. They can produce nonverbal expressions and choose a manner in which to interact with other participants. They may also choose how they will relate to the overall music with their sounds. With these basic conditions established, opportunities for dynamic expressions and encounters may be directed toward therapeutic goals.

Techniques

Music therapy improvisation techniques are described below in terms of the theoretical concepts of transitional objects and transitional phenomena—regressive adaptation and conflict-free ego involvement—and interpersonal approaches. As a reference point for these descriptions, a typical initial improvisation session with bulimic patients using a therapist-structured approach is described first.

Therapist-Structured Approach

During the early part of an initial group therapy session, patients are encouraged to experiment with making sounds with each of the instruments. This provides an opportunity for them to become aware of the expressive ranges of the instruments (e.g., loud, soft, harsh, gentle) and, of equal importance with bulimics, how to exercise control over each sound. A lack of control over a musical instrument may become a threatening experience and create regression, particularly for those who distort interpersonal feedback. During this time, friendly banter and free play are encouraged to create a setting where there are no rigid constraints regarding the use of these instruments for musical expression. This is also a time when the therapist begins to collect assessment data on each individual's ability to be spontaneous with instruments and with each other.

The participants then select their own seats and instruments. If the group on the whole seems anxious about making music, the therapist will structure, or lead, the initial improvisation. In this case, an arrangement of tones is prepared by the therapist on the xylophone, minimizing the possibility of dissonance. A pentatonic scale is an example of such a tonal arrangement. This tonal scale maximizes the possibility of creating a successful musical group experience. The therapist initiates a specific chord progression with clear tempo and rhythmic phrasing, with an unfixed melody to allow for a variety of melodic interpretations by the patients. Participants are invited to enter when they feel that they are able to synchronize with the music. At this point, the therapist can begin to work with the musical response of each participant. For example, the therapist can imitate by echoing, harmonize with the patient's melodies, add rhythmic subdivisions, and create antecedent and consequent "dialogues" with rhythms or melodic motifs. Following closure of the music, the therapist facilitates a discussion that deals with the perceptions of group members about the musical interaction, their own responses in terms of mood, and their perceptions of their roles within the group structure.

Tape Recording

A tape recorder greatly enhances the types of feedback available. The music is recorded during the playing of the instruments and then is played back during group processing. It is my experience that there is often a difference between the verbalized reaction to the music before listening to the tape and after. Particularly with bulimic patients, comments before listening to the playback often reflect low self-esteem and negative distortions in the effects of the individual's sound on the group. Comments such as, "It sounded fine until I began playing the tambourine too loud," and "I couldn't hear anyone but myself, I don't know if I fit in," are common. Following the playback, which is objective feedback, some patients will express great surprise over the difference between their perception of their function in the group and their actual effect.

Verbal Processing

Group processing after the musical experience is important because it allows the patients to verbalize their experiences in the improvisation. For example, a patient may experience that her role in the group changed from what she had intended. A simple, continuous pulse drumbeat, intended as a low-involvement form of participation, may be perceived by others as a steady, securing, rhythmic foundation that provides stability for others in the group. Reactions to being relied on by others may be discussed. Verbal processing offers an opportunity for patients to develop connections between interpersonal events experienced in the music and patterns that occur in their everyday relationships.

Reality testing is another important function of the group processing. Feedback from the group often differs from the experience of a particular patient. When this feedback occurs through the tape playback, the effect is less confrontational than when it is addressed by the therapist or another patient. The therapeutic effect is that a patient may begin to understand the distortion in her own terms. The group becomes available as a support rather than as an adversary. In this manner, the tape recorder, under favorable conditions of group cohesion, helps the patient to clarify treatment issues concerning reality testing through subsequent verbal processing.

CASE STUDIES

Music as a Transitional Object

Earlier in this chapter, a connection was drawn between the binge–purge cycle, employed as a means to reduce tension, and deficient operation of transitional phenomena, as described by Winnicott. Winnicott referred to the child's use of tunes or songs as a transitional object. The function of the transitional object is to bridge the inner state with the external world, especially in times of anxiety or stress.

As described earlier, musical experiences often give rise to imagery and associations relating to a person's inner world. When musical associations are anxiety related, flight mechanisms may block further awareness and disrupt the process of expression in achieving mastery. When emotional expression, or discharge, is maintained with group support, feelings from associations have a greater opportunity to reach expression with a sense of control. In this way, music as a transitional object encourages the patient to maintain musical contact with the group when diffuse sensations of anxiety appear.

The urge to withdraw in response to anxiety may lessen as the patient becomes more aware of the musical support. This process may provide an experience whereby the patient forfeits maladaptive behavior and becomes successful in controlling her tension.

Transitional phenomena involve a process whereby one's inner, subjective state successfully bridges with external, objective reality. This process helps the therapist to conceptualize the factors involved when, for example, emotional expression is maintained through the use of group support. The use of music serves as the transitional object so that the patient may remain in contact with her feelings, or subjective state, and simultaneously remain in contact with the musical support of the group, or external reality.

The following case study illustrates how musical expression functions as the transitional object to allow the patient to retain self-awareness and group contact as negative feelings arise.

Case 1

Tina, a 25-year-old single woman, had been bulimic for 4 years. Within the previous 6 months, her symptoms subsided to infrequent episodes of bingeing and purging. It had been reported by other treatment staff that she had perfectionistic tendencies, as well as ambivalence toward her father and relationships with men.

During an early music therapy session, Tina regularly appeared to be preoccupied with the control of her own sound, with little awareness of other members of the group. Her compulsively organized musical expressions were played very quietly. She stated that she did "not want to screw up the music." Her melodic playing contained only the highest pitched notes on the xylophone. When asked about this preference, she stated that she "doesn't like these low guys," referring to the lower-pitched tones. This reference was understood by the therapist as a possible association to men. In following through on this possibility, Tina was asked to lead an improvisation on the lower-pitched baritone xylophone to encourage further associations. Her instructions were to allow her mallets to find a sequence of notes that "sounded right" or made some sort of sense to her. The therapist and group gradually added a musical accompaniment in an attempt to support Tina's melodic theme. The therapist expanded the sound of her theme by adding a harmonizing melody on the guitar. The therapist and group then began to sing the theme on fixed syllables, providing empathic/supportive auditory feedback. Tina was verbally encouraged by the therapist to develop other musical options. She began to use the lowest-pitched tones on the xylophone and created a new, slower theme to which the group adjusted. As tears began to fall down Tina's face, she was verbally encouraged to stay with the music. The group began to hum her prayer-like theme, and Tina was able to maintain her involvement for an unusually long period. She later stated that prior to this occasion, she had not been able to cry for more than a few seconds without resorting to food. At the end of the piece, group members held and hugged Tina, but she was not asked to verbally disclose her response in specific terms.

Tina was able to speak with her primary therapist immediately following this session. Her therapist reported that, during the session, Tina was able to integrate previously diffuse feelings about her father and brothers. During a chance meeting later that day, Tina stated that at one point she wanted to stop the music and leave the room, but instead she told herself to "just let it go."

Discussion of Case 1

The empathic musical environment seemed to help Tina manage some control during a deeply felt experience. The statement, "just let it go," was understood as referring to her awareness of the supportive, comforting environment in which she could allow repressed feelings to surface with some degree of safety. Tina's use of the low-pitched musical themes appeared to stimulate associations or feelings that created some anxiety. The choice of musical tones served as both the vehicle of the associations and her link to the support of the group. The theme served as a transitional object in that it was her creation. Use of this theme illustrated a transitional phenomenon that linked Tina with the supportive foundation of the group.

The example also demonstrates how the therapist can explore a clinical hypothesis within the nonverbal process of the group. The therapist may develop improvisation experiences around specific clinical issues, such as Tina's feelings for male members of her family.

Referential Technique and Ego Psychology

The term "referential" describes the listener's relationship "to the extra-musical world of concepts, actions, emotional states, and character" in determining meaning from a musical work (Meyer, 1956, p. 1). In other words, the music refers to something other than the music itself. Or, put another way, something specific in the patient's world may be projected onto the music. In the preceding case study, there was a reference to "guys" through the low-pitched tones on the xylophone.

A referential approach may be used to explore a specific issue developed from a patient's subjective response to the music or from a patient's verbal disclosure. In this approach, a patient is asked to create a musical structure that refers to, or represents, a specific personal issue. The personal experience is reenacted musically with group support.

Because musical expression is unrelated to the world of objects, associative possibilities from rhythm, timbre, and other musical elements, as well as from the motoric action involved, remain subjective. A string of associations to the music may bring long-forgotten memories to the surface with their affective charge intact. On occasion, the affect from a formerly blocked event may emerge by itself. The referential approach may then be used to connect the blocked event with the emergent affect.

The therapist encourages the patient to continue a musical expression that connects her with the specific feeling state emerging as part of an association. This enables the patient to practice regressive adaptation on a conscious level while the therapist and group maintain musical support by providing a harmonic and rhythmic "ground" to the patient's musical "figure." Careful attention is paid to reproducing the patient's dynamics (volume of sound), timbre (tone color), melodic phrasing, and any other musical qualities that reflect her musical expression. Often, listening to the tape playback immediately afterward provides an opportunity for the patient to elaborate on the emerging feelings with specific events from the past. This experience may heighten awareness of feelings and thoughts that become available to the ego for controlled, safe expression.

The following case study describes how fantasy formation from musical associations can facilitate regressive adaptation as part of the ego's attempt to achieve mastery over a threatening situation. In this process, the stimulus (drum sounds) is transformed, in its symbolic representation, from "anticipated danger" to an "internalized strength made available for self-protection."

In this situation, theoretical constructs developed by Hartmann, Sullivan, and Horney are employed simultaneously. The case study also points to the importance of empathy in the group. Empathy in music is "established through affective communication" (Broucek, 1987, p. 103). Sullivan's concept of empathy as being primarily a nonverbal process is demonstrated through musical reflection and support as part of the group improvisational process.

Horney's description of the interpersonal attitude, moving toward others, fits the following example of compliant and passive interpersonal responses. As this case demonstrates, a patient's use of drumming in response to fantasy can alter her perception of herself within an interpersonal context. The patient in this case demonstrated a shift in her basic interpersonal attitude from passivity to an adaptive degree of domination. Horney wrote that the moving toward others attitude may mask strong inner needs to compete, to excel, and to dominate (Broucek, 1987), which, in this case, were made available to the ego and contributed toward mastery.

Case 2

Donna was a 27-year-old married woman who had been bulimic for 3 years. During a group session, she began to feel some anxiety from an association to the drums in the prior improvisation and stated that she would like to leave the room. Within moments, she confessed that she felt a need to purge. When asked about her associations and about what might have triggered her anxiety, Donna related her feelings to an event that occurred at home when she was alone with her husband's intoxicated male friend. The drums reminded her of the man ascending the basement stairs, in a manner that she felt was menacing to her. At the time, she had wished for the isolation of the bathroom, where she could purge to relieve the anxious feeling she felt in her stomach. However, she had thought that this act would increase her vulnerability because her husband had fallen asleep, and she felt afraid and unprotected. This conflict demonstrated to the therapist Donna's inability to turn aggressive energies toward her perceived potential threat. Her release of tension was understood as being additionally blocked by not having the purge as an outlet. This association was triggered by the aggressive drum playing of another participant during a prior musical improvisation. The therapist did not offer an interpretation at that time.

Donna was asked to recall her experience by using the drums to re-create the affective triggers of her experience. The group followed her drum pattern and began to increase their volume as Donna remained at her moderately quiet volume level. Group members began to verbally encourage her to "stay with it" as the overall sound increased in its intensity. Donna was able to gradually increase the volume and tension levels of her music, which took on a more spontaneous character than her usual compliant behavior in group. The drumming reached a peak of violent pounding and maintained this level with group support before Donna gradually returned to a calmer, repetitive rhythm. Donna decided to move to a xylophone and was able musically to influence the group to a quiet, dynamic level and slower tempo. The therapist used the guitar to provide support with melodic and harmonic improvised accompaniment. Donna maintained a serene melodic exploration, which included musical elements suggesting nurturance, peacefulness, and tender feelings.

Discussion of Case 2

In verbally processing this experience, Donna stated that the drums "fused" with the image of the threatening advances of the drunken man from her memory. Within the same drumming experience, the image changed to a sense of her own strength. She was aware of the pulsating support from the group and actually became aware of something "rising up" from her mid-section. She later interpreted this as her own power to defend herself and call off the threatening person within her reenactment.

The therapist understood this event as an attempt by Donna to achieve mastery over her mobilized aggression. In addition, Donna was able to adapt in a regressive process through the primitive beating of the drum; and, with the musical support and encouragement of the group and therapist, she was able to achieve a successful resolution of this conflict. Without a mode of expression, either in defense from a perceived threat or through the self-damaging act of purging, Donna maintained an easily aroused level of tension without an acceptable outlet for resolution. This may also describe a pattern in her life that was temporarily dealt with through purge behavior. However, in the therapy session, the physical act of drumming, within the memory reenactment, seemed to help her focus the aggressive energy into a controlled, outward expression. Her transformed musical expression was heard as containing a degree of confidence and self-assertion.

At the moment when Donna's aggressive drum pounding quieted, and she changed to a calm melodic expression on the xylophone, she maintained a musical direction which was easily followed by the group. Her prior attempts in leading a group improvisation consisted of scattered fragments of poorly organized sounds without a clear pulse. The melodic themes used following the expression of aggression appeared to reflect a gentle quality, yet they contained a clear pulse and retained the group's musical attention. This ability to present controlled musical expression across a wide range of feeling was understood by the therapist as a representation of the emergence of an increased range of available ego resources. That is, Donna's mastery over her aggressive drives increased the mobility of her ego toward a wider range of expression.

Contradicting Interpersonal Assumptions

In group music therapy improvisation, distorted interpersonal assumptions become apparent to the therapist during verbal processing, when patients offer their perceptions of the musical interactions. The use of the tape playback allows the distortion to become apparent to others in the group and, finally, to the patient. Interpersonal distortions function as a defense against anxiety. The therapeutic contradiction of the distortion must ultimately be understood by the patient in her own terms and only when she is capable of acknowledging group support. With the patient in control, she may utilize increased ego resources to deal with anxiety formerly binded by distortions.

At times, the distorted musical behavior may actually convey a different meaning to the group than it does to the patient. The musical expression may actually be understood by others as having an important function within the group musical expression. Thus, the patient may realize that she is not coming across to others as she thought; also, she may discover that her role, or function, in the group is seen as important by others.

Case 3

Kim had been relatively free of binge–purge symptoms for 2 years. However, she was struggling with her relationships, in which she felt passive. She was uninvolved in family decisions and complained about her lack of assertiveness. She did not believe that she was loved or wanted by her husband, children, or her mother. However, all of these relatives were reported to be close to the patient.

Within an improvisation, which could be characterized as quiet and controlled, Kim accidentally struck her metal triangle louder than planned.

She immediately grimaced and held her arms over her head, breaking musical and visual contact with the group. As soon as the music ended, she released from her protective posture and profusely apologized for "destroying the piece." The group participants did not understand Kim's comment until she recounted the incident to them, which they hardly remembered. What the group had not noticed before listening to the playback was that, immediately following Kim's loud triangle sound, the group music changed to a louder dynamic level and became less rigid and more expressive. The group members discussed that Kim's sound represented a "signal" or an "icebreaker" that introduced more spontaneity and less emphasis on control. At first Kim was unable to understand how her presumably destructive act could have such positive results. At this point, it was suggested to her by the therapist that she had cut off feedback from reality and was not objectively judging the effect of her sound. The discussion lead to Kim's statement that she "must have lost track of what was going on." Kim realized that she sometimes automatically assumes a negative expectation from interpersonal encounters. She traced this behavior back to when she was an active bulimic 2 years earlier.

Discussion of Case 3

The tape playback and resulting group discussion seemed to make Kim's assumption more difficult to maintain. The added component of social reward for her behavior, in fact, created anxiety for her. Kim was very surprised that her perception was so inaccurate; however, her anxiety provided a stimulus for change.

Music for Relaxation and Imagery

Music has been used throughout history to soothe and delight its listeners. Music-assisted relaxation and imagery techniques are methods used regularly by music therapists and others in health care. Helen Bonny (1978) developed the technique known as guided imagery and music, initially as a form of depth-oriented psychotherapy. The technique combines relaxation methods and meditative-like suggestion with programmed classical music to facilitate mental imagery. Within this form of treatment, the client verbally reports the contents of her imagery and her feeling responses to the music. The technique has been documented as an assessment tool and as a means for both insight-oriented and supportive therapy (Bonny, 1980; Kellog, Macrae, Bonny, & DiLeo, 1977; Nolan, 1983; Summer, 1981; Zwerling, 1979).

I developed a variation of this technique, which involves improvised music created intentionally for the purpose of facilitating a therapeutic relaxation and imagery experience. Patients are asked to focus on musical qualities that relate to their subjective impression of a state of relaxation. The musical qualities are often described as somewhat slow, mellow, light, carefree, simple, smooth, and pretty. The group and therapist play and record music using these descriptive guidelines. The group then moves from their chairs to mats and pillows on the floor, and the therapist directs the relaxation and induction instructions before playing back the music (Bonny, 1978). The listening lasts from 4 to 10 minutes and is followed by a gradual return to an alert state.

The intended therapeutic goals of this technique are for patients to experience a state of relaxation with syntonic imagery and for patients to recognize that this relaxation is a result of their own actions. The patients' mental representations, then, guide their musical productions. These musical productions are, in turn, used in a self-nurturing relaxation experience. This is a much more conscious and deliberate method of providing self-soothing than the unsuccessful impulse of food bingeing.

Group discussion often includes statements concerning the realization that a controlled, self-directed action can replace self-destructive behaviors. White (1985) found that strategies that reduce binge–purge behaviors include the administration of self-strokes. He offered examples of patients taking hot baths while listening to their favorite music. In a similar manner, this music therapy technique demonstrates through experience that the capacity to provide for one's own self-nurturance may be available in some form. Although these positive behaviors may not be actively used, the awareness of their existence seems to encourage hope and further motivation.

DISCUSSION

Group music therapy improvisation can be used with bulimic patients to bring about awareness of feelings and behaviors in the here-and-now. These awarenesses are then channeled into further improvisational experiences, which generate possibilities for behavioral experimentation with self and others. The use of an action-oriented treatment approach, specifically with an art form such as music, opens up both receptive and expressive levels of experiencing. The nonverbal exchange in music simultaneously effects physiological and emotional/cognitive processes. Music, as a creative arts therapy, "evokes responses more directly and more immediately than do any of the more traditional verbal therapies" (Zwerling, 1979, p. 843). Music therapy experiences may be symbolic, descriptive, and/or actual.

Therapists using music therapy improvisation need to have both musical and psychotherapeutic training and skills. Musical skills should include abilities within varied musical styles. The functional use of several instruments is helpful. Improvisational skills are essential and must be adapted to group interactions. This flexibility is fundamental for the use of interventions including empathy (musical reflecting), confrontation (increasing musical tension), and support (grounding musical statements). Psychotherapy training provides the foundation for dealing with countertransference, understanding psychopathology, and using verbal processing techniques. Integrating nonverbal material with verbal understanding is an important function of the therapist, although this task is not necessarily required for every musical experience. The therapist must be willing and able to assist the patient in organizing and clarifying feelings and thoughts within the patient's capacity for cognitive understanding. Also, the ability to utilize theoretical constructs such as those of Winnicott, Sullivan, Horney, and Hartmann separately, or in combination, further enriches the therapeutic process with bulimics.

The case studies used in this chapter were derived from treatment groups held within an outpatient eating-disorders treatment center. Treatment approaches vary between outpatient and inpatient treatment centers. Inpatient facilities foster a supportive therapy approach to bring about a rapid return to the community. Therefore, music therapy techniques that encourage the intensification of feelings as well as the use of uncovering methods may best be suited for outpatient treatment. Inpatient care is currently influenced by insurance payment limitations. Music therapy approaches within inpatient settings are therefore geared toward getting the patient "back together," which may require some adaptation of the methods described in this chapter. Outpatients generally demonstrate a high degree of motivation and possess the ego resources to tolerate the relatively high degrees of anxiety that may be generated during uncovering experiences.

Treatment concepts and methods for bulimia are still in early stages of development. Music therapy expands the range of viable treatment approaches. The model described in this chapter can be integrated with other treatment modalities and is adaptable for use in various treatment perspectives. The inclusion of music therapy into the available treatment armamentarium offers another means for establishing contact with the patient's healthy resources when dealing with the physical, emotional, and social effects of bulimia.

REFERENCES

American Psychiatric Association. (1980). *Diagnostic and statistical manual of mental disorders.* (3rd ed.). Washington, DC: Author.

Apel, W., & Daniel, R. (1974). *The Harvard brief dictionary of music.* New York: Pocket Books.

Barrett, M. J., & Schwartz, R. (1987). Couple therapy for bulimia. In J. E. Harkaway (Ed.), *Eating disorders* (pp. 25–39). Rockville, MD: Aspen.

Bonny, H. L. (1978). *Facilitating GIM sessions: GIM monograph no. 1.* Baltimore, MD: ICM Books.

Bonny, H. L. (1980). *GIM therapy: Past, present and future implications: GIM monograph no. 3.* Baltimore, MD: ICM Books.

Boxill, E. H. (1985). *Music therapy for the developmentally disabled.* Rockville, MD: Aspen.

Broucek, M. A. (1987). *An interactional model of music therapy improvisation based on interpersonal theories of psychotherapy.* Unpublished master's thesis, Hahnemann University, Philadelphia.

Bruscia, K. E. (1987). *Improvisational models of music therapy.* Springfield, IL: Charles C. Thomas.

Browning, W. N. (1985). Long-term dynamic/group therapy with bulimic patients: A clinical discussion. In S. W. Emmett, (Ed.), *Theory and treatment of anorexia nervosa and bulimia* (pp. 141–153). New York: Brunner/Mazel.

Cumming, J., & Cumming, E. (1962). *Ego and milieu.* New York: Aldine Publishing.

Goodsitt, A. (1985). Self psychology and the treatment of anorexia nervosa. In D. M. Garner & P. E. Garfinkle (Eds.), *Handbook of psychotherapy for anorexia nervosa and bulimia* (pp. 55–82). New York: Guilford Press.

Hartmann, H. (1958). *Ego psychology and the problem of adaptation.* (D. Rapaport, trans.). New York: International Universities Press.

Horney, K. (1945). *Our inner conflicts.* New York: W. W. Norton.

Kellog, J., Macrae, M., Bonny, H. L., & DiLeo, F. (1977). The use of the mandala in psychological evaluation and treatment. *American Journal of Art Therapy, 16,* 123–134.

Kohut, H. (1957). Observations on the psychological functions of music. *Journal of the American Psychoanalytic Association, 5,* 389–407.

Kreitler, H., & Kreitler, S. (1972). *Psychology of the arts.* Durham, NC: Duke University Press.

Kutash, S. B. (1976). Modified psychoanalytic therapies. In B. B. Wolman (Ed.), *The therapist's handbook* (pp. 87–116). New York: Van Nostrand Reinhold

Meyer, L. B. (1956). *Emotion and meaning in music.* Chicago: University of Chicago Press.

Mullahy, P. (Ed.). (1952). *The contribution of Harry Stack Sullivan: A symposium on interpersonal theory in psychiatry and social science.* New York: Science House.

Nolan, P. (1983). Insight therapy: Guided imagery and music in a forensic psychiatric setting. *Music Therapy, 3,*(2), 43–51.

Nordoff, P., & Robbins, C. (1977). *Creative music therapy.* New York: John Day.

Noy, P. (1966). The psychodynamic meaning of music. Part I. *Journal of Music Therapy, 3,* 123–126.

Noy, P. (1967). The psychodynamic meaning of music. Part II. *Journal of Music Therapy, 4,* 7–23.

Piazza, E. A. & Steiner-Adair, C. (1986). Recent trends in group therapy for anorexia nervosa and bulimia. In F. Sarocca (Ed.), *Eating disorders: Effective care and treatment* (pp. 25–51). St. Louis: Ishiyaku Euro-America.

Stephens, G. (1983). The use of improvisation for developing relatedness in the adult client, *Music Therapy, 3*(2), 29–42.

Summer, L. (1981). Guided imagery and music with the elderly. *Music Therapy, 1,* 39–43.

Vandereycken, W., & Meermann, R. (1984). *Anorexia nervosa.* New York: Walter de Gruyter.

White, W. D., Jr. (1985). Bulimarexia: Intervention strategies and outcome considerations. In S. W. Emmett (Ed.), *Theory and treatment of anorexia nervosa and bulimia* (pp. 216–267). New York: Brunner/ Mazel.

Winnicott, D. W. (1953) Transitional objects and transitional phenomena. *International Journal of Psycho-Analysis, 34,* 89–97.

Zwerling, I. (1979). The creative arts therapies as "real" therapies. *Hospital and Community Psychiatry, 30,* 841–844.

II

Anorexia Nervosa

10

The Use of Metaphor and Poetry Therapy in the Treatment of the Reticent Subgroup of Anorectic Patients

Camay Woodall
Arnold E. Andersen

Silence as a feature of the anorexic's behavior has been described by researchers in the eating-disorders field (Andersen, 1985; Bruch, 1973, 1978; Crisp, 1980; Gull, 1874; Selvini-Palazzoli, 1978). From the earliest descriptions of anorexia, it has been clear that the anorectic girl or woman strongly resists any intervention and, if anything, wishes only to be stabilized enough to go back to starving. Crisp (1980) referred to the anorexic's resistance as "a last ditch stance, her only and primitive resource, and potentially so unstable that she cannot allow any intrusion by others into her adjustment" (p. 13).

Charone (1982) described eating disorders as deriving from disturbed patterns of communications in early feeding relationships. She pointed out that one of the earliest determinants of the quality of mother–infant communication is mutual vocalization during nursing. Vocalization is the mode used by the infant to indicate her feelings (Osofsky & Danziger, 1974). Thus, the anorectic stance seems to be a despair in regard to communication—vocally and actively—expressed as a refusal to eat. Her reticence, her refusal to speak, thus seems an aspect of her general resistance to being influenced. This resistance seems to be composed of several facets, including an all but irresistible vulnerability to her parents' influence and a despair that, even when she does communicate with her parents, the results will not be supportive of her emerging self.

But it is not only the fear of parental interference that the anorexic experiences; a number of researchers have noted a broad and regulatory fear of maturation in these patients, a fear of life, for which the illness is a metaphor (Chernin, 1985; Crisp, 1980; Woodall, 1983). When one is afraid of life, to become afraid of *fat* makes the fear more controllable. Fear of life is too unmanageable; hence, the anorexic isolates one aspect of life—the management of food and fat—in which to experience fear and to control it. Indeed, the anorexic's fear of fat is manifested with the facial and bodily expressions of a threat to life, including wide eyes, rigidity, and/or trembling, tears, and an absence of any humor, except perhaps a kind of cynicism.

In contrast, the personal histories of anorexics reveal a significant feature of their growing up pre-anorectic years: compliance, indeed *over*-compliance. Sours (1974) described how "lifelong compliance to parental wishes" impoverishes the developing self; "experiences of the self through contact with strong affects are missed." He considered the symptoms of anorexia nervosa to be a desperate attempt to resist impulses to defer to the parents, who are ambivalently loved.

Refusing the parents, however, is fraught with difficulty for the pre-anorexic, especially because of guilt. With the onset of adolescence comes the universal requirement to evolve and establish the self. Yet the anorexic-to-be cannot refuse the parents. Indeed, if the parents do not regulate her, the daughter seeks them out and, in interesting and subtle ways, elicits their regulation (Minuchin, Rosman, & Gailer, 1978). It is the anorexic's illuminating discovery that, while she cannot comfortably refuse her parents, she can refuse their food. Food refusal thus becomes an equivalent for the resistance to being influenced. It is the first experience of the daughter's ability to withstand her parents' censure, without guilt. And she can maintain her estimation of herself as "good," since she is not doing anything to her parents, only to herself.

THE INTELLIGENT ANORECTIC PATIENT AND CREATIVITY

Bruch (1978) and others were impressed with the frequent finding of high IQs in anorectic patients as well as high levels of academic achievement. But there is a curious unevenness of development in these patients. They are intelligent, but often they are not creative. They are not divergent thinkers; that is, they are often unable to examine a problem for multiple options and solutions—but they can memorize and reproduce complex coursework.

When it comes to emotions, these young women show a dearth of words for mood, known as alexithymia (Sifneos, 1973). Or they show a repression of affect, feeling only "numbness." These two conditions may, of course, be the same thing, but the end result of either and both is that the patient will not or cannot consult herself for terms that will communicate her emotional experiences. Anorectic symptoms reflect a hatred of the body (Woodall, 1987), an abandonment of feeling, and a kind of victimization of the body in favor of a detached, controlled, intellectualized stance. This stance is experienced as a cognitive achievement by the anorexic rather than an inability to experience and express feelings. As such, this stance may be examined through the perceptual and cognitive steps in its development. Since body experience and the experience of feelings are preverbal in origin and often not conscious, they may best be approached through use of metaphor, which depends on body experience but is expressed verbally.

POETRY THERAPY

Poetry therapy was developed by J. J. Leedy (1969) as an outgrowth of bibliotherapy. He had been impressed by the observation that a certain poem read and interpreted by the therapist could help a patient formulate her problem more clearly, permitting new understanding and relief. Leedy proposed that a professional search for a fitting poem was a useful therapeutic technique. Contributors to his book (Leedy, 1969) substantiated this with examples of their own. A National Association of Poetry Therapists was formed, and a journal, *The Arts in Psychotherapy*, was started.

In the two books edited by Leedy (1969, 1973), however, there is no particular study of the mechanism by which poetry in psychotherapy works. That poetry is therapeutic says much about psychotherapy's examination of *meanings* in a patient's treatment (Lerner, 1978). Having the patient write her own poem based on a theme deemed important by the therapist was shown to be a valuable innovation (Goldstein, 1983; Woodall, 1983) for the patient's emotional growth.

POETRY IN THE TREATMENT OF
ANOREXIA NERVOSA

The rationale for using poetry therapy in the treatment of people with anorexia nervosa is twofold. First, as Bruch (1978) had repeatedly pointed out, anorexics suffer from a feeling of ineffectiveness. She linked this with their deficit in assertiveness. Second, many researchers, such as Crisp (1980), noted that anorexics, especially the younger ones, are quite reticent. Poetry therapy helps with both assertiveness and expressiveness. The reticence gives way to the interest in a cognitive task (which ends up full of feeling), and the spontaneous poem itself becomes an emergent self-assertion. Often a patient who finds it difficult to speak directly to the therapist will accept a writing task—which ends up relating her to the therapist. The therapist is then provided with substantial material to discuss and interpret, and the patient is gently confronted with original metaphors she can accept as coming from her own, perhaps previously buried, feelings.

The first author (C. W.) has found poems by Emily Dickinson particularly relevant for poetry therapy with anorexics. Emily Dickinson (1830–1885) was a college-educated woman who returned to her parents' home to live out her life. Although she had received several proposals for marriage, (Higgins, 1967), she did not marry, and she secluded herself in her home and garden. She did entertain and she carried on lively correspondence with friends and relatives (Higgins, 1967). She was perfectionistic and perhaps overly self-controlled. A number of her poems refer to feelings of loneliness and isolation. Several poems refer to depression and frightening images, while a few even refer to food restriction. It is these latter poems that were chosen by C. W. for poetry therapy with anorexics, along with poems about separation issues, anger, and disillusionment— also relevant themes for this population.

METHOD

"Priming" the Patient: The Dickinson Sequence

Emily Dickinson did not title her poems but instead used numbers. The poems that have been used in therapy with anorexics include the following:

- No. 486, about feeling unappreciated and ineffectual, afraid to say a word.
- No. 959, about loss, possibly the loss of a sense of self.
- No. 738, about submission and accommodation to a powerful and adored other; also about annoyance with this experience.
- No. 612, seems to be about Dickinson's experience with anorexia nervosa.
- No. 579, about yearning and longing for something, yet feeling a bit out of place when the goal is achieved.
- No. 508, about not belonging to parents anymore.
- No. 442, about struggling to accomplish something but failing and suffering humiliation—then coming back to "show them," this time

succeeding and subsequently feeling inexplicably shy and undeserving.

- No. 1331, about central human ambivalence, giving up the need for absolute certainty, and allowing oneself to be both ambivalent *and* comfortable.
- No. 1039, about feeling connected to life and at peace with oneself.

The therapist presents a poem about loneliness before one about anger, assuming that anger is a more threatening emotion for the anorexic than loneliness. A poem about psychological integration is not presented before the person has a chance to express grief. Also, a patient and therapist can spend more than one session with one of the poems. Indeed, this is indicated when the patient's original poem in response to one of Dickinson's is rich in detail or is so meaningful that both she and the therapist do not wish to go on to the next poem in the sequence. The meaning in the poem is often provided by the original metaphors that the patients produce. The metaphors structurally contain a known (to the reader) physical half and an unknown psychological half (Asch, 1956).

Of course, the Dickinson sequence suggested here does not have to be used at all. The therapist may prefer other authors. However, works that are too sophisticated or too long tend to discourage the reticent patient from the task of discovering and putting her own feelings into words. For poetry therapy, a poem should be concise, about deeply personal issues, and of an empowering tone. The work of Emily Dickinson is just such poetry, and so is that of Robert Frost. Political poetry is to be avoided in that it refers to broader social issues.

Types of Poetry Therapy

There are several ways to conduct poetry therapy, and new ways are certainly still evolving. In the group model (Goldstein, 1983), one or two poems of a published author are used in the beginning of a group session. The poems are read and interpreted by the therapist first and then by all the group members. Without further comment, each member is asked to write her own poem on that theme or a reaction to the theme. Group members read their poems aloud. Some people are inhibited in reading aloud, and some will decline. After each poem is read, the group acclaims the effort and is asked to comment on it. Participants are encouraged to take each other's comments seriously. In some groups, the therapist also writes a poem, which she or he shares; then the group reacts to it.

In another model, the therapist introduces a published poem, which the group members discuss as in the preceding model. However, in this model, they are invited to write a group poem. The therapist may write the first line. Each person then adds a line or two. As one may imagine, each person's contribution reflects her feeling state or defense against it. The completed poem is read aloud by the therapist. Group cohesiveness is often enhanced by this procedure; however, the resulting poem may be more threatening to some group members than in the preceding model. Both models require a fair amount of time, perhaps 1½ hours or longer. There are some similarities here to projective tests, which are also used to increase the therapist's understanding of patient's psychological functioning and defenses. Case studies follow to illustrate the use of poetry therapy with anorexics.

CASE STUDIES

Kathy

Kathy was a quiet 25-year-old woman who had been somewhat overweight, 140 pounds, at age 22. She dieted for a few months at 23 and became anorectic by age 24. Her lowest weight was 84 pounds at 5'6". Her parents insisted that she be hospitalized, which she finally was.

A detailed history was obtained. It was learned that, in college, Kathy had fallen in love with her young professor, but, although he enjoyed being with Kathy, he was engaged to someone else. They had a brief affair, then he left. Kathy began overexercising, dieting, and losing weight. Earlier in her life, when she was a senior in high school, her brother, one year older than she, had developed a progressive neurological disorder and had died within a year. Further questioning revealed that this brother had induced Kathy into sexual "games" from the time she was five years old to about age 12. Some of these games were painful to her, but she did not defy him or tell her parents. The whole family adored this brother.

At the beginning of Kathy's individual psychotherapy, three times a week with the first author (C. W.), Kathy was quiet and withdrawn. She stared at the floor throughout the session and bit her lip in order to control her tears. She answered questions in a monotone and as cryptically as she could. She accepted treatment but wanted it to be quick and neat, with as little real emotional involvement as possible. She would not permit any discussion of her feelings and often looked acutely uncomfortable. After several sessions with little response from Kathy, I suggested that perhaps she was aggrieved over the loss of her lover. This suggestion was based on the onset of the weight loss just after her college experience with the young professor. Kathy began to weep and was so uncomfortable that I agreed to end the session; however, I asked Kathy to write a poem about her sadness. At the next session, Kathy brought the following poem:

> Flowers crumbled, castles tumbled,
> All in disarray.
> Forgotten faces, mistaken places,
> Darkness come to stay.
> Never a time to sip of the wine
> Which flowed from fields so free.
> Paths untraveled, dreams unraveled
> Tomorrow never to be.

Kathy and I agreed that the poem needed no interpretation. She had found a way to communicate, and my appreciation of her poetic effort engendered trust. Perhaps when one's poetry is appreciated, one feels understood.

At this point, I decided to continue with Dickinson's poem No. 738 about submission and accommodation to an ambivalently loved other person. After the therapist read the poem aloud, Kathy said that it made her sad. She then allowed that sometimes accommodation was warranted, as with putting her health in the hands of experienced doctors. I agreed but suggested that the Dickinson poem seemed to be about overcompliance to overtly and covertly demanding parents. I asked Kathy how she felt about that. Kathy explained how hard it was to get through to her parents; anytime she tried, it would upset them so. She had never noticed that she was compliant. I suggested to her that while she was compliant to her parents, she did not want to realize that she had been giving in. She did not want to *be* that kind of person, and so she defended against seeing her overtly submissive behavior. Kathy responded with the following poem.

> The never of nothing survives alone
> In the dawn when the cold winds blow.
> It sways in the breeze and cries with the trees
> In the night when the rain turns to snow.
> Never happy, never sad
> Never thankful, never glad
> The never of nothing has a life of its own
> Never apart, yet never alone.

Kathy explained that the "never of nothing" refers to "something that is not good. It reminds me of the way I was in high school—family relationships weren't there. All evenings, even meals, were 'do your own thing.' I was devoted to school, friends, and library." I asked if she had been deliberately isolating herself from her parents. She answered, "Yes. I could work on my own things." This period was important for her in the evolution of her personhood. I asked why she had given it a negative name, "the never of nothing?" Kathy became thoughtful. "It was good for me," she said. "But my parents saw this time as negative. Still they never did anything but complain." It became clear that Kathy's efforts to find her own way were unacceptable to her parents. This fact made Kathy sad and angry. "I wouldn't let them interfere with school. I did this by making school things sound unimportant. It had to be unimportant to be free of their interference."

This self-diminishment actually applied to all aspects of her life at that time. She developed an emotionless demeanor. "Never happy, never sad, never thankful, never glad" refers to the importance of hiding her emotional life from her parents—happiness or sadness. The last line of the poem, "The never of nothing has a life of its own," refers to compromising. Kathy explained, "I agreed to live with them bodily but mentally I was always someplace else." We discussed the evolution of this hiding, starting with secrecy as a child about being molested by her brother, then later pulling back from all family relationships in a struggle to minimize her parents' intrusiveness. But even then, she was "never apart, never alone."

At this point in Kathy's hospital treatment, she still felt uneasy with her parents, although her assertiveness with others had developed along with a significantly increased self-esteem and steady weight restoration. We began to talk about her eating. I asked what had happened to permit her to gain weight. Kathy laughed softly, "I don't know. It used to be like the most important thing. It was like the worse I felt the better I felt. It's weird. Now I feel so much better energy-wise."

During the next two sessions, we worked with a Dickinson poem (No. 612) about the poet's own anorexia, about not being able to eat despite the fact that there is plenty of food present. The poem discusses the pain of hunger, which was, in Dickinson's graphic phrase, "upon me like a claw." The daily frustration of living with this hunger and at the same time being afraid to eat became so oppressive to Dickinson that she began to think of death—and yet she felt incapable of that as well. I pointed out that this seemed like a torment. Dickinson seemed trapped between hunger and suicidal urges. Although we discussed the trap of anorexia nervosa, Kathy seemed to produce a poem that was about another kind of trap.

> Nothing grows in winter's snows
> When the iceman comes to call
> People die and children lie
> As the snow begins to fall
> Bleeding bed of brown and red
> Cries out beneath the ground
> Wasted in the death of life
> When the iceman comes around.

Kathy explained that the first line was literal. The third line, "People die and children lie," she could not explain. It was suggested that perhaps the line should be reversed. "Children lie" could refer to her and her brother's secrecy, while "people die" could refer to his subsequent death. Her association to when "the snow begins to fall" was "snow covers up a lot of things." The line "bleeding bed of brown and red" left her puzzled. I suggested that brown and red are the colors of blood and earth, and the line "cries out beneath the ground" might refer to her brother's demandingness and oppression, which would not die. At this Kathy winced. " 'Wasted in the death of life' meant 'living but not really living,' " she said. "Everything was wasted—our whole childhood was not right. Our [sexual] relationship interfered with everything. We didn't have a childhood like other children." The "iceman" in her poem refers to death, she said. She had always felt that their relationship was so problematic, one of them would have to die.

As Kathy's poems improved in clarity, cohesiveness, and insight, her weight approached normal. She became more self-reflective. In one poem, she spoke of "darkness as the only friend." I asked what this meant. Kathy explained, "That's the place where all my poems come from. It's like a foreign language." Both Kathy and I were surprised by this last statement. Asked why she thought her poetry was a foreign language, she thought a while and said, "It's not very happy poetry—at times I have to stop writing it, it gets so confusing." I suggested that her poetry *was* sad, but it was not a foreign language. I told her that her original poetry was the language of the *real* Kathy, while the "foreign language" could refer to the way she communicated with her parents. Kathy was impressed with this hypothesis and asked to think about it a while. She wrote one last poem, which needed no interpretation.

> There never was a rainbow that ever came to stay
> There never was a storm cloud that ever stayed away
> But showers end and rainbows send their colors home to play.
> Then sun returns and quickly burns away the shades of gray.
> Shine on, sun, your warmth so strong and teach us now to see
> That rain and sun can dwell as one in skies harmoniously.

Tina: An Anorectic Only Child

Tina was a serious, studious, silent girl of 16, who was brought for therapy by her concerned grandmother. Tina was 5'4" and weighed 99 pounds. The year before she had weighed 113 pounds and was running regularly. She had ceased menstruating at 113 pounds, but she was not concerned enough about this to stop running. She kept her grades at the honors' level. After 3 months of strict dieting, she weighed 99 pounds. Her grandmother explained that Tina was her parents' only child. The parents had separated four or five times during her childhood, and now, although they lived together, they were not happy. There were many arguments. Tina had always been a sad child and rarely smiled.

When Tina began losing weight, Tina's mother initially commended her, but as her weight loss continued, both parents fought with her to eat more. Much later, during her outpatient psychotherapy, Tina agreed with her therapist (C. W.) that this represented the first time that her parents' attention was focused on her in a supportive way. The illness, she said "did give me an edge. I was always shy, and couldn't open my mouth to either of them."

At the beginning of therapy, Tina said almost nothing, but stared at the therapist with large, sad eyes. She answered all questions in soft monosyllables. She often felt lightheaded and weak, and she had been asked by school officials not to partake in gym classes. She had not menstruated in more than 10 months. Asked what her goals in therapy would be, she shrugged her shoulders. When gently encouraged to speak of her life at home, she became tearful and stared at the floor. This is the familiar impasse that therapists are confronted with in treating reticent anorectic patients.

Tina was handed a copy of the Dickinson poem No. 486, which expressed feelings of ineffectualness and fearfulness at saying a word. Tina read the poem aloud. She then slowly handed it back. Asked how she was feeling, she said, "It sounds like me." She was then encouraged to write a poem of her own on this theme. Without hesitating, this silent girl took pen in hand and wrote the following poem in 9 minutes.

> In the screaming, silent dark
> I drown in seas of red and black
> singing sobs of who is there
> (if anyone at all) and
> grabbing fistfuls of
> air to package my
> raging thoughts and
> seal them
> (for the moment)
> deep inside.

The therapist read her poem aloud carefully and reverently, commending the effort. Tina was encouraged to explain her symbolism. She said that the "screaming, silent dark"—note the logical impossibility of having both conditions at the same time—referred to her frequent experience of lying in bed in the dark, weeping in rage and grief, but trying not to let her parents hear her cry. They would be arguing in the next room. "I drown in seas of red and black," she explained as her experience when she squeezed her eyes shut. "Singing sobs" referred to her small, high-pitched whimpers, which were involuntary when she cried, and which she tried to stifle. "Of who is there (if anyone at all)" was her clear expression of longing for her parent's affection while they were always involved with each other. "Grabbing fistfuls of air to package my raging thoughts" referred to her silently pounding her pillow in frustration at their hours-long arguments. Her therapist agreed there wasn't much to smile about if a girl had to cry herself to sleep each night. Tina looked at her therapist and managed a slight smile.

A few weeks later, Tina's weight had gone up to 103 pounds; during the next few months, her weight hovered between 105 and 109. She had agreed to stop at her grandmother's regularly after school for a late lunch, but she still refused to have supper with her parents. This impasse was resolved with continued therapy, during which Tina wrote more rich, descriptive poetry.

Dee: An Anorectic Parent Advocate

Dee was a Southern girl with an ever-present smile, the daughter of an alcoholic mother and a successful ambitious father. At 15, she began dieting, weighing 130 pounds at 5'2", and she soon moved on to semi-starvation. Once or twice a week, she would binge; afterward, she would induce vomiting. She was also a compulsive exerciser. She continued this pattern for 2 years, reaching a low of 95 pounds. She arrived at therapy with her mother, who wore the same smile, and who said Dee had been a joy to raise. When asked about Dee's refusal to eat, her mother began talking about her own alcoholism.

During the first two individual sessions, Dee smiled constantly, and answered questions with "maybe." Asked about her feelings about being in therapy, she blushed. At the third session, Dee was handed the Dickinson poem No. 738, which expressed feelings of submission as well as the joy of pleasing others. Asked to write her own poem about submission, she produced the following in 16 minutes:

> I gave when others needed,
> And even when they didn't.
> They would take and be happy,
> Pleasing me greatly.
>
> I seemed to be the go-between
> Whenever two had problems.
> I always seemed to work things out
> Pleasing me greatly.

I stand in the background
Stepping out only when called
And always willing to help when asked
Pleasing me greatly.

I'd like to know what others
Actually think about me.
Wondering if they like me,
Wanting to please them.

Is this my goal in life,
Always giving up what
I want,
Only to please them?

This poem was a clear statement, almost devoid of metaphor, containing no personal symbolism. The last two stanzas contained a change in mood, as Dee questioned if people could respect her for being so accommodating. Finally, she began to question her methods: "Is this my goal in life?" We discussed the reciprocal nature of her actions, "always giving up what I want." For the first time, she suddenly looked sad. "I always thought what I wanted was the same as what others wanted for me," she said. The therapist suggested that the poem said otherwise.

Dee continued in therapy, gaining some weight, and relinquishing much of her compulsive exercising. She took a part-time job that required making decisions. As of this writing, she is in outpatient therapy, where she continues to write about her vulnerability to other's demands and her pleasure in her increasing spontaneity.

DISCUSSION

The patient's original poem usually provides rich experiential data. It often contains images from her early life and of her family. The poem can reveal feelings of excitement, grief, longing, fear, and guilt. The production is the patient's; it is not a theory, a technique, or a bias. The poem is born in a moment of deep introspection, primed by the experience of another writer with whom the patient can identify. This approach lessens the patient's fear of being controlled from without. The procedure helps her to transcend her fear of being influenced, and her poem becomes the vehicle for enhanced self-esteem.

The use of poetry in psychotherapy avoids the intellectualized discussions that may characterize psychotherapeutic efforts with anorectic patients. It also attempts to bypass the censoring and self-interrupting style of these patients, which, in other circumstances, inhibits the ability to identify and express basic emotional states.

There are several advantages to the use of poetry in psychotherapy. First, poetry therapy can be a form of short-term psychotherapy; significant change was found in anorexics—but not in obese patients—in as few as ten sessions (Woodall, 1983). Second, poetry therapy can be used as an adjunct to conventional insight-oriented psychotherapy, providing a way to break through initial resistance. Third, poetry therapy often helps the patient to formulate and focus her thoughts; her creations are often a surprise to her and provide new connections. Finally, poetry therapy has no obvious toxicity. As Leedy (1969) wrote, no one has ever died from too much poetry.

At the present time, it is not possible to specify why poetry therapy works, although this observation is often made of many forms of psychotherapy. Also, not all patients benefit from poetry therapy; some refuse the task completely, although most of them do try. Further, poetry therapy ultimately relies on the skill and training of the therapist, who must use original metaphors to formulate questions and interpretations in therapy. As such, poetry therapy is a technique rather than a therapy, but it is a potentially very effective technique nonetheless.

Individual Sessions for Reticent Anorectic Patients

The poetry therapy model used at the Johns Hopkins Hospital Eating and Weight Disorders Unit, developed by the first author, uses one Dickinson poem per session in the previously noted sequence. It is used primarily for the reticent subgroup of anorectic patients, constituting about 25% of the anorexia nervosa inpatient population at Johns Hopkins. The therapist asks the patient to read the poem aloud and then to read it again to herself. The patient is then asked what the poem is about and what the writer is trying to say. The patient offers interpretations of her own and then the therapist offers interpretations as well. Together they discuss these interpretations, taking perhaps 15 minutes.

Next, the patient is asked to write a poem of her own—a minimum of four to six lines, more if she wishes—about the same theme or her reaction to it. She is told that the poem does not need to rhyme, that poetry has a natural rhythm that will emerge from her feelings. She is given 10–15 minutes for this task. When the patient has finished writing, her poem is read aloud slowly and respectfully by her therapist. The patient is sometimes shy about reading it herself, but, if she wishes, she may read it first. However, it is important that the therapist also read the poem out loud, so that the patient hears her production and can experience hearing her work valued and taken seriously. The therapist then asks the patient what her poem refers to and how each metaphor relates to the context. Each line is considered in detail, the therapist informing the patient of Archibald MacLeish's notion (1974) that the poet writes in order to find out what he means. If the poem has not been titled, the patient is asked if she can now name it; sometimes a name emerges that had not occurred to her before. This may be an initial step in overcoming alexithymia.

In the remaining minutes, the therapist offers his or her own interpretation of possible meanings of the patient's poem but in a Aristotelian manner—that is, as a question: Is it possible that you may have been referring to X when you said Y? The patient then responds to each question, approving or denying the interpretation. All of her comments are respected by the therapist. The patient is considered the authority in regard to her own poem.

How Poetry Therapy Works

At this point, it may be possible to propose several explanations about what may occur in poetry therapy. First, a poem is invariably a communication and, therefore, contact with another person. For the reticent anorexic, communication and contact by traditional means has often been problematic and anxiety provoking. Contact with the therapist is no exception to this, and indeed may be even more difficult for the patient. Using a published poem represents contact with a communicator not present, which is nonthreatening. The patient often is relieved not to have to talk to the therapist directly. The published poem may remind her of school work, a task with which she is already familiar.

Second, communication and contact with feelings may occur because the task of writing a poem may render the patient's conscious defenses nonoperational (Edgar, Hazley, & Levitt, 1969). This meeting ground between therapist and patient then loses the aura of authority and control.

Third, a well-chosen poem of a published writer can evoke an identification with the conflict stated in the poem; it can also allow the patient to experience vicarious relief. This relief and identification hearten the patient and encourage her to attempt a formulation of her own issues.

Fourth, there is a similarity between symptom formation and the poetic process: "Like symptoms, initial ideas and inspirations represent an impulse or a conflict and its defense together. In this light, the poetic process and the work of psychotherapy follow an analogous sequence" (Rothenberg, 1972, p. 244). Symptom formation is a "solution" that does not permit growth because, although it relieves some of the person's tension and anxiety in the short run, it does not communicate and reach out for true resolution. The meaning of the symptom is unknown to both the sufferer and those around her. But the act of making a poem *always* communicates. That is, there is always a presumed listener, even if it is limited to the observing self. Rothenberg's work (1972) provides clarification and extension of these comparisons.

Fifth, the patient becomes proud of her poem as she often has been proud of her academic accomplishment. This pleasure in accomplishment and her increase in self-esteem hearten and sustain her while she endures the examination of the symbolism and metaphors in therapy. Potentially painful realizations are mitigated by the pride of accomplishment.

Sixth, the patient's poem is *not* an interpretation of her behavior or a part of a theory. The patient recognizes the poem as her own creation and a bridge from the reticent self to the therapist and to her own healthy self.

As Winnicott (1971, p. 85) wrote, "A poem is layer upon layer of meaning . . . and always about the self." Poetry therapy provides a means of transforming into words what is communicated physically through the symptoms of anorexia nervosa.

REFERENCES

Andersen, A. E. (1985). *Practical comprehensive treatment of anorexia nervosa and bulimia.* Baltimore: Johns Hopkins University Press.

Asch, S. (1956). On the use of metaphor in the description of persons. In H. Werner (Ed.), *On expressive language.* Worcester, MA: Clark University Press.

Bruch, H. (1973). *Eating disorders: Obesity, anorexia nervosa and the person within.* New York: Basic Books.

Bruch, H. (1978). *The golden cage: The enigma of anorexia nervosa.* Cambridge: Harvard University Press.

Charone, J. K. (1982). Eating disorders: Their genesis in the mother-infant relationship. *International Journal of Eating Disorders, 1*(4), 15–42.

Chernin, K. (1985). *The hungry self.* New York: Times Books.

Crisp, A. H. (1980). *Anorexia nervosa: Let me be.* New York: Grune & Stratton.

Edgar, M. F., Hazley, R., & Levitt, H. I. (1969). Poetry therapy with hospitalized schizophrenics. In J. J. Leedy (Ed.), *Poetry therapy.* Philadelphia: J. B. Lippincott.

Goldstein, M. (1983). The production of metaphor in poetry therapy as a means of achieving insight. *The Arts in Psychotherapy, 10,* 167–173.

Gull, W. W. (1874). Anorexia nervosa. *Transactions of Clinical Society of London, 7,* 22–28.

Higgins, D. (1967). *Portrait of Emily Dickinson. The poet and her prose.* New Brunswick: Rutgers University Press.

Johnson, T. H. (Ed.). (1960). *The complete poems of Emily Dickinson.* Boston: Little, Brown & Co.

Leedy, J. J. (1969). *Poetry therapy: The uses of poetry in the treatment of emotional disorders.* Philadelphia: J. B. Lippincott.

Leedy, J. J. (Ed.). (1973). *Poetry the healer.* Philadelphia: J. B. Lippincott.

Lerner, A. (Ed.). (1978). *Poetry in the therapeutic experience.* New York: Pergamon Press.

MacLeish, A. (1974). *Poetry and experience.* Baltimore: Penguin Books.

Minuchin, S., Rosman, B. L., & Gailer, L. (1978) *Psychosomatic families: Anorexia nervosa in context*. Cambridge: Harvard University Press.

Osofsky, J., & Danziger, B. (1974). Relationships between neonatal characteristics and mother-infant interaction. *Developmental Psychology, 10*(1), 124–130.

Rothenberg, A. (1972). Poetic process and psychotherapy. *Psychiatry, 35*, 238–254.

Selvini-Palazzoli, M. (1978). *Self-starvation*. New York: Jason Aronson.

Sifneos, P. (1973). The prevalence of "alexithymia" characteristics in psychosomatic patients. *Psychotherapy and Psychosomatics, 22*, 255–262.

Sours, J. A. (1974). The anorexia nervosa syndrome. *International Journal of Psychoanalysis, 55*, 567–576.

Winnicott, D. W. (1971). *Playing and reality*. London: Tavistock Publications.

Woodall, C. (1983). *Eating disorders, body image and self-hate*. Unpublished doctoral dissertation, Rutgers State University, Newark, NJ.

Woodall, C. (1987). The body as a transitional object in bulimia: A critique of the concept. In S. C. Feinstein (Ed.), *Adolescent psychiatry* (Vol. 14; pp. 179–184). Chicago: University of Chicago Press.

11

Structured Eating Experiences in the Inpatient Treatment of Anorexia Nervosa

Jane L. Sparnon
Lynne M. Hornyak

The failure to eat enough to maintain a minimally healthy body weight is the target symptom of anorexia nervosa and results in the tragically emaciated state associated with hospitalization. Subsequent refusal to maintain goal weight after being discharged and persistent distortion regarding nutritional needs contribute to the high recidivism rate seen with this patient population. A dilemma facing the inpatient treatment team is that expedient weight gain, against the patient's will, often results in negligible long-term weight restoration. It appears that patients who are allowed to maintain a passive stance during nutritional rehabilitation will gain weight rapidly under close supervision but fail to continue to adequately nourish themselves independently. In addition, focusing on the physical aspects of the disorder may lead to inadequate evaluation and treatment of the underlying psychological disorder, contributing to relapse.

One of the most challenging tasks facing the recovering anorexic prior to discharge from the hospital involves the transition to self-directed eating. Andersen (1985) and others recognized the importance of stabilizing weight before discharge and recommended a minimum period of at least 2 weeks for this phase. Patients who leave during the active weight-gain phase of treatment may generalize that all eating leads to weight gain and become fearful of exceeding initial weight goals. Thus, as nutritional rehabilitation reaches the weight-stabilization phase, attention must be directed toward identifying and teaching the patient her caloric needs for weight maintenance.

Opportunities for practicing self-controlled eating in a variety of situations, and experience with realistic stressors during meals, can also provide patients with successful coping skills to carry outside the hospital. These practices can help patients to achieve confidence in their ability to control weight through healthy eating. Furthermore, patients often need to be reintroduced to the social aspects of eating, since fears of eating in public may have resulted in social isolation. A supervised cooking group provides a rich opportunity for patients to practice planning, cooking, and eating meals with others in a structured manner.

There are few references in the eating disorders literature regarding the use of structured eating activities in comprehensive inpatient treatment programs for people with anorexia nervosa. In light of this lack, this chapter provides an overview of structured eating activities in inpatient settings; the theoretical background of this approach; a description of the structured eating treatment component developed at Dominion Hospital in Falls Church, VA, specifically the Cooking Group; and considerations in the use of structured eating activities, based on the experience of the first author (J. L. S.).

Material in this chapter refers specifically to anorexic patients, although bulimic patients also participate in the Cooking Group at Dominion Hospital. Also, the group leader is referred to as the "dietitian" since that is the first author's profession; we recognize, however, that leaders of groups at other institutions may be from different disciplines.

OVERVIEW

Definition

Structured eating activities may take a variety of forms. For the purposes of this chapter, we limit our comments to the Cooking Group. We define the Cooking Group as a therapeutic activity that allows patients to actively participate in the planning, cooking, serving, and eating of a meal with other patients under the supervision of the program dietitian.

The Literature

Some references on the use of structured eating activities in inpatient eating-disorders programs are included in the occupational therapy literature. For example, Martin (1985) reported on cooking as an occupational therapy activity in the eating-disorders program at St. George's Hospital

in London. Giles and Allen (1986), in their practical article on the rehabilitation of anorectic patients, included shopping, cooking, and eating
practice as functional therapeutic activities that can be used by occupational therapists.

Other references are found in the psychological and medical literature on comprehensive inpatient eating-disorders programs. For example, Andersen (1985) reported that aspects of desensitization are involved in the last (maintenance) phase of the Johns Hopkins Hospital
program in Baltimore. Meals are prepared and eaten with the occupational therapist, and patients are encouraged to go out to restaurants to
"practice eating normally and in a social context" (p. 335). Roth (1986)
briefly described similar *in vivo* eating practices included in the Shep-
phard and Enoch Pratt Hospital program in Towson, MD. Larocca (1984)
reported on the use of BRUNCH (Basic Recovery Utilizing Normal Col-
lation in Hospital) at St. John's Mercy Medical Center in St. Louis. Inpatients, outpatients, and staff eat together once a week at lunch with the
emphasis being on comfortable social interaction during meals. Larocca
noted that patients often cite BRUNCH as one of the most valuable tools
in their recovery. Johnson and Connors (1987) wrote about the Sunday
Supper Group, which is an activity in the eating-disorders program at
Northwestern University Medical School in Chicago. Patients plan, shop
for, and prepare a meal that they then eat together. Patients explore and
discuss their experiences after the meal; the authors reported that patients find the group to be quite helpful.

THEORETICAL BACKGROUND

It is generally recognized that anorexia nervosa is a multidetermined disorder (e.g., Garner & Garfinkel, 1985). Once the condition is established,
a variety of factors, including some that may not have been causative, can
serve to maintain unhealthy eating patterns. As Giles and Allen (1986)
pointed out, one critical factor can be

> the anorexic individual's changing reactions to food and eating arising as a
> consequence of the initial dieting behavior. These factors might include the
> effects of classical conditioning, differentiation of the inner states of hunger
> and satiety, and the tendency to binge which may be present in almost all
> "restrained" eaters. (p. 53)

In other words, anorexics may become sensitized to a variety of internal
and external cues related to food and eating. These cues may not be salient for nonanorectic or nondieting individuals. Furthermore, these cues
may be unique to a particular patient.

Two concepts from the behavioral and cognitive–behavioral literature are useful when considering factors that might maintain anorectic behavior (i.e., restrictive and inappropriate eating behaviors, maladaptive emotional reactions to food). First, anorectic behavior may be maintained by both positive and negative reinforcement. Harris and Phelps (1987) explained this concept as follows:

> Subjective feelings of anxiety are experienced in response to the fear of weight gain brought on by urges to eat. Food refusal . . . become[s] negatively reinforced by decreasing the possibility of gaining weight and consequently decreasing subjective feelings of anxiety. Food refusal . . . subsequently [is] employed to reduce anxiety arising from *other* sources (e.g., interpersonal conflict). Additionally, eating- or weight-related responses such as frequent weighing, [and] food refusal . . . may be positively reinforced when the patient is rewarded for losing weight or "being ill." (p. 492)

Thus, a variety of behaviors that an anorectic individual might include in her dieting repertoire or associate with weight loss could be maintained by positive and negative reinforcement.

The second concept relates to the role of the cognitive variables. As delineated by Garner and Bemis (1982, 1985), it is important to take into account that an individual's attitudes, beliefs, and assumptions about the meaning of weight may maintain maladaptive eating patterns. These cognitive variables should be assessed and attended to in treatment since they affect eating behavior.

The implications are that treatment should emphasize the modification of faulty sensitization to internal and external cues; reduction of subjective feelings of anxiety; and modification of misperceptions, attitudes, and assumptions that serve to maintain maladaptive eating patterns. Several authors (Andersen, 1985; Garner, 1986; Garner & Bemis, 1982, 1985; Garner, Garfinkel, & Bemis, 1982; Roth, 1986) have provided detailed descriptions of cognitive–behavioral principles that they consider essential in their comprehensive treatment approaches. The use of behavioral rehearsal and reinforcement of adaptive, competent behavior are often recommended. However, substantive details for utilizing structured eating experiences, which serve as such behavioral rehearsal, are sparse.

Garner (1986) mentioned meal planning as an intervention to address the anorexic's confusion about appropriate eating. Meal planning can involve "establishing precise guidelines for the quality, quantity and spacing of meals," minimizing choices, and "monitoring of food intake through detailed records . . . gradually replaced by more natural eating behavior" (p. 308). Garner recommended the introduction of avoided foods in reasonable quantities, complemented by cognitive interventions to challenge dichotomous thinking (e.g., "good" versus "bad" foods). Further-

more, Garner noted that "resistance and fear of deviating from symptomatic behavior provide valuable opportunities to examine dysfunctional
attitudes" (p. 309).

Principles of *In Vivo* Practices

Structured eating activities may be considered similar to "exposure *in vivo*"
practice sessions. Exposure *in vivo* involves accompanying an individual in
real-life situations that arouse anxiety for her. The individual typically
avoids or escapes from such situations in order to avoid or reduce anxiety.
While approaching or remaining in the real-life situation with the client,
the therapist or trained paraprofessional can guide her in becoming aware
of what she is thinking, feeling, and doing to improve or worsen her distress. Interventions can be initiated immediately. Thus, the individual can
experiment with alternative behaviors and cognitions and note any accompanying reduction of anxiety or arousal.

Exposure *in vivo* is commonly used in the treatment of anxiety disorders to address the behavioral, cognitive, and affective components of
these conditions. While anorexia and anxiety disorders are not equivalent
problems (Garner & Bemis, 1982), some of the objectives of *in vivo* experiences are pertinent to changing maladaptive eating patterns. Handling
and eating food, particularly in the company of others, can arouse considerable anxiety and emotional reactivity for anorectic patients. During
structured eating activities, the patient and therapist together can observe
the patient's thoughts, feelings, and behavior while engaging in eating or
food-related situations. The therapist can intervene to guide the client in
coping more effectively with her reactions. Interventions may address
maladaptive eating behaviors as well as cognitions (thoughts, attitudes, beliefs, and assumptions) regarding food, eating, and nutrition.

There are three areas that the first author (J. L. S.) has found to be
critical in treating maladaptive eating patterns: nutritional disorganization, oversensitization to problematic food cues, and maladaptive emotional responses to food and eating. Methods for addressing these areas
follow a brief description of the treatment structure of Dominion Hospital's Eating Disorders Unit, of which the Cooking Group is one component.

TREATMENT STRUCTURE

Providing education and practice for healthy eating involves the team efforts of the dietitian and other psychotherapeutic professionals. Education begins at admission, as the patient is oriented to the protocol for meal

service on the ward, and continues throughout hospitalization. The dietitian teaches weekly nutrition classes with lectures, discussions, and projects. The sessions focus on the physiological adaptations and alterations in nutritional status resulting from impaired eating patterns and weight fluctuations. Each patient is placed on a carefully calculated diet once the initial nutritional assessment is completed. The diet is calculated to provide for maximal weight gain while avoiding symptoms of medical distress related to refeeding. Nursing personnel monitor and record each patient's intake, noting any bizarre or ritualistic eating behaviors. Eventually, trips taken off the unit allow patients to test food situations that have caused stress in the past.

The structured eating treatment component was specifically designed to gradually and systematically allow patients to resume control over selecting and eating food, prior to discharge. Treatment is divided into three phases: a first phase in which the patient is medically stabilized and begins to gain weight; a second phase in which the patient is granted partial independence around eating; and a third phase in which the patient eats entirely independently in a variety of situations. The patient cooks and eats a meal with peers once a week beginning in the second stage of treatment. Most patients accomplish this after two to three weeks in the hospital.

The Cooking Group is designed to be educational as well as interpretive; patients practice planning, cooking, and eating meals according to standards learned in nutrition education classes and then discuss their reactions in the context of an actual dining experience. Each Cooking Group lasts 2 hours to allow time for preparing and eating the meal and processing the feelings generated by the experience. The session is coordinated and supervised by the staff dietitian, who also approves the menu. The meal replaces a regularly scheduled lunch and must provide all of the calories and nutrients required for each participant in the group.

Eligibility Requirements for the Cooking Group

In order to attend the Cooking Group, a patient must meet specific eligibility criteria. The clinical staff must assess her as physically and emotionally stable as defined by the following:

1. The patient must make a commitment to handle all items used in preparation of foods safely, including knives, which could be used self-destructively.
2. The patient must comply with the established meal protocol, eating her entire prescribed diet in the allotted time period of 30 minutes.

3. The patient must show no evidence of bingeing, purging, avoiding meals, or compulsively exercising.
4. The patient must have shown evidence of intent to comply with established weight goal by gaining at least 25% of the difference between admission weight and goal weight.
5. The patient must have successfully completed the steps of contracting with the staff for the privilege of selecting her own meals on the ward from written menus, following a pattern established by the dietitian.
6. The patient must demonstrate behavioral changes in tolerating a wide variety of foods, including previously restricted items, and reducing and/or controlling rituals and/or bizarre eating patterns.
7. The patient must show evidence of the development of a therapeutic alliance with staff members through open communication and acceptance of feedback.

Meal Planning Phase

Planning for the Cooking Group beings at least 2 days prior to the day on which the session is held. The dietitian meets with eligible participants to orient them to the Cooking Group experience and to provide them with guidelines for planning the menu. Patients are provided with a "Cooking Group Request Form," which outlines the procedure for ordering food, supplies, and equipment for the session.

Individual nutritional needs and food preferences must be coordinated into one single menu because the emphasis is on joint effort, to reinforce the social–interactional aspects of eating. The menu is approved by the dietitian for nutritional adequacy and availability of foods. Conflicts over menu items are referred back to the planners for resolution. Once the menu is approved, no changes or substitutions are allowed. Attention is directed toward patients working together to salvage the meal if it becomes apparent that the recipe is faulty or items are missing. Errors are viewed as an opportunity for the dietitian to point out to patients their dichotomous thinking patterns (e.g., good versus bad, success versus failure) and to assist them with the task of working together to cope with and adapt to the unexpected.

The meal planning phase also emphasizes planning realistically for eating after discharge. Most patients need to adjust the timing and spacing of meals near the end of their hospitalization to develop a pattern more consistent with their home schedule. Planning and preparing meals together on the unit provides an opportunity to integrate their nutritional needs with their lifestyles, including an honest estimation of their time and talents for cooking. Patients are encouraged to use convenience items and shortcuts to expedite meal preparation and to avoid getting bogged down in the logistics of cooking.

Patients are provided realistic tasks to test their control over eating in situations determined by them to be stressful. For example, patients who attend school full time may be encouraged by the dietitian to plan and prepare portable lunches suitable for consumption in the school cafeteria, along with nutritious after-school snacks that are consistent with their calorie requirements. Patients who will eat alone after discharge need assistance learning how to purchase quantities of food consistent with their needs from supermarkets geared to serve families. Busy professionals are guided to plan ahead for meals to avoid the consequences of haphazard and poorly planned last-minute meals. Expectations of preparing a balanced meal without preplanning can set one up for failure.

A theme, such as "weekend meal at home with parents," is selected by the patients for each session in order to practice eating in a potentially stressful situation. Themes vary according to the needs of the eligible patients from casual lunches to meals at school to simple but elegant dinner parties with friends. Patients may elect to role play a situation that they have previously avoided or one in which they recall having failed to eat adequately despite good intentions. The dietitian may suggest a theme related to a predominant issue identified in patient sessions during the week, including issues of competition, dependency, loss, control, and anger. Separation themes are common due to the inevitability of leaving the security of the hospital.

TREATMENT METHODS

A brief description of the physical setting used during cooking sessions may help the reader to visualize the process. The Eating Disorders Unit includes a self-contained kitchen that is used regularly as the dining room for these patients. It can be physically closed off from the remainder of the Eating Disorders Unit for privacy. Patients are instructed in basic cooking and sanitation techniques prior to the session and use standard equipment to measure foods.

Techniques for Addressing
Nutritional Disorganization

Most anorexics present with significant "nutritional disorganization." This phrase describes anorexics' difficulty in identifying or responding appropriately to their bodies' signals of hunger and satiety. Anorexics may eat or refuse food according to emotional rather than physiological stimuli, so it is both unsafe and unrealistic for patients to rely on their bodily signals for hunger and satiety early in treatment. Anorexics typically deny their hunger to the extent that they can feel full with minuscule amounts of food or even vicariously full from watching others eat. The major objectives of the educational process during treatment are to teach accurate nutritional principles and to establish clear guidelines for food intake.

Quantitative Distortions

Nutritional disorganization centers around two quantitative themes: how much to eat and how much time to spend eating. Issues relating to how much to eat stem from conflicts between the patient's desire to eat (appetite) and her actual nutritional needs. Confusion regarding portioning of foods is addressed through instruction on, and consistent use of, a simple but adaptable food-selection system to plan meals. This system, which was developed by the first author (J. L. S.), categorizes food into six groups: dairy foods, high-protein foods, fruit, vegetables, starches, and fats. Patients are taught how to order desserts, casseroles, sandwiches, and other complex items using a combination of allowable foods groups to meet caloric requirements and achieve adequate levels of other nutrients. It has been the first author's experience that patients include more variety in their diet, and show greater propensity to include foods previously feared or avoided, when they are provided concrete guidelines to use for planning. Focusing on food groups rather than calories can provide an opportunity for patients to let go of the distrust of specific foods. For example, using the food group system, a patient can safely plan to eat a piece of apple pie once she realizes how to break the item into components of the food group system. In this manner, a dessert can come to be viewed as part of the overall balanced diet, rather than a sinful caloric extra. This system also encourages variety while assuring nutritional adequacy, as long as the correct number of portions are selected from each group. Thus, patients learn how to use many different items in planning a balanced diet.

Disorganization around timing often leads to prolonged periods between meals and very slow eating patterns that preclude eating sufficient quantities to satisfy caloric requirements. The time distortion is first addressed while patients are eating all meals on the ward. Structure is provided by serving meals at regular intervals with specific amounts of time allotted for eating. Typically, 30 minutes are allowed for meals, with 15 minutes for snacks. As the quantity of food increases to satisfy caloric requirements, patients learn to eat faster in order to finish on time. They may learn to recognize and avoid behaviors that interfere with completion of meals, such as cutting foods into small pieces, separating all foods on the plate, and talking too much during the meal.

In Cooking Group, the strict time limits are removed to test the patients' ability to eat the prescribed meal with less structure. In the first author's experience, patients typically finish the meal in about 30 minutes. This suggests that external control over timing, which is introduced and reinforced through meal service on the unit, gradually becomes internalized by the patient.

Intervention for addressing the quantitative distortions around eating involves using the following techniques:

1. The patient is provided written and verbal education in nutrition group.
2. The patient practices by selecting menus on the ward and portioning foods in Cooking Group.
3. The patient is confronted with faulty perceptions and distortions through comparison of estimated portions with actual standard portions in Cooking Group (reality testing).
4. The patient and dietitian evaluate the session in terms of learning experiences provided and feelings generated.

The following example illustrates how these steps are applied for a patient, Susan, who is struggling with her distortions around quantity in preparing a cold salad plate.

1. Susan is first taught in nutrition education sessions that, according to the food group system, an appropriate portion of cottage cheese is half a cup. She learns how this quantity looks on a plate from observing the item on trays on the unit and comparing the size with the menu slip, which states "half a cup of cottage cheese." Susan eats the cheese to recognize how many bites it takes to eat and how full she feels with this quantity of cheese in her stomach.

2. Susan then practices portioning cheese. First, she serves what she perceives as an accurate portion without measuring. Then she selects and uses the correct size measuring cup. Susan is also helped to recognize how many tablespoons half a cup contains and to experiment with viewing the cheese in differently shaped and sized plates and bowls.

3. Susan then compares her concept of what a serving should be to the portion measured out with standard measuring equipment. This comparison allows her to test the reality of her perceptions.

4. With the assistance of the dietitian, Susan evaluates the accuracy of her portioning and discusses feelings generated by the experience. They also discuss how she can apply this learning to planning meals after discharge.

Bizarre Eating Patterns

Nutritional disorganization may also be manifested by bizarre eating patterns. Examples of bizarre patterns seen in Cooking Group include eating only one specific kind of food; eating only one color of food at a time; eating only foods beginning with a certain letter; endless rearrangement of items on the plate; manipulation of foods by mashing, mincing, cutting, or mixing items together or inappropriate use of condiments; dawdling over meals by hesitating before each bite or chewing extremely slowly; and/or becoming distressed with food combinations in the meal. Based on the assumption that issues of control and avoidance often underlie these behaviors, therapeutic intervention for bizarre eating patterns involves use of the following techniques:

Limit Setting. The patient is confronted by staff and peers with the inappropriateness of her eating habits. Negative consequences of the destructive eating behavior are identified. The nurse or dietitian provides guidelines for eliminating the behavior.

Discrimination. Behavior is discussed privately with the patient to help her discriminate between emotional reactions to food and bodily sensations arising from eating the food. Attitudes toward and associations with foods are identified and challenged immediately after the Cooking Group.

Establishing Responsibility. Control over eating is transferred back to the patient gradually as she shows evidence of her desire and readiness for this. Planning meals and selecting food items provide healthy outlets for control and may lessen the need to manipulate foods at mealtimes.

Learning and Practicing Coping Skills. It is often difficult for the patient to let go of an established behavior until a new one is learned to fill the gap. The patient is requested to reconstruct a particularly difficult eating experience and to think of ways she could cope with the situation using newly learned coping skills. For example, if a patient relates that she has great difficulty eating when she is angry, she may be helped to separate the feeling (anger) from the behavior (avoidance of food), while planning for more direct expression of her feelings.

Stimulus Control. This technique involves completely eliminating foods identified by the patient as provoking strong fears until the patient demonstrates improved impulse control at mealtimes. This technique is most often used on the ward with newly admitted patients. Occasionally, patients regress during treatment as structure is reduced, and they may benefit from temporarily avoiding specific foods. An example of this is to avoid visible fats, such as margarine, on the tray and to incorporate foods containing unnoticeable fat, such as nuts, in the meal.

Desensitization Techniques

A purpose of the Cooking Group is to help patients establish self-control over eating as opposed to avoidance and starvation behavior. As stated earlier, many patients become overly sensitized to cues related to food and eating. Consequently, two types of desensitization may be helpful: desensitization to the presence of foods and desensitization to feelings of fullness from increased quantities of food.

Frequently, patients present with strong resistance to eating specific foods and must be desensitized to the presence of these items. In order to prioritize the foods that cause negative reactions, the dietitian does an assessment hierarchy of avoided foods for each patient as part of the initial interview. Patients are permitted to eliminate three specific foods during their hospitalization, but other previously avoided foods will be included in meals. In the initial phase of treatment, the dietitian writes all menus for the patient, using the avoidance hierarchy as a guide. Restricted items are reintroduced gradually, with emphasis on the nutritional contribution of the item and avoidance of idiosyncratic eating patterns. Total refusal to eat, as in fasting, is not an issue by the time a patient qualifies for Cooking Group. A more typical reaction is fear of or refusal to eat specific foods that were eaten in the past but refused as the dietary restriction progressed. These fears often emerge concurrent with the increased responsibility and decreased structure associated with the second phase of treatment. True physical reactions to foods, such as allergies, are respected and are not counted toward the individual's three most-disliked foods.

A specific application may best illustrate this method. Amy, a 17-year-old anorexic, had eliminated all animal foods from her diet during the previous year. She did not claim to be a vegetarian but avoided meat because it made her feel "too full" and contained fat, which she considered highly threatening. Amy listed her avoided foods as follows: red meats, desserts, eggs, fish, poultry, and milk. According to unit rules, she was allowed to eliminate the first three items from all meals. Therefore, her trays on the ward contained small amounts of fish, poultry, and dairy foods for protein. In nutrition classes, Amy learned to plan balanced meals avoiding red meats, desserts, and eggs. She practiced ordering small amounts of these items when eligible to select her own menus and ate them with other accepted foods. In the planning session for Cooking Group, Amy was chosen to prepare the entrée because her eating habits remained more restrictive than those of her peers and she was unwilling to eat some of the foods they suggested. Amy decided to prepare a poultry dish. As discussed above, she had been partially desensitized to poultry through inclusion of the item on her trays, but she had never prepared it. A further step in desensitization was for Amy to actually touch the poultry during the process of cooking. Amy selected a recipe for stir-fried chicken and vegetables that she had enjoyed eating in the past. It combined small amounts of chicken with a variety of vegetables that Amy liked. The dietitian assisted Amy with the preparation of the entrée on her first session and encouraged her to attempt other recipes in subsequent Cooking Groups. An additional step for Amy was to prepare and eat poultry in a less disguised manner, such as broiled, in which the flavor is more apparent.

A second type of desensitization involves tolerating fullness from increased quantities of foods without reverting to avoidance techniques such as skipping meals or snacks. This sensitization refers to the amount of food eaten and not to specific foods as in the above example. During the initial phase of treatment, the amount of food gradually increases to meet the patients' nutritional needs and to provide sufficient calories for weight restoration. Desensitization thus begins on the ward and continues throughout treatment. In Cooking Group, patients practice preparing foods that provide adequate levels of nutrients without undue bulk.

Methods to address the issue of tolerating fullness include education about the physiology of weight gain and metabolic adjustment, gradual increase in calories, and careful spacing of meals and snacks. The dietitian intervenes by educating the patient about the physical effects of her progressively increasing dietary intake. Physical discomfort related to fullness is very distressful to patients unaccustomed to eating or retaining large quantities of food and may result in impulses to restrict or purge in a vulnerable individual. The processes of ingesting, digesting, absorbing, and eliminating food from the body are studied in nutrition classes in order to dispel myths and to clarify the physiological impact of starvation and refeeding on the body. Patients learn that metabolic adjustments and sluggish bowels are troubling, but not dangerous, components of recovery. It has been the first author's experience that this education is invaluable in allaying fears and enabling patients to tolerate their discomfort.

Several problems are frequently encountered during refeeding. First, since patients are usually constipated early in treatment, it is difficult for them to accept increasing quantities of food. They may falsely assume that they are retaining all the food they have eaten and therefore have no room for more. They may be truly fearful of eating until they eliminate previously eaten meals. At this point, a discussion on bowel adjustments to changes in dietary patterns may diminish their concerns. Also, patients may question the large quantities of food needed to restore lost weight, as their experience has been that any increase in intake prior to admission led to swift weight gain. In response to this, the dietitian explains that metabolic adjustment to changes in dietary intake is a gradual process. Temporary changes in intake do result in weight variance. If one continues to eat more, however, the body gradually senses that more energy is available and becomes less conservative in using calories, and the metabolic rate rises. In order to sustain progressive weight gain, the calorie intake must remain ahead of the rising metabolic needs. Thus, it is usually necessary to provide in excess of 3,000 calories daily to anorexics. A common side effect of this rapid rise in metabolic rate is the potential for "thermogenesis" or calories wasted in heat production. Patients may show symptoms of sweating or feeling hot, especially at night.

Second, patients often inaccurately label fullness as the sensation felt once the initial, ravenous hunger is diminished. In severely restricting patients, this may occur after the first few bites of food. In nutrition class, the dietitian points out how signals for hunger and satiety are poorly interpreted by patients due to their habitual denial of these signals before admission. Education focuses on the need to adopt external guidelines for fullness based on measured amounts of food provided at regular intervals until the body becomes more self-regulated. Patients are reassured that their discomfort will be minimized through careful attention to the bulkiness of meals.

A third goal is helping patients to evaluate fullness after meals in order to draw connections between the degree of discomfort and the type of foods eaten. Many anorexics insist on eating a salad and fresh fruit at each meal. As the quantity of food increases to meet caloric demands, inclusion of these foods may result in very full trays. The dietitian explains this dilemma to patients and then helps them to select more calorically dense foods. Patients are informed that when adequate weight is gained, their calories will be dropped back down to a stabilization level. Once reassured, patients may be able to accept a serving of apple pie, trusting that it can replace two fresh fruits and some bread.

As mentioned earlier, patients may manifest impulses to destroy or manipulate foods as meal structure is reduced. In Cooking Group, these urges to control food are channeled into physical tasks such as measuring, beating, whipping, mixing, and cutting foods during the preparation phase. Additionally, patients assert control over eating patterns through establishing and following a menu pattern.

Techniques Addressing Emotional Responses to Eating

The first author has identified four stages that the anorexic typically passes through on her way to independent eating. These stages have been noted during work with hospitalized as well as outpatient anorexics: refusal (avoidance), "make me" (resistance), "help me" (dependence), and "let me" (independence). Commonly, the emotional responses and accompanying anxieties that characterize these stages are manifested indirectly. Thus, familiarity with the stages can help the group leader to accurately identify and respond to these verbal and behavioral cues.

The first stage involves a refusal to eat, which permits avoidance of the "feared object" (i.e., food). An individual in this stage remains in denial of the severity of her illness and verbally minimizes her symptoms. Typical behaviors include skipping meals, severely restricting the variety of foods eaten, chewing gum compulsively, fluid loading with noncaloric beverages such as diet colas or coffee, and lying about food intake. This anorexic will go to great lengths to hide the extent of her illness from others and will often refuse treatment.

An individual has usually reached the second stage, or "make me," by the time of admission to the hospital. She may still resist eating but will do so in a highly structured environment. She may be able to identify how the eating disorder negatively affects her life, but she is helpless to change her behavior. The patient reports persistent fears about eating and gaining weight, a sense of guilt from "giving in" to those who urge her to seek help, and frustration related to her inability to tolerate stress. Behaviors typically seen at this stage include dawdling and crying at mealtimes; somatic complaints of dizziness, headache, or gastric upset; obsessive eating behaviors, such as cutting or mashing foods; and making disparaging remarks regarding the quantity or quality of food served to her. At this stage, most of the intervention is provided on the ward by the dietitian and nursing staff. Techniques used include providing education regarding physical adjustments to refeeding with emphasis on the temporary nature of the weight-gain phase, setting limits on destructive and manipulative eating behaviors, and applying logical consequences to maladaptive eating patterns (e.g., if meals are not eaten, the patient is required to eat a snack providing the missing calories).

A patient qualifying for Cooking Group is most often entering the third stage, "help me." This stage is characterized by the development of trust in one's caregivers and a diminished resistance to eating. The patient begins to identify and work on stressors related to eating. She may experience a temporary sense of dependence on the hospital staff to provide guidance and structure as she begins to eat restricted foods and gain weight. At this third stage, the patient continues to experience strong emotional responses to eating but shows improved control over dysfunctional eating behaviors. Specifically, she will verbalize her reactions, rather than acting them out by destroying or refusing a food. As the struggle over eating lessens, the patient usually becomes very interested in learning and practicing improved eating patterns. The dietitian provides nutrition education focusing on portion sizes, food groups, and appropriate combinations of foods. Appropriate short-term goals for this stage include finishing all meals on time and expanding the variety of foods in the diet. Longer term goals include weight gain, demonstration of the ability to plan a balanced diet, reduction of idiosyncratic eating patterns, and the reintroduction of the social component of eating.

The last stage, "let me," represents a genuine move toward independence. The patient must have successfully performed the tasks described above, both on the ward and in Cooking Group, and must have contracted for advanced status with minimal structure. Interventions at this point are aimed at preparing the patient to live outside of the hospital. In Cooking Group, the "let me" individual is expected to assume leadership in the planning and production of the meal. She is encouraged to challenge herself to eat previously avoided foods and items similar to those she will eat after discharge. The dietitian may also assign other structured eating activities, such as planning meals to be prepared home while on a therapeutic pass and out-of-hospital trips to buy groceries or eat in restaurants. These activities test self-control in a variety of eating situations.

Intervention Techniques

The dietitian's role is twofold. First, he or she must recognize and respond to each patient's verbalizations and behavior patterns in planning tasks appropriate to their stage of treatment. Second, he or she must attend to cues indicating readiness for movement into the next stage in order to provide appropriate feedback. The following case study illustrates how the stage model is used to understand a patient's behavior and to respond to her particular needs, as well as the use of nutritional intervention techniques.

CASE STUDY

The patient, Tanya, was selected for the case study because her significant denial, supported by her high intelligence, allowed her to minimize her illness in verbal discussions. Her intellectualization provided an impervious veil behind which she maintained her resistance to change. This pattern is commonly observed in anorexics. Tanya was unable, however, to use these defenses against her emotional reactions evoked in Cooking Group, where she was encouraged to experience and process her emotions. Thus, the general approach used with Tanya in cooking sessions may be useful for readers when working with this type of patient. Tanya remained on the unit for almost 4 months and provided great challenges to those working with her. She attended Cooking Group during her last month of hospitalization. This discussion focuses on techniques used during the Cooking Group sessions.

Description

Tanya, a 41-year-old, married, professional, was admitted to the hospital at the insistence of her outpatient therapist due to profound and continuous weight loss. Tanya had been unsuccessful in complying with requirements to gain weight as an outpatient. Prior to admission, her weight plunged to 76 pounds at 5'4".

Tanya developed severe symptoms of anorexia comparatively late in life. Although she admitted to a lifelong preoccupation with her weight and had maintained a chronically low weight of 90–95 pounds throughout most of her adult life, her symptoms did not worsen until 18 months prior to admission. Significant precipitating events included despondency over her 40th birthday, declining work performance, marital conflicts, financial stress, and a sudden weight gain up to 108 pounds. As she perceived a loss of control in other areas of her life, Tanya focused on adhering to an extremely restrictive diet to lose weight. Initially, her efforts produced substantial weight loss. Then she reached a plateau of 86 pounds 6 months prior to admission, which Tanya still perceived as too high. In a desperate attempt to lose more weight, Tanya began to experiment with stimulant-type laxatives and diuretic pills with increasing frequency. In addition, she began a frenetic exercise schedule of aerobics, walking, and stretching, but she denied that she felt fatigued from this regimen.

Concurrent with the onset of severe anorexic symptoms, Tanya developed a potentially serious alcohol problem and compulsively bought excessive amounts of clothing and jewelry. Tanya typically drank two 12-ounce bottles of beer daily, but as her diet diminished to a mere 500–600 calories a day, the impact of the alcohol increased. In the months preceding hospitalization, the alcohol frequently provided over half of her daily calories, with no usable nutrients. Thus, she exacerbated her degree of malnutrition and often became moderately intoxicated in the evenings. Also, her compulsive shopping patterns were resulting in significant debt despite Tanya and her husband's substantial joint income. In order to earn more money, Tanya took on a part-time job in addition to her full-time employment.

At the time of admission, Tanya's denial was profound. She rationalized that since she could work two jobs without fatigue, never caught colds, could exercise better than women half her age, and maintained menstrual cycles despite catastrophic weight loss, she could not be anorectic. Indeed, she claimed that she had never felt stronger in her life. She denied any ill effects of the weight loss but admitted that she had noticed that it was slightly harder to concentrate recently.

There were also significant developmental precipitants to her eating disorder. Tanya was hospitalized frequently during the early years of her life for surgery and convalescence related to a birth defect. This may have interfered to some degree with parental bonding and resulted in Tanya viewing herself as somewhat fragile. Tanya described herself as "small and delicate" as a child and recalled her parents being very concerned that she ate sufficiently. She was bright and capable in an academic setting but suffered from social isolation due to her sense of being different from other children. Tanya described her parents as capable but undemonstrative. Possibly due to frequent separations related to her medical treatments, Tanya became self-reliant at a young age. She recalled priding herself on her ability to please others by anticipating their expectations and complying with their wishes. She recalled being referred to as a "model patient" by nurses.

Eligibility

In order to qualify for Cooking Group, Tanya was required to meet the criteria outlined earlier in the text. Due to her emaciated state, she was required to gain 8 pounds (one fourth of the difference between admission weight and goal weight). Additionally, Tanya was required to comply with the protocol regarding meal service, to refrain from inappropriate eating behaviors, to discontinue unsupervised exercising, and to elicit support and feedback from her peers and caregivers.

Tanya's resistance to eating and gaining weight was a substantial barrier to her progress and eligibility for Cooking Group. Her disruptive behaviors at mealtimes on the unit alienated her peers to the extent that they were unsupportive of her request for reduced structure. Her disparaging comments about the foods and her obsession with her bones was upsetting the other patients who were struggling to eat. Tanya initially resisted participating in the nonverbal therapies, such as art therapy, occupational therapy, and leisure education, by arriving late to meetings and discussing extraneous matters during sessions. Tanya openly expressed her distaste for Cooking Group and resisted selecting her own menus. She verbalized her recognition of how difficult such activities would be for her. With significant effort and support from staff members, Tanya accomplished the tasks required to advance to Cooking Group during her final 4 weeks of treatment.

Goals in Cooking Group

In establishing Tanya's goals for Cooking Group, it became evident that she needed to work on developing coping skills in the following areas:

Social Eating. Tanya needed to be reintroduced to the social–interactional component of eating. Due to her tendency to avoid social engagements and her self-consciousness about eating in public, Tanya seldom ate meals with others. Tanya recalled that even as a child she did not enjoy eating. As Tanya progressively restricted her diet, she learned the art of appearing to eat without ingesting much food by moving foods around on her plate. Recently, with the addition of her part-time job, Tanya was able to avoid eating dinner entirely as she was not at home with her husband.

Nutritional Disorganization. Despite her apparent preference for "natural and health foods," Tanya really had no idea what constituted a balanced diet. She was unable to accurately identify or respond to physiological cues of hunger or satiety. She ignored stomach growls and was always surprised that others seemed to eat regularly while she had "no need to do so." Tanya would frequently fast for long periods of time and claimed the experience left her "refreshed." She unfailingly overestimated portions served to her by others and accused them of trying to make her fat.

Idiosyncratic Behavior. As mentioned above, Tanya had developed some specific techniques for avoiding eating. She would express her aversion to foods through facial grimaces, disparaging remarks, manipulation of food items (mashing, mincing, mixing, and seasoning foods inappropriately), and would feel her bones during mealtimes to reassure herself that they were still very apparent. She described losing weight as making her feel clean and pure.

Inexperience with Cooking. Due to her aversion to foods and her reluctance to assume the responsibility for cooking in her home, Tanya did not know how to prepare many items. She lacked basic cooking expertise to the point that her meals consisted almost entirely of canned soup, plain yogurt, coffee, beer, and salad with no dressing. On the few occasions she ate with her husband, he cooked and she washed the dishes.

In summary, goals for Tanya in Cooking Group included the reintroduction of the social component of eating, correction of quantitative distortions around nutrition, reduction of idiosyncratic eating patterns, and development of basic cooking skills.

Behavior in the Meal Planning Phase

As Tanya became eligible to order her own meals on the ward, her discomfort with the self-selection of foods became apparent. When counseled by the dietitian regarding her caloric needs, Tanya burst into tears and refused to write her menus. After a period of time, she was once again presented the privilege of ordering menus. This time she listened and appeared to understand the food group system, but she balked at the quantities required for her meals. She also showed her fears through procrastination when requested to help plan the menu for Cooking Group. Tanya found it difficult to coordinate her preferences with the others eligible for Cooking Group. Eventually, she stated that she would eat whatever the others planned, thus avoiding any responsibility for the meal. Due to her high level of anxiety, the group leader allowed Tanya to maintain a passive role in selection during her first planning session. In subsequent sessions, Tanya was required to play a more prominent role in the selections of foods. In addition, she was required to plan meals featuring foods she would be likely to eat, and suitable to her busy schedule, once she left the hospital.

Treatment

Nutritional Disorganization. Tanya presented with significant nutritional disorganization around portioning foods and timing meals. Her quantitative distortion regarding appropriate amounts of foods was confronted and corrected in the following manner. In each cooking session Tanya was required to estimate sizes and amounts by serving herself portions that she felt were consistent with her food plan. Then she was directed to measure these portions with standard utensils to compare her estimates with the measured amount and to correct her error by adding more food. Attention was directed toward helping her correlate her perception of the portion size with the actual portion as measured. She was encouraged to visualize the foods on the plate, remembering the appearance of her trays on the ward, to aid her in discerning the proper quantity of food. At first, the concept of a half-cup was meaningless, but gradually she began to associate to quantity of foods she received in half-cup portions (e.g., vegetables, starches) with the idea "half-cup."

Her disorganization around the timing of meals presented problems in Cooking Group. Tanya was unable or unwilling to organize the preparation phase of the session to allow herself a full 30 minutes to eat. For example, on an occasion when she cooked alone with the dietitian, she dawdled and played with the ingredients for her pizza until she had only 10 minutes left to eat. With her difficulty in chewing, this behavior proved disastrous. The intervention was to allow consequences (e.g., Tanya having to rush through the meal to finish, resulting in anxiety and stomach discomfort) and then to evaluate which behaviors (e.g., dawdling, procrastination, manipulation of ingredients) led to the outcome.

Idiosyncratic Behavior. Tanya's refusal to cook with meat was addressed by desensitization. The intervention with Tanya was similar to that described earlier.

Cooking Skills. Tanya's inexperience with food preparation was addressed by helping her to select simple recipes with few ingredients and providing guidance and practice in Cooking Group. Specifically, Tanya was taught to use standard measuring utensils, to read recipes, and to plan the preparation of food items so that all elements of the meal are done at the same time. Tanya prepared foods such as sandwiches, hearty casseroles, and soups, which are consistent with her busy life-style.

Over the course of treatment, the dietitian assessed which stage of treatment Tanya was functioning within and responded with appropriate interventions. Input from other members of the treatment team was considered. Initially, in the second stage, Tanya was allowed to avoid preparing the entrée by convincing her peers to do the task. At her second Cooking Group, however, she was again confronted by peers with the fact that she had been unwilling to help them plan the meal. Additionally, they encouraged her to take a turn stirring the meat and to portion out the meat for her own taco after preparation. The interventions used in this situation were to allow consequences; to help Tanya discriminate how her behaviors led to a disagreeable outcome; to establish responsibility by not rescuing Tanya from the confrontation with her peers and by allowing her to portion her own meal; and to help her to develop coping skills by practicing new ways of dealing with stress rather than avoidance.

During the third and fourth Cooking Group sessions, Tanya had gained better control over her disruptive eating behaviors, so more time was directed toward helping her develop confidence in her cooking skills. She was promoted to "Chief Cook" and was required to prepare the entree. At this point Tanya was in the third stage, or "help me." She was still fearful of gaining weight, but she was able to eat her meals more easily. Tanya selected chicken as her entrée and was astounded to see raw chicken arrive for the session. Tanya showed her aversion to touching the chicken through facial grimaces, crying, and holding the item far away from her body. As she was clearly uncomfortable with the process, Tanya was encouraged to discuss her feelings, but she was not allowed to pass the task of preparation to a peer. The main intervention was to set the limit that Tanya could not avoid the task, and she was given supportive feedback for her efforts. Her vulnerability was noticed by peers, who responded in a supportive manner, drawing her into their circle for the first time.

In this session, Tanya identified that she was able to eat cooked meat at this point but still had difficulty seeing and touching raw meat. The dietitian educated her about the various ways meat is packaged and sold in stores and encouraged Tanya to use time on a therapeutic pass to go to a grocery store to investigate. She was encouraged to use shortcuts to facilitate her cooking and to ease her discomfort. Specifically, she was taught that she could purchase poultry already cut up and boneless for use in her favorite stir-fried dishes. She was cautioned, however, about the additional cost of such convenience items. Tanya was also directed to very simple cookbooks that describe and show pictures of food during the preparation and meal service phase.

It so happened that Tanya was the only individual eligible for Cooking Group during her final cooking session. She had learned to recognize and work with her limited cooking skills. She was able to plan, prepare, and eat a simple meal quite successfully and was moving into stage four, or "let me." Rather than planning a fancy meal, Tanya realistically decided to prepare a grilled cheese sandwich, soup, fresh fruit, milk, and purchased cookies. She was able to coordinate her preparations so that all the foods were ready on time, and she was able to eat within time constraints. Consequently, Tanya stated that she felt less rushed and uncomfortable after the meal and more likely to duplicate the meal after discharge. Education focused on developing and implementing consistent patterns for meals once Tanya left the hospital. She established a goal of preparing and eating at least one meal a week with her husband, and she acknowledged the destructiveness of using his absence at mealtimes as permission to avoid eating. The dietitian discussed with Tanya the special problems inherent in planning and eating meals alone.

DISCUSSION

Much of the anorexic's success in maintaining her illness revolves around uncorrected distortions regarding nutritional needs and body image concerns. When a patient is "re-fed" rather than participates in feeding herself, she has the option of rejecting the weight goals and nutritional recommendations of her caregivers. For example, the most expedient path to weight restoration may be delivering a concentrated, high-calorie diet to a patient restricted to total bed rest. However, this system is so contrary to the dietary principles and control issues of the anorexic that she would be unlikely to willingly submit to such a regimen. When this is carried out against her will, she is perfectly capable of undoing the "damage" (i.e., weight gain) at her earliest convenience. Her anger and indignation with such a program is likely to further fuel her resistance to recovery. Many times, a patient is so firmly entrenched in dysfunctional eating patterns by the time she is hospitalized that she sees her identity as being an anorexic. She may remain incapable of change until this is challenged in therapy and she learns other, healthier outlets for control over her life. A structured Cooking Group provides a therapeutic means for linking the theoretical with the practical aspects of treatment. Patients are provided valuable hands-on experience in preparing and eating meals with others who share their concerns under the direction of an experienced clinician.

It also provides an opportunity to facilitate the progress a patient makes toward the resumption of healthy and independent eating patterns.

As elaborated earlier, the patient needs to develop trust in her caregivers in order to risk possible failure as she attempts unfamiliar tasks. She needs to learn to tolerate the inevitable sense of panic associated with giving up an established behavior pattern in order to benefit from therapy. The patient should be at a place in treatment where she is developing a cognitive understanding of her normal nutritional needs for weight restoration and maintenance. She needs to understand the food group system for planning meals on the ward and in Cooking Group, and she must be ready to accept a change in her lifestyle. Regardless of treatment style, only the patient who really desires recovery can be helped.

Client Selection and Eligibility

The Cooking Group described in this chapter is an integral part of an inpatient eating-disorders program. Therefore, patient selection for this therapy is determined jointly by representatives of all disciplines working with these patients. The eligibility criteria outlined earlier in the chapter are adhered to except in special situations in which the patient is to leave before fully qualifying for inclusion in the group. An example of this is the patient who meets most of the criteria but has not gained sufficient weight. If the patient must leave for reasons other than noncompliance (e.g., financial reasons, return to work or school), she will be granted permission to attend Cooking Group and will be instructed how to select her own menus.

Patients who plan to leave the program earlier than medically recommended would not be allowed to participate, as they seldom demonstrate investment in their treatment. Also, Cooking Group is part of the gradual restoration of control to patients and is perceived as a privilege. Consequently, allowing a resistant patient to participate could seriously undermine the progress of patients who struggled to qualify. Because of the length of time required to provide nutritional rehabilitation to a seriously malnourished anorexic, many patients attend this therapy for a month or more on a weekly basis before discharge. In this ideal situation, the patient and group leader can identify and set goals for Cooking Group consistent with her stage of progress in treatment.

Patient Reactions

Due to the combination of reduced structure and heightened responsibility, patients' reactions to the Cooking Group tend to be strong, particularly in the first session attended. In the first author's experience, patients have cried, shouted, walked out of the session, refused to participate, became nauseated, appeared very angry, and, on one occasion, choked violently during the session. It is imperative that the group leader have a backup support system available for coping with these potentially dangerous situations. The leader cannot leave several patients alone with knives and food in order to attend to a patient who has fled the session. Also, labile emotions can lead to volatile acting out, which may require immediate intervention to avoid potentially serious consequences.

As a safety precaution, the group leader should be well acquainted with the Heimlich maneuver for disengaging food stuck in the throat in case of choking. In addition, at least one person on the premises must be proficient in cardiopulmonary resuscitation (CPR) in case of serious choking that results in loss of breathing, as in the accidental ingestion of a fish bone.

Cooking Group is an emotional experience for the patients, and the group leader must recognize and respond appropriately to possible transference issues. Many patients associate cooking and eating with their mothers or other authority figures and may harbor hostile feelings toward or show evidence of feeling threatened by the leader. This may present as aggressive or passive behavior in the group. Reconstructing the experience and exploring feelings elicited by the experience can be a valuable therapeutic tool but requires skillful intervention by the leader. In some cases, the first author has found that having patients role play emotional scenes, such as mother–daughter interactions in the kitchen, can be an effective intervention.

Most patients enter the session with some degree of trepidation, but with practice and structure they emerge more confident in their ability to eat independently after discharge from the hospital. Patients often share that their initial resistances to attending the cooking session were based on fears of failure related to their lack of confidence in themselves and false assumptions regarding what the session would be like. With education, practice, and a healthy sense of humor about the results of the meal, they learn to put eating into a different perspective. Many patients eventually grow to enjoy the sessions as they master control over their fears.

Therapist Qualifications

Ideally, the group leader should be a skilled counselor, a proficient cook, and a knowledgeable nutritionist. It is of foremost importance, however, that the group leader understand the dynamics of eating disorders, that is, what is happening experientially for the patients. When education and practice with healthy eating patterns is the primary focus, the leader should be a registered dietitian with substantial experience working with eating-disordered patients. (A registered dietitian, by definition, has had supervised training beyond an educational degree and has passed a national registration examination.) If the focus of the group is to be primarily recreational and creative, an activity therapist would be appropriate for leading the session. If processing patient reactions is of utmost importance, then a trained mental health professional (e.g., psychologist, social worker) would be suitable. If the individual leading the session is not a registered dietitian, one should be consulted for guidance.

Also, the group leader must be acquainted with and observe basic safety and sanitation rules for food preparation and service, including any certification requirements of the local jurisdiction. For example, in the state of Virginia where Dominion Hospital is located, persons cooking or preparing food for others need special training to qualify as "Certified Food Service Managers." As noted in the client reactions section, there is a potential for injury from choking or dysfunctional eating behaviors. Consequently, one needs to be trained to react quickly and appropriately in an emergency. Finally, in addition to the obvious educational training, the group leader needs to be warm and empathic as patients tend to have difficulty opening up about their feelings and may be intimidated or put off by a reserved individual.

Adaptability for Outpatient Practice

It may be feasible to use the Cooking Group for outpatient treatment if certain essential criteria can be met. Specifically, the group leader must assess the client carefully for potentially self-destructive behaviors and must have developed a sense of rapport with the individual. At a minimum, all individuals considered for this therapy should be medically cleared by a physician experienced with eating disorders, with the patient being judged by a mental health professional as emotionally stable. Whenever a therapist works independently with a client, the subjective assessment of suitability for a particular intervention carries a degree of risk. As mentioned in the previous section, there is a potential risk of injury or illness whenever food preparation or eating is involved. However, from a therapeutic viewpoint, the greater risk encountered in using this therapy involves the potentially negative impact on the client–therapist relationship. This is related to the heightened emotional tone of these sessions, in which a client struggles to do difficult tasks under the supervision of the group leader. If the therapeutic relationship is weak, it may collapse under the stress of this experience. A client may feel vulnerable and exposed as she risks failure in her attempt to achieve control over her impulses around food. Conversely, the relationship may be strengthened if the client feels the group leader is empathic and views the experience as a "shared triumph." It is valuable to diminish the risks through careful collaboration with other qualified individuals working with this population. It may be possible to contact other individuals who have worked with the client if permission is granted. As a measure of investment in treatment, anorexics should have begun to gain weight as directed by a physician or dietitian. In addition, it may be wise for the therapist to draw up a contract outlining the goals and expected results of the Cooking Group. This contract should be signed by the client and group leader. If a client appears resistant to attending a cooking session, it seems advisable to not include this individual in the group.

Planning must also include attention to the size of the group. From the first author's personal experience, a workable number is four to five participants. With more people in the group, it becomes difficult to direct attention to everyone.

Another consideration is the significant financial investment required to rent and outfit a suitable kitchen and dining area. Minimal equipment would include a range and oven, sink, refrigerator, work area, and a table with chairs. Also, the expense of food supplies for the sessions can be very high. In the first author's experience, anorexics want to prepare seafood, exotic salads, and expensive entrées.

There are several alternatives to conducting a structured eating group. One is to work individually with a client. The therapist may assist the client in planning menus, accompany her to a grocery store to supervise her purchases, and then observe her cooking in her own home. This is extremely time-consuming and difficult to make cost-effective. For instance, if the cooking session replaced a regularly scheduled session, would the usual fee be charged even though the time spent was longer? Another alternative is to accompany the client to a restaurant for a meal. Again, the financial and logistical arrangements need to be clearly defined in advance. For instance, does the client's fee for the therapy session include the cost of her meal? Third, the primary therapist may refer the client to a registered dietitian for this aspect of her recovery if the primary therapist has no training in nutrition.

CONCLUSION

In order to correct quantitative distortions and improve eating patterns in anorexics, it is essential that patients' nutritional needs and maladaptive behaviors be addressed prior to discharge from an eating-disorders program. A supervised Cooking Group provides practice eating in situations that replicate problematic ones for these patients. The experiential nature of this approach allows one to get below the "intellectual defenses" that prove such substantial barriers to recovery and lead to chronicity of symptoms. The Cooking Group also allows patients and staff to clearly observe progress toward independent eating patterns. For some anorexics, the introduction of an element of risk encourages them to test their reactions in other difficult situations. Finally, the experience has the potential to deepen the therapeutic alliance, which can be very rewarding for both the patient and the therapist.

REFERENCES

Andersen, A. E. (1985). *Practical comprehensive treatment of anorexia nervosa.* Baltimore: Johns Hopkins University Press.

Garner, D. M. (1986). Cognitive therapy for anorexia nervosa. In K. D. Brownell & J. P. Foreyt (Eds.), *Handbook of eating disorders: Physiology, psychology, and treatment of obesity, anorexia, and bulimia.* New York: Basic Books.

Garner, D. M., & Bemis, K. M. (1982). A cognitive-behavioral approach to anorexia nervosa. *Cognitive Therapy and Research, 6,* 123–150.

Garner, D. M., & Bemis, K. M. (1985). Cognitive therapy for anorexia nervosa. In D. M. Garner & P. E. Garfinkel (Eds.), *Handbook of psychotherapy for anorexia nervosa and bulimia* (pp.107–146). New York: Guilford Press.

Garner, D. M., & Garfinkel, P. E. (Eds.). (1985). *Handbook of psychotherapy for anorexia nervosa and bulimia.* New York: Guilford Press.

Garner, D. M., Garfinkel, P. E., & Bemis, K. M. (1982). A multidimensional psychotherapy for anorexia nervosa. *International Journal of Eating Disorders, 1,* 3–46.

Giles, G. M., & Allen, M. E. (1986). Occupational therapy in the rehabilitation of the patient with anorexia nervosa. *Occupational Therapy in Mental Health, 6,* 47–65.

Harris, F. C., & Phelps, C. F. (1987). Eating disorders. In L. Michelson & L. M. Ascher (Eds.), *Anxiety and stress disorders: Cognitive–behavioral assessment and treatment.* New York: Guilford Press.

Johnson, C., & Connors, M. E. (1987). *The etiology and treatment of bulimia nervosa.* New York: Basic Books.

Larocca, F. E. (1984). An inpatient model for the treatment of eating disorders. *Psychiatric Clinics of North America, 7,* 287–298.

Martin, J. E. (1985). Occupational therapy in anorexia nervosa. *Journal of Psychiatric Research, 19,* 459–463.

Roth, D. (1986). Treatment of the hospitalized eating disorder patient. *Occupational Therapy in Mental Health, 6,* 67–87.

12

Experiencing the Self through Psychodrama and Gestalt Therapy in Anorexia Nervosa

M. Katherine Hudgins

Anorexia nervosa, with its confusing array of psychosomatic symptoms, often presents both conceptual and treatment challenges to the practicing clinician. The particular clinical configuration of anorexia nervosa—denial of body sensations, distorted perceptual processes, and reliance on external support—points to the use of experiential psychotherapy as a treatment method of choice for patients with anorexia nervosa. Experiential psychotherapy targets interventions directly at the somatic, nonverbal level of dysfunction, which is of primary importance in these patients.

This chapter presents psychodrama and gestalt therapy interventions in the treatment of people with anorexia nervosa. Theoretical constructs from self-psychology (Kohut, 1971), object relations (Winnicott, 1965), and family systems theory (Humphrey, 1987a, 1987b) are integrated in a stage process model that targets treatment at both individual and interpersonal levels of dysfunction.

A number of recent studies have supported use of stage process treatment for more difficult disorders, such as patients with borderline personality disorders (Forssmann-Falck & Hudgins, 1988) and dysthymic patients (McCullough & Carr, 1987). Conceptualizing the therapeutic process in stages provides a structure for the long and often difficult treatment of developmentally delayed patients, and therefore seems applicable to the treatment of anorexia nervosa. In the model presented in this chapter, stage 1 targets increased awareness of the patient's nonverbal, experiential self through empathic bonding with the therapist. In stage 2, the patient learns to discriminate reliably between self and others for competent decision making. Stage 3 provides the patient a chance to individuate successfully from the therapist, despite a vulnerability to separation anxiety.

THEORETICAL ORIENTATION

Contributions from Self-Psychology and Object Relations

From a self-psychology perspective, the physical symptomatology of anorexia nervosa represents a disruption in the internal organization of the self structure (Goodsitt, 1985; Kohut, 1971; Sours, 1980; Swift & Stern, 1986). Goodsitt (1985) wrote that, "The symptoms of anorexia nervosa represent both a disruption of the self and the defensive measures against further disruption" (p. 55). Both Goodsitt and Kohut (1971) described the anorexic's denial of internal sensations, even ones as severe as self-starvation, as an attempt to stay in control of a chaotic, fragmented self-organization. These patients show developmental deficits in a consistent sense of self, both in the experiencing self and in the ability to observe the self. Bruch (1979) detailed the now-familiar triad of distorted body image, inaccurate perceptual processes, and helplessness.

As a result of this developmental arrest in an experiential sense of self, the ego functions suffer and become defective. A vulnerable self faces the external world with primitive defense mechanisms—denial, splitting, and projective identification—to preclude awareness of separation out of fear of the "annihilation terror" (Winnicott, 1965) that often arises when anorexic patients are alone.

Winnicott (1965) addressed the etiology of the false self that the anorexic patient adopts, or introjects, from significant others. Introjection is a normal psychological process whereby individuals internalize the beliefs, structures, and images of others to guide their own behavior. However, with anorexics, a true sense of an experiential self is missing or distorted, leaving them vulnerable to internalizing beliefs of significant others that are destructive to their development. Anorectic patients have no reliable internal criteria, so they rely on the beliefs of others, and they are unable to discriminate their own wants and needs from what they are told. Thus, anorexics often present for treatment as delayed in self-development and inexperienced in self-reliance, making therapeutic change a formidable task.

Contributions from Family Systems

Given the anorectic patient's tendency to depend on significant others for decision making, the family structure becomes important when considering therapeutic change. The family structure of the anorexic contributes to both the development and maintainence of dysfunctional psychological patterns. Humphrey (1987a, 1987b) described the internalizing of family patterns by women with eating disorders. Commonly, the family has its own dysfunctional patterns, leaving the patient without adequate role modeling of adaptive strategies for normal developmental tasks such as separation and individuation. It is as if the patient psychologically "eats" the family structure and dysfunction, internalizes it, and repeats the patterns intrapsychically.

This eating metaphor can be continually used throughout treatment by both therapist and patient to address the similarities between the patient's intrapsychic self-deficits and the family-wide rigidity. I believe that both intrapsychic and family issues needs to be addressed for patient change to occur.

Anorexia nervosa most often appears in adolescents or young adult women facing the developmental tasks of separating and individuating from their families. Unfortunately, the anorexic faces these tasks with a fragmented sense of self, developmentally arrested defense mechanisms and a family structure that often functions with rigid control. Being developmentally stuck, with little ability to differentiate self and others, many anorectic patients sacrifice any sense of autonomy to stay within the confines of an enmeshed family, since they have no internal sense of self-support or protection to rely on for decision making.

Contributions from Psychodrama and Gestalt Therapy

Research literature on gestalt therapy indicates that this treatment approach is effective with a wide variety of disorders (Elliott, 1987, Greenberg & Rice, 1981). Psychodrama has also been found to be an effective adjunctive tool to traditional individual psychotherapy (Hudgins & Kiesler, 1984, 1987; Stein & Callahan, 1982). While there are conceptual and practical differences between psychodrama (Moreno, 1947, 1977) and gestalt therapy (Perls, 1969, 1975; Polster & Polster, 1974) both systems of psychotherapy speak the same experiential language philosophically. Psychodrama and gestalt therapy alike respect the subjective, individual experience of self and include psychotherapeutic interventions to increase awareness at the somatic level. Both psychodrama and gestalt therapy bring the physical and mental experiences of self into focus through use of action-oriented interventions by the therapist. In this way, the patient can become aware of her actual experiences and thereby access her dependence on internal support in decision making.

Three constructs are used to guide clinical treatment of anorexia with the stage process model of psychodrama and gestalt therapy; they are described in the following section of this chapter: active experiencing; surplus reality; and empathic bonding.

Active Experiencing

In both psychodrama and gestalt therapy, a theoretical emphasis on active experiencing distinguishes these action methods from their more traditional verbal counterparts. While verbal psychotherapy often focuses on cognitive meanings and strategies leading to cognitive insight by the patient, experiential psychotherapies involve active experiencing by the patient as the primary goal of psychotherapy, believing that it is necessary for successful treatment. As Moreno and Moreno (1969) wrote, "Interpretation may be questioned, rejected or totally ineffective, but the act speaks for itself" (p. 108). Starr (1977) wrote that the goal of psychodrama is "action insight." Action insight relies on experiential awareness based on experimentation with new behaviors, not merely cognitive understanding.

For the anorectic patient, active experiencing helps develop an experiential sense of self that can be trusted. Psychodrama and gestalt interventions increase body awareness and provide the opportunity for the patient to correct distorted perceptions and rely on her own sensations. In turn, a solid sense of self allows anorectic patients effectively to discriminate introjected images of the false self from the active experience of real self, thereby building a larger experiential foundation for decision making.

Surplus Reality

All psychotherapies seek to increase the patient's awareness of thoughts, feelings, and behaviors. Moreno (1977) developed his interventions with the goal of making the patient's internal reality overtly visible between the therapist and patient. Moreno (1965) wrote that, "There is, in psychodrama, a mode of experiencing that goes beyond reality, which provides the subject with a new and more exhaustive experience, a surplus reality" (p. 212). According to Buchanan (1984), surplus reality is the extension of the patient's perception of reality, that is, dramatizing and concretizing the patient's internal reality through psychodramatic enactment.

With anorectic patients, the concept of surplus reality helps the patient to move beyond rigid control and denial of sensation simply by enacting images in a way that makes them larger than life. Surplus reality is accomplished through the use of psychodramatic techniques that allow the patient to concretize the images, perceptions, and expectations that she has in everyday life. For example, rather than the patient reporting about an interaction with a significant other, she could actually portray both sides of the interaction.

Empathic Bonding

All psychotherapies emphasize establishing a therapeutic alliance and a trusting relationship with the patient. Bruch (1973) observed that standard interpretations do not work with anorexics because they are developmentally arrested and have difficulty establishing a working alliance. She wrote that the therapist needs to be more active with anorectic patients. Goodsitt (1985) suggested the therapist's role to be a "mode of action intervention . . . he is acting as external auxiliary ego" (p. 63). Both suggestions rely on increased empathic bonding as the first step in successful treatment of anorexia nervosa.

Within psychodrama and gestalt therapy, the therapist may physically "mirror" the patient's nonverbal behavior, which tends to further strengthen the alliance. The therapeutic experience of empathically bonding with the therapist is developmentally necessary and reparative for anorectic patients.

STAGE PROCESS MODEL OF PSYCHODRAMA AND GESTALT INTERVENTIONS

The stage process model of treatment with anorectic patients is divided into three stages. Each stage has specific goals, therapist guidelines, clinical interventions, and predicted patient change. Each stage builds on previous developments and occurs in a particular sequence. Predicted patient changes are detailed to guide the therapist in knowing when to change the specific stage emphasis.

To present the model clearly, a composite clinical case is used. Clinical material is taken from sessions where the principles and interventions of psychodrama and gestalt therapy were integrated into ongoing, long-term individual psychotherapy. Each case includes the therapist's process (i.e., reasoning for interventions of interpretation of what is happening) when appropriate.

Stage One: Bonding with the Experiential Self

Goals

In stage 1 with the anorectic patient, the therapeutic goal is to bond with the patient's healthy self in a trusting therapeutic alliance.

In addition to bonding with patients, the therapist's task during stage 1 is to teach them to look inwardly for a sense of self for reference to questions. Klein, Mathieu-Coughlin, and Kiesler (1984) referred to this ability to identify internal experience as a necessary precondition to effective psychotherapy. The task is in itself antidotal to the pathological reliance of most anorexics on external figures.

Therapist Guidelines

During stage 1, the therapist's primary guidelines are to bond with the patient's healthy, experiential self and to provide the structure and support for the patient to begin to do experiential work.

Interventions

Two specific interventions that I standardly use in stage 1 for both assessment and treatment are doubling (Hudgins & Kiesler, 1984, 1987; Moreno & Moreno, 1969; Taylor, 1986) and focusing (Grendlin, 1981).

Doubling is a psychodramatic technique in which the therapist or a group member sits next to the patient and adopts her nonverbal posture. The doubler speaks in the first person, as though he or she is part of the patient's internal awareness. The therapist's task as double is to verbalize hypotheses about the patient's internal state. This role relationship between patient and therapist allows the therapist to test hypotheses from a fairly nonconfrontative position, thus decreasing resistance. Traditionally, doubling has been used in group psychodrama (Buchanan, 1984), and it has only recently been adapted to the individual psychotherapy relationship (Hudgins & Kiesler 1984, 1987).

Doubling increases the patient's awareness of internal cognitive, affective, and motivational states. During stage 1, doubling is most often implemented when the patient needs support and is learning the process of introspection. The following case demonstrates the use of doubling to promote bonding and to increase experiential self-awareness during stage 1.

In this case, the patient was a 23-year-old female anorexic with a 5-year history of hospitalizations and sporadic outpatient psychotherapy. The material here was taken from an early session. The patient had previously been withholding information concerning her history, thoughts, and feelings. Doubling was implemented in an effort to work around her resistance.

THERAPIST: Andrea, to understand you better, today I'd like to come over and sit next to you and be your double. Doubling involves my sitting like you and talking out loud as though I am your inner voice. If what I say fits your experience, then repeat it in your own words. If what I say is wrong, then please correct me. Is that OK?

PATIENT: *(Compliantly.)* OK.

THERAPIST: *(As double, takes patient's bent-over posture, head down, hands in lap.)* I feel like I have the weight of the world on my shoulders. I get so tired of carrying around everyone's problems.

PATIENT: *(Silence.)*

THERAPIST: *(As double.)* I'm tired of carrying around Mama's problems, Daddy's drinking, and my own problems, but I feel guilty even thinking that, much less saying it out loud.

PATIENT: Yes, that's right. I am tired of that. I'm so tired I almost want to give up. No, I don't want to give up. I don't want to give up, but I don't know what else to do.

THERAPIST: *(As double, to increase patient's self-awareness.)* I feel walked on, like I can't push them off my back. Sometimes I feel too worn out to push them off.

PATIENT: I am tired of people walking on me, and I guess, I'm gonna have to stand up for myself.

THERAPIST: *(As double.)* I want to stand up for myself, but this weight is holding me down. I wonder if I would feel different if I held my body differently? *[This direction was given to encourage the patient to experiment with new behavior.]*

PATIENT: *(Raising her head and adjusting her shoulders.)* Yeah, I'd like to stand up for myself, not take it anymore, but I'm too scared.

THERAPIST: *(As double.)* I'm scared, but I still want to learn how to stand up for myself, how to get out of the mess in this family.

After the doubling intervention, the therapist moved back to her role as therapist and initiated discussion of the experience to assist the patient to become more aware of her own wants and needs. I have observed that the empathic bonding provided by the nonverbal component of doubling helps provide the patient with the safety needed to experiment with new behavior.

Focusing is a clinical intervention, designed by Gendlin (1981), that teaches introspective skills. The therapist teaches the patient to focus—in other words, to pay attention to a set of internal referents in order to increase self-awareness and thus expand the basis for decision making.

Focusing is a prerequisite to effective psychotherapy for the anorectic patient. Turning one's attention inward and beginning to experience a sense of autonomous self is in itself antithetical to the pathological inter-personal patterns (e.g., relying on other's opinions and views) that the anorectic patient normally uses to establish safety and reduce anxiety. While focusing is not a gestalt therapy intervention *per se,* it incorporates many of the theoretical concepts found in Perls' writing (1969) about experiencing the world from an intrapsychic perspective.

After Andrea read Gendlin's 1981 book *Focusing*, she was willing to use this experiential intervention. Although Andrea, like many anorectic patients, was initially scared of looking inside and finding only emptiness—Winnicott's "annihilation terror" (1965)—reading the book provided cognitive explanations that relieved some of her fear. This example was taken from the seventh session, as the therapist began to teach the patient to introspect.

THERAPIST: Andrea, I know you're scared about looking at your self, inside your self, so let's begin the focusing work slowly. Let's begin by allotting just five minutes to looking inside. You can begin by either closing your eyes or just staring into space—the contact is with yourself, not with me, though I am here to support you. If you get scared, we can stop at any time. OK?

PATIENT: OK *(Compliantly and quietly, closing her eyes, slumped into chair.)*

THERAPIST: Now, just begin by noticing anything at all about your internal experience. It can be a sensation, an image, a feeling, a thought, anything that grabs your attention when you think of going inside and finding a safe place.

PATIENT: I see one of the little kids where I work.

THERAPIST: *[To help patient deepen her experience.]* Can you see the child's face? The expression, the look in her eyes?

PATIENT: Yeah, she looks kind of happy and free, just, you know, playing.

THERAPIST: Good, now let yourself notice how your body feels as you look at the feeling on the little girl's face. How do you experience feeling happy and free inside of you? Where in your body?

PATIENT: *(Points across chest, keeping eyes closed.)*

THERAPIST: OK. Take a couple more deep breaths and let that feeling of happy, free, and safe expand inside, just a little, so that with each breath you can feel yourself getting a little happier.

In this example, focusing was used to teach the process of introspection and to help the patient experience a sense of safety inside herself. In later stages, focusing is expanded, as discussed later in this chapter.

Patient Changes

The following patient changes signal the end of stage 1 and the transition to stage 2: (1) the patient verbally acknowledges bonding with the therapist; (2) there is a commitment to psychotherapy as shown by collaborative goal setting as verbalized between patient and therapist; and (3) the patient participates in the doubling intervention and is able to focus for at least 10 minutes at a time. At the point in therapy at which the patient attains these predicted changes, the therapist redirects the therapeutic emphasis. Stage 1 targets increases in intrapsychic awareness, while stage 2 emphasizes interpersonal awareness.

Stage 2: The Real Self

Goals

The goal of stage 2 with the anorectic patient is to teach her to discriminate between the experience of the "real self" and of the "false self," which has been internalized from interactions with significant others. During stage 2, the therapist focuses on the parallels between the patient's individual symptoms and the family dysfunctions to develop treatment interventions. Thus, a successful outcome would be the patient's increased awareness about the strategies she has developed to cope with a dysfunctional family so that she can make more effective decisions on her own. The therapeutic alliance established by this point allows the working through of the pain and disappointment resulting from this increased awareness in such a manner as to facilitate development and prevent regression.

Therapist Guidelines

During stage 2, the therapist's goals are (1) to help increase patient's awareness of the parallels between eating-disordered behavior and the family structure; (2) to facilitate the patient's working through of feelings that accompany increased awareness of how the family structure has contributed to the development and maintenance of the patient's disease; and (3) to support the patient in developing new defensive structures.

During stage 2, the patient must develop more age-appropriate coping strategies. New cognitive structures that support autonomy and individuation must be developed. One example might be changing the belief that many anorexics have that they must be in control of their feelings no matter what the cost to a belief that emotions are a normal part of being human. Changes in cognitive structure allow the release of primitive emotions that have been repressed through the extreme measure of self-starvation and permit the development of healthier defenses.

The main task of the therapist is to facilitate active experiencing to strengthen the observing ego. At this point, the patient not only learns to recognize her own cues for decision making, but she also learns to discriminate her behavior in interaction with significant others.

Interventions

Two interventions I regularly use in stage 2 are gestalt two-chair work to increase intrapsychic awareness of the self (Greenberg & Rice, 1981), and psychodramatic role reversal to increase interpersonal awareness (Moreno & Moreno, 1969). In both experiential techniques, the primary goal is to make concrete the patient's internal reality in action, so as to increase awareness. The therapeutic relationship supports the addition of more intensive experiential work at this point in treatment.

Two-chair work (Greenberg & Rice, 1981; Perls, 1969) is one of the primary experiential interventions used in gestalt therapy. Two-chair work facilitates contact and discrimination between parts of the self and targets intrapsychic awareness. For example, two-chair work is often used to make concrete the child-like and punitive adult parts of the self during a decision-making process. Then an internal dialogue is facilitated between these two parts of the self so the patient can explore a new resolution.

The following example, which also provides a good picture of the use of surplus reality, was taken from stage 2 with Andrea. She had been in psychotherapy for 9 months at this point. She had been consciously addressing the issue of separation from her alcoholic family for several weeks prior to this session.

PATIENT: I'm confused about what to do, whether to try and get a job or to stay on disability. I'm afraid to do anything. Part of me says it's time to get a job so I can move out on my own, but the other part says I won't make it, so why bother.

THERAPIST: Let's work on this confusion, OK? *(Patient nods.)* Let's put the part of you that wants to get a job, who really knows she can, in this chair. *(Pulls up an empty chair.)* What does she look like, the woman that wants to get a job and knows she can? What is she wearing? How old is she?

PATIENT: She's my age, about 25. She has on a dress and knows she looks good. She feels confident. She knows she can handle anything.

THERAPIST: OK, good, now sit in that chair so you can more fully experience that confident part of yourself. *(Patient moves into chair.)* Sit like you feel confident. Notice how your body feels as you breathe, open up your shoulders, look straight ahead. Now, look back at this other part of yourself—the part that feels she can't make it. What do you want to say to her as your confident self?

PATIENT: *(Confident self.)* You know, you really are such a baby. You can do it. You can go get that job. Just go to the interview. You'll do fine.

THERAPIST: So, you know she can do it. How old does she look? You called her a baby. Does she look like a baby? I wonder if you can continue to talk to this scared, child-like part of yourself and remind her of how confident you feel. Give yourself the reassurance your own parents never could.

PATIENT: *(Confident self.)* You are such a baby, but I guess you can't help it. No one ever taught you any differently. Sometimes I get so frustrated with your fears, how you hold me back. I know I can do it. I know it's time to get out and take care of myself.

THERAPIST: Can you take care of her too?

PATIENT: I don't know.

THERAPIST: Well, come sit back over here and tell your confident self what you need.

PATIENT: *(Moves to other chair as scared self.)* I just want to feel OK. I want you to like me, to tell me I'm OK. You never pay me any attention.

THERAPIST: Good, now reverse roles and answer from your confident self.

PATIENT: *(Moves to confident chair.)* I'll take care of you, if you'll just let me know what you need.

THERAPIST: Now, move back and tell her what you need when you're scared.

PATIENT: *(Moves to scared chair.)* I need you to like me, to let me be me even when I'm scared. Sometimes you push so hard. I can't move so fast.

THERAPIST: So, you're asking her to slow down and pay attention to you, reassure you when you are scared, not ignore you? *(Patient nods.)* OK, now come back to your confident self and speak to this kid inside you one more time before we end today. What do you want to make sure she hears today?

PATIENT: *(Confident self.)* I'll take care of you. I'll try to listen to your fears and just tell you it'll be all right. You are OK—just like you are.

THERAPIST: OK, now come back to your child self and take in the reassurance.

PATIENT: *(Moves to scared chair.)* OK. That feels good. I feel OK—just don't leave me.

THERAPIST: Good work. Let's discuss that confusion, now that you've had this experience with the two parts of you that are involved in the decision to get a job.

While the two-chair intervention targets intrapsychic conflict resolution, role reversal targets interpersonal awareness. Role reversal is a psychodramatic intervention whereby the patient reverses roles with actual or imagined significant others so as to increase the patient's experiential awareness of herself and others (Moreno, 1965). Role reversal helps the patient test perceptions of herself and others for experiential accuracy, to discriminate self boundaries, and to practice new behaviors within a safe environment (Buchanan, 1984). Rosen (1985) proposed that an inability to reverse roles demonstrates separation–individuation difficulties, making this a valuable assessment tool.

Role reversal during stage 2 was employed to help Andrea discriminate boundaries between herself and her abusive, alcoholic father. Initially, Andrea vehemently defended the integrity of her father, a man who had repeatedly beaten her into submission for showing any spark of self, but also a man she was empathically bonded to. Not only could she feel his pain, but she could also not separate her sense of self from her concerns about him. This enmeshment between Andrea and her father was shown most clearly in the hallucinations she experienced, specifically that he was laughing at her and ridiculing her whenever she would say something about herself.

The following example of role reversal was taken from a session in the middle of Andrea's psychotherapy, about 10 months into treatment.

THERAPIST: Andrea, I notice that as we talk about you and your dad, you don't seem clear what you're feeling and what he's feeling as you work on separating from him. I wonder if you'd like to experiment with an exercise to clarify that boundary?

PATIENT: I guess so. What do you want to do?

THERAPIST: Well, let's put two chairs here face to face. One of the chairs is your dad and one of the chairs is you. First, I want you to be your dad and talk about how you feel as Andrea separates from you—what you think, what you want to do. Then you can reverse roles and speak from your own feelings as Andrea. Understand?

PATIENT: *(Sits down in father chair.)* OK. I think Andrea is making a big mistake living in town. She should come home and let us take care of the finances while she goes to college. I never have understood that girl. *(Pauses, looks uncertain.)*

THERAPIST: OK, now move to the self chair and express what you're feeling.

PATIENT: *(Hesitantly.)* I can't go home again. *(Begins to cry.)* I'm scared of living all alone and having all this responsibility, but I know I can't go back to all that craziness again. Why doesn't he see?

THERAPIST: Tell him directly, tell your father in the chair.

PATIENT: *(Angrily.)* Why can't you see what you're doing? Can't you see that you're destroying yourself and everyone around you? Your drinking makes you and everyone else crazy. I will not return to that! I wish you would stop. I wish you would stop this drinking and leave me alone.

THERAPIST: Now, reverse roles and answer yourself from your father's position.

PATIENT: *(Moves to father chair.)* Andrea, I need you. You're the only one who cares about me. I'm scared if I stop drinking, I won't have anything. Please don't go.

THERAPIST: Reverse roles again and tell your dad how you feel about him wanting you to take care of him again.

PATIENT: *(Moves to self chair.)* Dad, I just can't do it anymore. It's killing me. I can't eat. I can't get to work. I can barely get by. I have to take care of myself. I love you, but I have to take care of myself.

   This example of role reversal demonstrates the power of psychodramatic interventions to work through the guilt that is so pervasive in anorectic patients (Goodsitt, 1985). Andrea experienced extreme feelings of guilt from attempts toward individuating because she empathically understood the needs of her lonely, alcoholic father so well. Experiential role reversal allowed her the opportunity to separate her healthy sense of self from the hostile and limiting messages from her father. She experienced the difference in their positions and could feel her self-support and, thus, trust her own experiential learning.

Patient Changes

At the end of stage 2, the patient may be expected to demonstrate a more cohesive sense of self. Her behavior, both in and out of session, should show increased tolerance for separation and individuation. The following changes show readiness for stage 3: (1) the patient has a clear self-concept grounded in an experiential sense of self; (2) she is able to discriminate her beliefs from other people's; (3) she demonstrates the ability to make decisions based on her own needs and wants; and (4) she sets a date for termination.

Stage 3: The Autonomous Self

Goals

The goal of stage 3 is for the patient to terminate psychotherapy successfully. For psychotherapy to be effective, the patient will move toward a clear sense of autonomy, separate from significant others. After developing a sense of self, the anorectic patient can also separate from the therapist without a great deal of regression. She is able to grieve the ending of the relationship with the therapist, while also expressing a sense of competency in an ability to individuate.

Therapist Guidelines

During stage 3, the therapist's main focus is on the impending termination. After having set a termination date, the patient and therapist look at the evolution of the therapeutic relationship while labeling intrapsychic and behavioral changes in the patient. Therapist guidelines for stage 3 are as follows: (1) to facilitate awareness and expression of the patient's feelings about termination; (2) to cognitively label behavioral, structural, and familial changes; and (3) to discuss preventive coping strategies for facing separations in the future.

Stage 3 allows the patient an opportunity to practice separation within a safe setting. Anorectic patients may remain vulnerable to anxiety about separation, but stage 3 emphasizes preventative coping strategies to prevent regression into anorectic eating as a response to future terminations.

Interventions

To facilitate expression of the feelings surrounding termination, I often utilize gestalt empty-chair work. This clinical intervention consists of the patient placing an image of the therapist in an empty chair and expressing feelings about termination to the image. Empty-chair work allows the therapist and patient to facilitate full expression of feelings and to make final discriminations between the real relationship and the remaining transference, thereby strengthening the patient's boundaries. This intervention is most useful when the patient is reluctant to express negative emotions directly to the therapist, and it allows the therapist to role train the patient.

This session took place about 6 weeks before actual termination. The patient had set a termination date about 1 month before this session, and the therapist and patient had briefly discussed termination.

PATIENT: I feel stuck today. I don't want to be here. I want to be done with this termination stuff. If we're going to end therapy, then let's just do it. Why do we have to obsessively make meaning out of all this?

THERAPIST: You sound angry with me today.

PATIENT: I'm not angry, I'm just tired of talking about all of this

THERAPIST: Well, I'm wondering about that, about what is going on with you, and with you and me. So, if you're willing, I'd like to use the empty chair and put an image of me in it. See what I have on. What time of year is it? What am I saying to you?

PATIENT: You're saying that it's time to go—that I'm ready.

THERAPIST: And, as you sit here, seeing that image of me, what are you feeling? What's happening inside your body? Inside yourself?

PATIENT: I feel tight. I don't want to talk to you.

THERAPIST: OK, again, if you're willing . . . just say that much to the image and see what happens, OK?

PATIENT: (*Turns to image.*) I don't want to talk to you anymore. (*Starts crying.*) It hurts too much. I feel like I'll never see you again.

THERAPIST: Well, try it out. Sit back and see if you can close your eyes and see this image of me—the image you formed of me telling you that you're ready. I trust you. I know you can take care of yourself now. And now, you can always carry that image of me around to support you.

PATIENT: *(Still crying.)* I know I can too, most of the time.

THERAPIST: So, if you're interested, let yourself sit back and focus on that now, today with me, so it will stay with you when I'm not there.

PATIENT: OK. I can see you smiling and I feel your trust in me. I can take care of myself now. I sure will miss you, but I know I'll be OK without you.

During stage 3, focusing seems to be helpful as a primary intervention because it is ideally suited for cognitively making meaning out of experiential awareness (Gendlin, 1981). Focusing facilitates autonomy because the patient is able to focus with minimal help from the therapist at this point, strengthening the patient's sense of competency.

The following clinical example was taken from a session in the last 3 weeks of psychotherapy, during which time Andrea and the therapist were directly discussing the termination process.

THERAPIST: Andrea, you seem pleased with your accomplishments today. You can see the changes in your eating. You are also, equally importantly, able to set limits with your dad—to tell him no, I won't take care of you anymore. No, I don't deserve your abuse. If you're willing, I'd like you to focus on that sense of accomplishment and see how it feels in your body, OK?

PATIENT: *(Closes eyes.)* OK. As I go inside, I'm finding . . . finding a feeling of electricity in my arms. My arms feel alive . . . they feel like dancing. I see an image of myself dancing . . . in a white tutu . . . and the feeling is one of freedom. I am dancing with a friend—a woman friend—and we both feel good. There is no audience. Just the sense of joy. That's what I found.

THERAPIST: OK, still with your eyes closed, ask yourself the question, "What is all this about? What does dancing, feeling free, and feeling joy with a friend mean for me?"

PATIENT: Well, my sense is that you are the woman. We are friends and you are helping me celebrate my freedom. There are no strings between us, just the joy. I guess that's how I would have liked my own mother to be.

THERAPIST: Take a moment and breathe that in and then come back and let's talk a little more about your ideas.

Focusing in stage 3 is used to facilitate cognitive understanding of experiential awareness. One of the main principles of experiential psychotherapy is that experiencing occurs prior to cognitive labeling, which is accomplished in the example presented above.

Patient Changes

At the end of stage 3, the patient will have successfully terminated psychotherapy. The following criteria suggest successful termination: (1) The patient is more comfortable with a concrete sense of her experiencing self; (2) the patient demonstrates the ability to reliably discriminate between herself and others during decisions made in psychotherapy; and (3) the patient separates from the therapist with appropriate expression of emotion and without regression to behavioral symptoms.

DISCUSSION

This chapter has presented my stage process model of psychodrama and gestalt therapy for the treatment of developmentally delayed anorectic patients. One of the major strengths of this model is its flexibility in providing structure for the therapist, while also allowing individual differences in patients. No time limits were suggested for each stage. The therapist guidelines and predicted patient changes provide a clear indication of progress across time.

Patients must be willing to begin to engage in the therapeutic process. This is often difficult for the anorectic patient who is in an acute stage of physical deterioration and suffering from cognitive deficits and perceptual distortions. This stage process model of psychodrama and gestalt therapy has the advantage over traditional verbal psychotherapy of emphasizing nonverbal communication. This allows the therapist to begin clinical intervention, even at the point when the patient is still in acute distress. As described in this chapter, many of the experiential interventions involve empathic bonding. This increases trust between the patient and therapist, allowing the patient to take greater risks in actively experiencing new behaviors.

This model of treatment for people with anorexia nervosa can be applied to both inpatient and outpatient settings. Given the flexibility of the stage process model, treatment could begin while the patient is hospitalized and continue into long-term outpatient psychotherapy. Stage 1 could begin in the hospital where the patient feels safe and is willing to explore internal awareness. After discharge, stage 2 could be implemented to aid the patient in dealing with family relationships, while stage 3 would start as the patient faces separation and individuation within the therapeutic relationship.

While this stage process model of treatment has many possible uses, caution needs to be applied. As Stein and Callahan (1982) pointed out, action interventions need to be thoroughly processed within the individual therapy relationship. The therapist's role-playing involvement has an effect on transference and, possibly, on the patient's struggles with dependency. A thorough understanding of the theoretical underpinnings of experiential psychotherapy is necessary to utilize this treatment method most effectively. Both theory and clinical examples have been included in this chapter to give readers adequate information with which to apply this model to their clinical practice.

REFERENCES

Bruch, H. (1973). *Eating disorders*. New York: Basic Books.
Bruch, H. (1979). *The golden cage: The enigma of anorexia nervosa*. New York: Vintage Books.
Buchanan, D. R. (1984). Psychodrama. In T. B. Karasu (Ed.), *The psychosocial therapies: Part II of the psychiatric therapies*. Washington, DC: American Psychiatric Association.
Elliott, R. (1987). *The experiential therapy depression project: Initial report*. Paper presented at Society for Psychotherapy Research Annual Meeting, Germany.
Forssmann-Falck, R., & Hudgins, M. K. (1988). The stage process model: Operationalization of the psychotherapy process with the borderline patient. *Annals of Clinical Research*, 73–83.
Gendlin, E. T. (1981). *Focusing*. New York: Bantam Books.
Goodsitt, A. (1985). Self psychology and the treatment of anorexia nervosa. In D. M. Garner & P. E. Garfinkel (Eds.), *Handbook of psychotherapy for anorexia nervosa and bulimia* (pp. 55–82). New York: Guilford Press.
Greenberg, L. S., & Rice, L. N. (1981). The specific effects of a gestalt intervention. *Psychotherapy: Theory, Research and Practice, 1*, 31–37.
Hudgins, M. K., & Kiesler, D. J. (1984). *Instructional manual for doubling in individual psychotherapy*. Richmond, VA: Virginia Commonwealth University.
Hudgins, M. K., & Kiesler, D. J. (1987). Individual experiential psychotherapy: An analogue validation of the intervention module of psychodramatic doubling. *Psychotherapy, 24*(2), 245–255.
Humphrey, L. L. (1987a). Comparisons of bulimic-anorexic and non-distressed families using structural analysis of social behavior. *American Journal of Child and Adolescent Psychiatry, 26*(2), 248–255.
Humphrey, L. L. (1987b). Family-wide distress in bulimia. In Baber & Canon (Eds.), *Addictive disorders: Psychological assessment and treatment*. New York: Pergamon Press.
Klein, M. J., Mathieu-Coughlin, E., & Kiesler, D. J. (1984). The experiencing scales. In L. S. Greenberg & W. M. Pinsof (Eds.), *The psychotherapeutic process: A research handbook*. New York: Wiley.
Kohut, H. (1971). *The analysis of the self*. New York: International Universities Press.
McCullough, J. P., & Carr, K. F. (1987). Stage process design: A predictive confirmation structure of the single case. *Psychotherapy, 24*(4), 759–768.
Moreno, J. L. (1947). *The theater of spontaneity*. Beacon, NY: Beacon House.
Moreno, J. L. (1965). Therapeutic vehicles and the concept of surplus reality. *Group Psychotherapy, Psychodrama and Sociometry, 18*(4), 211–216.
Moreno, J. L. (1977). *Psychodrama* (Vol. 1). Beacon, NY: Beacon House.
Moreno, J. L., & Moreno, Z. T. (1969). *Psychodrama: Action therapy and principles of practice*. Beacon, NY: Beacon House.

Perls, F. S. (1969). Theory of the self. In J. O. Stevens (Ed.), *Gestalt therapy verbatim*. Lafayette, CA: Real People Press.

Perls, F. S. (1975). Theory and technique of personality integration. In J. O. Stevens (Ed.), *Gestalt is*. Moab, UT: Real People Press.

Polster, E. & Polster, M. (1974). *Gestalt therapy integrated: Contours of theory and practice*. New York: Vintage Books, Inc.

Rosen, M. (1985). Gifts to the self: The development of new roles in the young adult's experience of separation and individuation. *Journal of Group Psychotherapy, Psychodrama and Sociometry, 37*(4), 167–175.

Sours, J. A. (1980). *Starving to death in a sea of objects*. New York: Jason Aronson.

Starr, A. (1977). *Psychodrama: Rehearsal for living*. Chicago: Nelson-Hall.

Stein, M. B., & Callahan, M. L. (1982). The use of psychodrama in individual psychotherapy. *Journal of Group Psychotherapy, Psychodrama and Sociometry, 35*(3), 118–129.

Swift, W. J., & Stern, S. (1986). The psychodynamic diversity of anorexia nervosa. *International Journal of Eating Disorders, 2* (1), 17–34.

Taylor, G. S. (1986). The effect of nonverbal doubling on the emotional response of the double. *Journal of Group Psychotherapy, Psychodrama and Sociometry, 36*(2), 61–68.

Winnicott, D. W. (1965). *The motivational process and the facilitating environment*. New York: International Universities Press.

13

Disturbed Body Image in Anorexia Nervosa: Dance/Movement Therapy Interventions

Julia B. Rice
Marylee Hardenbergh
Lynne M. Hornyak

The physical body is the vehicle we use to explore, understand, and experience the world. The body is our most basic communication tool. We form and maintain attachments to others on a body level. Furthermore, the body is simultaneously the container of the "self" and an object with which the self has a relationship.

In anorexia nervosa, the body is not only the vehicle in which the disorder is played out, but it is in itself the feared or hated object. Therefore, the physical body needs to be attended to as a whole, that is, on emotional, movement, spiritual, and medical levels, when treating anorexics.

Dance/movement therapy is a type of psychotherapy that focuses on the interrelationship of psyche and soma. The body itself is the tool, and movement is the process used to effect integration and growth of the individual. This approach has been used successfully with a broad range of populations, including children and the elderly, as well as with people with physical and emotional problems that vary in degree of severity. As with other forms of psychotherapy, dance/movement therapy can be used in group or individual formats.

Given the central position of the body in this approach, body image is a primary area that dance/movement therapists attend to in working with individuals. While the dance/movement therapy addresses other areas such as self-esteem, creativity, and relationships, this chapter focuses specifically on treatment of body image disturbances; the other areas are addressed only indirectly. In the first section of this chapter, we discuss the concept of body image as related to dance/movement theory. We next present the beliefs that guide our methods and identify characteristic movement patterns that we have observed in our clinical work with anorectic clients. We then present our treatment model, with techniques applicable to anorectic clients. Finally, we discuss several issues that are important to consider in applying dance/movement methods.*

THEORETICAL BACKGROUND

Body and Self Concept

As Freud (1961) stated, the ego "is first and foremost a bodily ego" (p. 26). The infant's earliest sense of self is thought to be conveyed through sensations with her own body, a process known as proprioception (Mahler & McDevitt, 1982). Schilder (1935), a pioneer in the area of body image, proposed that the body schema develops and is maintained by impressions or stimuli through the body senses—sight, taste, smell, hearing, and the kinesthetic senses of touch and movement; there is ever-changing, continual interplay between the body and the environment. Schilder's work has served as a foundation for many dance therapy theoreticians' writings on body image.

Five dance therapy theoreticians who have addressed the concept of body image are Penny Bernstein (1972), Marian Chace (cited in Chaiklin, 1975), Liljan Espenak (1981), Diane Fletcher (1979), and Elaine Siegel (1979, 1984). Their contributions to understanding the concept of body image are noted in the following.

The Concept of Body Image

Body image is a very complex concept. Bernstein (1972) wrote that body image includes "libidinal investment in the body, awareness of the body and its functions, effective control of primary process material and others' opinion of the self including cultural norms concerning physical attractiveness" (p. 90). In other words, body image has conscious and unconscious components, which include positive investment in, awareness of,

*In reference to dance theory and clinical material, the term "we" refers to authors Julia B. Rice and Marylee Hardenbergh.

and control of the body. In addition, these components may vary in the importance they hold for each individual's body image development.

Fletcher (1979) wrote of the body scheme, which is an individual's constant representation of her body. Over that, there are "moment to moment images of the body which are continually changing, forming, reforming, being torn down, fragmenting, multiplying, and superimposing themselves on the next image. The moment to moment representations of the body do not change the more constant body scheme" (p. 135). Dance/movement therapy, however, works to alter those aspects that are amenable to change.

Siegel (1979, 1984) included both outer and inner aspects of body image in her theoretical position. The outer aspect is a felt, conscious knowledge of one's physical body, which is integral to the processes of differentiation and acquiring a sense of the body self as an entity. Siegel identified two components of this outer aspect, body boundary and body space. Body boundary is the awareness of where one begins and ends; for example, awareness of body boundaries allows an individual to know if she will fit into a chair. Body space is the felt, experienced knowledge of where one is spatially comfortable in relation to other persons and things; for example, it is the sense of comfort a person feels at various distances from a parent versus from a new acquaintance. In reference to the inner aspect of body image, Siegel (1979) emphasized the fluidity of this representation, that it is able to be influenced by both internal and external factors. Siegel also contended that this internal representation exists at any given moment on both conscious and unconscious levels.

While there are many components to body image, three qualities in particular seem to characterize a healthy body image. First, a healthy body image is flexible. As discussed above, body representations can change, influenced by inner sensations, intrapsychic events, and external events; a core body scheme remains constant, however, providing a sense of stability and cohesiveness. By contrast, individuals with body control issues do not seem to allow new or discrepant information into their body schemata, resulting in rigid images. Second, as Chace (cited in Chaiklin, 1975) proposed, a healthy body image is connected with the reality of the world and healthy aspects of the personality. The mental image of the body coincides with what the body actually looks like, that is, as others objectively perceive it. In addition, the image that the individual holds is realistic, rather than an ideal to be lived up to. Third, body image is three-dimensional. In other words, the "picture" of one's body is experienced fully, as compared with the two-dimensional picture of the body front observed in a mirror. The picture is also a complete picture, including and accepting all parts. Each piece of the body's structure feels alive and is available to consciousness simply by turning one's attention to it. By contrast, if a part feels "frozen" or "out of touch" to the individual, her body image tends to be more fixed, unrealistic, and missing a sense of aliveness. This quality of three-dimensional experience includes the dimension of movement, which is uniquely dealt within dance/movement work and may not be as available in forms of body image treatment that focus on perceptions and attitudes.

Body Image Formation

One of the avenues by which we form and influence body image is sensory information. Siegel (1979) stated that body image is "dependent upon the visual and tactile exploration of the surface of one's body as well as the sensations derived from inner organs, skeleto-muscular systems and the skin" (p. 93). Espenak (1981) proposed that one's body image is formed by the organization of sensory information at that moment. Furthermore, these various moments, over the course of development, eventually evolve into a relatively constant body image.

Movement also influences body image formation. As Chace (cited in Chaiklin, 1975) proposed, body image is influenced by perceptions of gravity and of body motion. Movement provides sensory stimuli as well as a process (i.e., action) by which to interpret and integrate these sensations. In addition, movement of the body has an impact on both internal and external environments. For example, walking firmly across the floor can arouse feelings of strength and confidence; moving closer to another person can evoke a response from him or her.

Chace (cited in Chaiklin, 1975), Bernstein (1972), and Espenak (1981) discusses the influence of others' responses to, and interest in, one's body on the development of body image. Early experiences of being touched and held are viewed as essential means by which infants develop their internal sense of momentum as well as pleasure (cathexis) with their bodies. The emphasis here is on the nonverbal messages communicated to the infant through the quality of the other's presence. For example, if an infant is held tentatively, she has a qualitatively different experience from an infant who is held firmly and confidently. Furthermore, both verbal and nonverbal responses from others' continue to influence body image throughout one's life.

Development of Body Image

Bernstein (1972) proposed that body image formation occurs through a sequential progression of phases that parallel the formation of self-image. Each developmental phase has a series of movement tasks that correspond to tasks of psychological development. Later phases build on the experiences and mastery of previous tasks, although the themes may continue into later years. Margaret Mahler provides one model of psychological development (Mahler, Pine, & Bergman, 1975).

Bernstein (1972) identified six phases of body image development. These phases are investment of positive affect in the body, differentiation of body from environment, recognition of body parts and their interrelationship, movement of the body through space, sexual identity, and the aging process.

Investment of positive affect in the body refers to developing body cathexis and is reflected in basic care for one's body, such as providing food and sleep. Given that this phase begins in early infancy, the infant's sense of body pleasure derives from the parents' attitudes toward the infant's body, which she senses on a physical level. This phase parallels the events of symbiosis (Mahler et al., 1975), during which time the infant gradually differentiates sensations of pleasure and pain. Experiences of inner and outer, self and other are not yet differentiated.

Differentiation of body from environment refers to the development of body boundaries and sense of body space discussed earlier. These tasks parallel the initial tasks of the separation–individuation phase (Mahler et al., 1975), during which the infant begins to differentiate herself from other.

Recognition of body parts, and their interrelationships is the third phase, and it is an essential precursor to being able to move through space. At this time, the infant gains awareness that her body parts work together and operate in an organized fashion.

The fourth phase, movement of the body through space, is an important step in individuation, and parallels Mahler's practicing subphase. This achievement provides the infant with the sense that she can successfully regulate her own interactions. At this time, the child's ability to stop her own action, as well as initiate the action, helps to establish a healthy sense of control and mastery.

In the fifth phase, elements of one's sexual identity are incorporated into the body image. The body comes to be valued on yet another level, that of procreation. Incorporation of sexual identity elements into body image also influences one's ability to be intimate with others. These tasks seem to parallel Mahler's concept of consolidating individuality, which she perceives as a task of the fourth subphase of the separation–individuation period; this subphase does not have a definite ending point.

Finally, the phase of aging refers to the experiences of mortality, which are integrated into body image. These experiences include awareness of changes happening to the body through natural aging processes, as well as one's attitudes (e.g., acceptance) about these processes. Tasks of these last two phases, in particular, can span many years of one's life, and they can influence body image in various ways, depending on one's circumstances.

As indicated in the concepts above, body and self are intricately connected in the body image. It is our position that there is a close connection between how we feel about our bodies and how we feel about ourselves. This position provides the rationale for our approach, as discussed later.

Body Image Disturbances in Anorexia Nervosa

Hilde Bruch (1962, 1973) was the first to propose that distortion of body image, specifically overestimation, was a central component of anorexia nervosa and that correction of the distortion was necessary for recovery. Distorted body image has since been included as an essential feature for the diagnosis of anorexia nervosa according to DSM-III-R (American Psychiatric Association, 1987).

Body image disturbance, however, involves much more than the perceptual distortion noted by Bruch. While our understanding of the body image construct is still evolving, we identify six core issues in anorexia nervosa that are important to address in the treatment of body image disturbance, based on the interrelationship between body and mind mentioned earlier.

These issues, which are typically addressed in verbal forms of psychotherapy as well, include working toward (1) positive cathexis with the body (experiencing pleasure); (2) sensory awareness (developing sensory capacity, as well as overcoming denial or detachment from the body); (3) differentiation from the environment (developing body boundaries); (4) body integration (perceiving parts as forming a whole); (5) sense of personal impact (initiating movement in space); and (6) individuation (developing internal locus of control).

DANCE/MOVEMENT THERAPY WITH ANOREXICS

Dance/Movement Therapy: Beliefs

The profession of dance/movement therapy has been developing over the past 45 years. A language and notation system, known as Laban Movement Analysis (formerly known as Effort/Shape Analysis), was designed, which enabled dance professionals to observe, analyze, and record body movements in a systematic way (e.g., Bartenieff, 1980). Dance therapists believe that every movement has meaning, whether conscious or unconscious. Movement also has intention, whether it be to express, hold in, or cover up the meaning. In light of this, we present several beliefs that we have found to be particularly influential in guiding our treatment of anorexic individuals.

1. Everyday gestures and emotional expressions share the same neuromuscular pathways (Schmais, 1985). Also, movement/posture patterns have thought correlates (Schmais, 1985). For example, an individual who holds fixed, rigid beliefs manifests body postures that tend to be more rigid. As a result, when the range of movement/posture options increases for an individual, the extent of her coping skills also increases (Dulicai, 1984). Specifically, by creating new movements, the mover can also tap into new ways of experiencing the world or expressing emotions.

2. In the organization of the self, body (soma) and mind (psyche) are interrelated parts that form a cohesive whole (Bartenieff, 1980; Bernstein, 1972). This relationship between body and mind is reciprocal. Body movements are influenced by thoughts, attitudes, and feelings; thoughts, attitudes, and feelings are influenced by the rhythm and movements of the body. Hence, the physical body serves as a bridge between internal and external experiences. Alterations in movement patterns can result in alterations in internal perceptions, such as body image or feelings about the self. Similarly, changes in one's internal environment can result in movement changes.

3. Initial bonds between the infant and primary caretaker are established physically through rhythmical body movements, including sensations such as the mother's heartbeat (Kestenberg, 1965a). Rhythm continues to be a potent force in relationships throughout life, creating a sense of rapport and bonding on a nonverbal, usually unconscious, level (Kestenberg, 1965a, 1965b, 1967; Schmais, 1985). Consequently, the dance therapist can make use of this element, which is basic to dance or movement, in order to establish a bond with an individual.

4. Dance/movement is a primary process activity; that is, it comes directly out of unconscious material and does not use symbols, such as language, to represent itself (Bernstein, 1972). Through movement, body issues are addressed on a physical level without translation into words, which require secondary thought processes. The body is focused on in an immediate way, reinforcing the body's reality, rather than talking about it.

5. Dance/movement therapy can create corrective body experiences (Bartenieff, 1980; Bernstein, 1972). First of all, the body is useful and active, and dance/movement methods can emphasize these qualities. Also, creation of pleasant body experiences through dance and movement can modulate negative affects related to prior experiences. Furthermore, an individual can internalize this experience in therapy and eventually seek out such situations on her own.

6. Resistance, based on underlying fears and misperceptions, is ex-

perienced in the physical form of energy blocks or tension (Bernstein, 1972; Lowen, 1971; Reich, 1949). This resistance can be experienced and challenged through dance/movement activities.

7. Each person possesses a healthy, internal creative force. Dance/ movement therapy attempts to expand on this creative force; therefore, the focus of treatment is positive and growth-oriented. The healthier the individual's ego strength—in other words, the greater her emotional stability and capacity to cope with emotional difficulties—the less active the therapist is in dance/movement activities. In this way, the individual is able to more clearly experience her own ideas and choices, separate from the therapist.

Movement Patterns of Clients with Anorexia Nervosa

We have observed several characteristic movement patterns in working with anorectic clients. While research is lacking to substantiate the meanings of these patterns, we offer our working hypotheses, based on the preceding beliefs about the interrelationship of body and mind.

1. Anorexics often display rigidly controlled postural/movement patterns. Their trunks appear undifferentiated, with various parts operating as a unit rather than moving sequentially. By contrast, healthy movement includes elements of both control and fluidity. We propose that this pattern reflects the anorexic's attempt to keep rigid control. For example, a flexible trunk movement, such as a ripple through the spine, might increase the "danger" of producing bodily sensations or emotions—particularly sexual feelings in the pelvic area—which anorexics typically fear and/or avoid.

2. Anorexics often breathe shallowly. Shallow breathing decreases the flow of emotional and sensory experiences through the body (Bartenieff, 1980; Bernstein, 1972). This tendency also suggests attempts at control of feelings and sensations. For example, shallow breathing can dampen the body's awareness of hunger pains. In addition, holding one's breath produces the desirable side of effect of keeping the stomach flat, since the stomach tends to be held tightly in when the diaphragm is contracted. Third, shallow breathing can be a factor in some clients assuming soft, breathy, high-pitched voices. This voice tone suggests a sense of helplessness, which paradoxically can be a very powerful means of controlling others and situations.

3. Anorectic clients often groom themselves meticulously and place an emphasis on their overall physical presentation. This appears to reflect not only a compliance to cultural standards of attractiveness, but also a belief that "if I look good, then I *am* good." This pattern may also reflect control issues, in that an individual can control her presentation more easily than her interactions with others.

4. Symmetrical movement is rigidly imposed; that is, when a movement is done on one side of the body, anorexics repeat it equally on the other side. Unilateral movements are rare. We propose that these patterns reflect perfectionistic tendencies. They may be these individuals' attempts to impose order on themselves, as if to compensate in a physical way for an internal lack of balance.

5. Movements tend to be initiated in the peripheral body parts, as opposed to centrally in the trunk. These peripheral movements do not travel in a natural flow. They remain gestures, separate from full involvement with the body. Thus, we propose that peripheral initiations reflect distant involvement with or detachment from the self. This pattern also suggests that anorexics may lack a sense of internal locus of control, since a bodily sense of control is experienced when turning or moving through the trunk.

6. Anorexics often engage in compulsive or punitive exercise, which can stem from, as well as contribute to, body dissatisfaction. This rigorous exercise tends to isolate body parts, such as the thighs, rather than focusing on how one's body moves as a whole. In addition, the goal of such exercise typically is to change or reduce size, which exacerbates nonacceptance of the body as a whole. This pattern reflects the anorexic's attempt to gain control by controlling her body. It may also reflect a lack of self-integration, in which the body is treated as an object to be perfected and controlled, rather than part of the whole self to be enjoyed and treated respectfully. Unreasonably stringent exercise can also result in chronic pain or tension. The tendency to disregard this pain and mistreat the body may result in pain becoming the norm. The anhedonia, or limited experience of body pleasure, typically noted with anorexics can result from experiencing the body as naturally painful.

7. Anorexics often exhibit "cheerleader arms," which move in flat planes, in spoke-like or arc-like movements. These movements have "bound flow," which is a restricted flow of energy and often lack inflections, similar to a bland, monotone voice. These directional movements are thought to reflect a goal-oriented attitude, in contrast to allowing one's self to be involved in the process of movement (Dell, 1970). We also suggest that this pattern is the movement complement of a superficial, "everything is fine" attitude, as expressed by many anorexic clients.

8. Anorexics often do not experience an internalized sense of the force of their body weight. Their movements tend to lack the resilience, "jauntiness," and solidness observed in a person with a sense of her own active weight or strength. We propose that difficulty or inability to produce active weight is characteristic of individuals who have difficulty asserting themselves.

9. Anorexics seem to have little sense of kinesphere, or space surrounding their body. This tendency is exhibited by a preference for

movements within a narrow confine; broad, sweeping gestures are un-common. In other words, anorexics do not seem to have a clear sense that they have a "personal space," which they deserve to have, and that this space can create a sense of safety or protection when they are out in the world. This pattern may indicate both a poor sense of body boundaries and low self-esteem. Bartenieff (1980) suggests that development of kinesphere increases self-esteem.

In working with clients, anorexic or otherwise, we assume that the movement patterns that these individuals develop are initially functional for them. However, these patterns become dysfunctional as other alter-natives are excluded and the patterns become rigid. Thus, expanding the client's repertoire of movement can increase her sense of control as well as her respect for herself.

APPLICATIONS

Just as body image develops progressively, it is our observation that treat-ment of body image disturbance progresses through predictable stages. We have identified three stages: "What Body?" "Who Owns This Body?" "What Can My Body Do?" We follow this developmental model and ad-dress the therapeutic tasks of each step whether working on a short-term basis, such as two or three sessions, or over a longer period of time. We have used this model with inpatient and outpatient populations, in indi-vidual and in group sessions. Throughout this section, we use the term "body" to refer to the physical body and "body image" to refer to the client's mental representation of her body.

Stage 1: What Body?

At this stage, the anorexic tends to focus almost exclusively on her body size. Thus, one goal of stage 1 is to increase the client's general body awareness. We teach her an expanded vocabulary, based on the body's sensory capabilities, including touch and kinesthetic sense. In this way, the client can learn to perceive and interpret her own body cues. It may be necessary to educate a client about the various sensory and proprioceptive channels through which humans receive body signals (e.g., heat/cold, pressure, tension/relaxation). It may also be necessary to provide specific information about body functions if the client has misperceptions or idio-syncratic ideas about how her body functions.

A second goal is for the client to attend to the individual qualities of her own body and to identify basic reactions (i.e., like/dislike) to these parts. This can occur in a number of ways. For one, using specific com-plaints about physical discomfort can be an initial way to introduce a client to more specific terms for her body and its sensations. This more detailed attention to body cues can serve to "lower the pain threshold"—in other words, to help her identify more subtle body cues. Second, the client can be asked to name the specific parts of her body that she likes and dislikes. Third, the therapist and client can closely observe and compare parts of their bodies, commenting on unique features. It is our experience that focusing on peripheral body parts tends to be less threatening than focusing on central body parts such as the trunk. Consequently, we often begin with the hands or feet at this stage. The following are several techniques we use to address the issues in stage 1:

Chair Exercise. This exercise provides a rough estimation of body size distortion and can be an introduction to body awareness. The client is asked to gauge her girth at her widest point, usually the hips, by placing two chairs to frame that distance. Then she physically checks out her perceptions by standing between the two chairs. In discussing the exercise, we talk about the difference between the way the client feels, which is large, and the way she looks, which is small. We generally explain that she has "trained" her eyes to be inaccurate and suggest that she can learn to retrain her eyes, as well as to rely on other more accurate senses, such as touch, to estimate her body size. If the client's size has fluctuated over time, her sense of her body outline may be unclear. She may experience a phantom fat phenomenon. "Phantom fat" is an experience parallel to phantom limbs, in which physical sensations are experienced in an area of the body that no longer exists. We have noticed that clients find this explanation helpful for them to make sense of their distorted sensations and perceptions in a nonjudgmental way.

Self-Touch Exercise. This exercise is used to initiate sensory awareness. Since the anorexic tends to use sight as the primary sense for judging her body, emphasis is on development of increased kinesthetic and tactile awareness. The therapist guides the client in exploring her body from top to bottom through touch. Generally, the client closes her eyes, although a mistrustful client can be instructed to "use a soft focus" and to note stimuli through other senses as well as sight. The therapist can guide the exploration with instructions such as

> I want you to touch your hair with your fingers, noting its texture and temperature. Is it curly? Straight? Wavy? Thick? Thin? Trace your hairline with your fingers. This line helps define the shape of your face. What does it feel like? How would something that feels like that look? Now continue your exploration by touching your forehead . . . wrinkle it . . . feel it. Now let it be smooth and feel it. Notice how the shape changes.

Exploration can be carried further to locate areas of bone, muscle, and fat. The client can be encouraged to feel the differences among these. She can be asked to determine which side of her body is more muscular and to explore the changes in muscle shape as she flexes and relaxes various body parts. When this body exploration is completed, we usually discuss what the client noticed about herself. Often a client will notice differences between the way she feels and how she looks.

Mirror. The goal of this exercise is to help the client focus on her whole body rather than just the negatively charged regions. The client is asked to walk quickly to a full-length mirror and observe her whole body simultaneously, noticing the outline in particular rather than specific parts. The client is instructed to look at her image for just a few seconds, then to look away. She is again asked to look at her image, but this time to come up with one word for what she sees. In discussing the exercise, the emphasis is on defining a "whole body" sense.

Sensing. The client is instructed to lie down, with her eyes closed. She is asked to direct her focus to her toes and to notice any body sensations. She is guided slowly up through various body parts, with the instructions to notice any differences in temperature, tension level, and awareness in various body parts. The client is told, "Note any specific messages your body might have for you, such as 'I am cold,' 'I am hungry,' or 'I am tense.'" This exercise can be expanded, either in movement or in the discussion, to learning ways to respond to these body cues or messages. For some clients, however, focusing on being in their body is a terrifying experience. In these cases, we create a game in which we time how long the client can comfortably focus on her body, with the goal of gradually achieving longer periods of time in body sensing.

Body Map. The client lies down on a large piece of paper while her outline is traced by the therapist. This tracing results in a concrete representation of her size. (Readers should note that they should hold the pen or marker perpendicular and flush with the client's body when tracing, in order to minimize distortion.) The client then personalizes her body map by drawing and writing on it. Instructions can vary from client to client, depending on the client's needs and concerns. For example, some clients may make notes on body parts that have memories associated with them or body parts they do and do not like. These notes serve to create a concrete representation of the client's body experiences and to validate these experiences. If a client has difficulty with self-care, she can practice touching and caring for her body map in the way she would like to care for herself. She may be encouraged to hang up her body map in a favorite or safe place in her room.

The body map technique can be applied in many different ways. One application is as a concrete measure of changes in the client's size over time, by retracing the client's outline on the same map each week. In this way the client can see how weight gain or loss affects her body map. This can be used to allay a client's fear that she will become obese, or that one part of her body will become massive, as she regains weight.

Self-Care. A client who has been abused, or who abuses herself, can be instructed to gently touch and care for the part or parts of her body that have been hurt. For example, a client can gently stroke a scar, saying, "This is a part of me that has been hurt and I can care for it." Often the therapist first demonstrates how to use gentle self-touch on herself. In this way, the therapist models that touching can feel good and demonstrates caring, valuing ways to touch one's self.

Rocking. This exercise, which is particularly useful for clients with early life traumas, is intended to create a sense of safety and comfort in the body as well as an experience of mastery. The client sits on the floor and is instructed to rock back and forth until she finds a comfortable rocking rhythm. This exercise can be extended to help the client experience synchrony with another person in a safe way; with the client's permission, the therapist can join her, sitting back to back, and rocking in the client's rhythm.

Body Awareness. This exercise is useful for a client who relies on sight rather than body sensations to tell whether she is being touched. An example would be a client who is only aware of firm touch; with her eyes closed she has difficulty sensing touch at all. It is also a good exercise for identifying different parts of the body that are deadened to sensations. It is important to explain this exercise thoroughly to the client before starting because being touched with one's eyes closed can produce intense fear. We tell clients that they have the right to say no to, or to stop, any exercise if they feel afraid or unwilling to do it. The client is instructed to close her eyes and tell the therapist when she feels that she is being touched. Initially, the therapist touches the client's arm or hand firmly; gradually she lightens the pressure. For variation, the therapist can ask the client to say whether her touch is moving toward the center of her body or toward the edge of her body. We have noted that incest and abuse victims typically prefer touch that goes away from the body's center, perceiving it as safer.

Videotape. This method provides a concrete record of shape, and helps to objectify the process of looking at one's body. When a client is videotaped, she is asked to bring "fat clothes," "thin clothes," and a bathing suit to wear during the session. She is instructed to move around the room as she is taped, in order to record the changes that her body makes during movement. Instructions may vary; a very fearful client can be asked to move from a front to a side view of her body. A less threatened client can be asked to move around the room in a way that expresses her feelings. The client and therapist then view the tape together, looking at proportions and distinguishing bones and muscles. The goal is to see what happens during movement, how body shape can change in response to different movements. Videotaping the client in different types of clothes can be useful to challenge distorted beliefs. For example, a client may believe that certain clothes can magically change her body shape (i.e., make her look very slender or heavy). We recommend that this technique be used only after a trusting relationship has been established, since clients may feel exposed and threatened when they see themselves on tape.

Stage 2: Who Owns This Body?

After having gained an internal sense of her own body and a vocabulary for describing her experiences, the client is ready to learn how to differentiate herself from influences in her environment. The goal of body ownership involves learning about boundaries. That is, while a person exists within a context (e.g., family, culture), she is not synonymous with that context. Ego boundaries are related to having a sense of her own kinesphere, a sense of "containment" in her body, and the experience of her body as a "whole." In learning that she is a separate person, an individual develops a clearer sense of spatial boundaries. Reciprocally, when she moves and learns about spatial boundaries, these experiences can enhance a firmer sense of ego and of separateness from others.

Boundaries occur at different levels. The skin forms one body boundary, between the self and the world. Another boundary is that of "personal space" between the self and other persons. Often clients are not aware that they have a natural right to their separateness and self-protection. Thus, these methods focus on forming and exploring various body boundaries.

This stage also involves learning about choices. That is, a person has choices about how she relates to her environment. Consequently, methods focus on movements as a way to expand one's options for responding to the environment. Vocabulary continues to be added to, allowing the client to talk about a variety of topics with more complex shades of meaning.

Coping skills are augmented to deal with more external situations that arise as well as internal stimuli (feelings).

Family and sociocultural influence on one's development are discussed verbally and explored through body movement. The impact of these factors on the formation of body image are specifically examined.

In this stage, the client moves more in sessions; there is less talking. The therapist's role as an educator diminishes, and the client explores her increasing autonomy through movement expression. The processes of self-exploration and sensory awareness, begun in the first stage, are deepened.

The techniques described below can be enhanced by encouraging a client to create her own "Owner's Manual" for her body. The Owner's Manual is a tool for recording her body image work in a visible, tangible fashion, by writing or drawing her responses to therapeutic exercises. A typical Owner's Manual might contain drawings of areas of the body that are or are not safe to touch, with instructions on the types of touch that are acceptable. The goal is to make as concrete and explicit as possible the boundary exploration that the client is undertaking. In addition, the authorship of her manual implicitly highlights the fact that she is owner of her body. The following are several techniques we use to address the issues in stage 2:

Touch Exercises. These exercises deepen the sensory awareness begun in stage 1; the goal is for the client to discover the quality of touch that does or does not feel good to her. Starting with the body parts that she feels safest with, the client is asked to note, for example, if she prefers a soft or a firm touch, if the touch feels nurturing, and so forth. The therapist should discuss with the client that this exercise is meant to be nonsexual. If she does have sexual feelings, the client is asked to speak about them, and the exercise is stopped for discussion of the experience. A client may need to be educated and to experience the range of touch quality, particularly if she has difficulty distinguishing sexual from nonsexual touch. After self-touch, the client is asked to instruct the therapist how to touch her in ways that seem safe and respectful of her body boundaries. Again, we do not touch sexual areas, and if a client has difficulty distinguishing sexual from nonsexual touch, the therapist may choose to listen to the client's description rather than to touch her directly.

Proximity Exercises. This exercise is used to increase a client's awareness of her comfort level in physical proximity to others. The client begins by instructing the therapist to sit in a particular place in the room. Next, the client approaches and moves away from the therapist, noticing distances that feel comfortable. She is asked to imagine doing the exercise with various family members and friends and to note the distances with which she might feel most comfortable with these individuals.

Rolling. This exercise can be used to define the entire outside surface of the body, as well as to develop a sense of mastery over movement. While many variations are possible, the first step is teaching the client to roll. The client lies on her back and starts to roll, using her hips to initiate movement. If done correctly, the roll's momentum will perpetuate the movement, and the client can experience her body moving her. Contact with the floor on the length of her body creates tactile stimulation, which can strengthen awareness of her body's surface.

Safe Space/Bubble. This exercise is used to create an internalized experience of a protective, external boundary. The client is asked to find a safe space in the room and to close her eyes. The client is instructed to create, or mold with her hands, a bubble around her. The instructions should be open-ended so that the client creates a bubble of the size, shape, and texture that suits her. Creating this boundary beyond her skin can allow the client to feel less vulnerable and more assertive, and she can gradually develop other ways to protect herself than by retreating inward.

Addressing Sociocultural Influences. Since culture influences beliefs about the ideal body image, this exercise helps the client become more aware of the ideal image she holds. The client is instructed to imagine her picture of an ideal body. Then she is asked to put on this image as a "costume" and to move around the room "dressed" in this fashion. The client is instructed to notice changes in her posture and movement as she takes on this ideal body, as well as her reactions. She can be asked to compare these movements to her usual movements and posture.

Mother's Body. This exercise is designed to give the female client insight into the nonverbal messages she may have received from her mother. As in the above exercise, the client is asked to move around the room, but as her mother moved. Discussion of this exercise can include questions such as, "What does it feel like to stand, sit, and walk in this body?" and "What messages is this body giving you, and giving me, as the observer?" Choices and boundaries are key concepts here. Discussion often revolves around the idea that the way a person moves influences the way she feels about her body—as well as the way others respond to her. Another theme is that there are ways to move that one may not have learned in one's family. Discussion can evolve into exploring various alternatives.

Stage 3: What Can My Body Do?

When a client is at this stage, she experiences her body as a part of her self, rather than as an object. The decision of whether to accept her body is no longer a daily struggle, reflecting that her body is being integrated as a positive part of her self-image. She experiences herself as a person, differentiated from others.

The goal of this stage is to increase the client's sense of mastery in her own body, as well as in relationship to others. This goal involves developing a repertoire of positive body experiences through movement expression. It involves strengthening the client's trust in her body's ability to move and balance, parallel to learning to trust her body with food.

A related goal of this stage is to achieve a more fully developed sense of individuality and uniqueness, along with the power and autonomy that accompany it. Movement expression can help the client to tap into her own creative potential, with the client exploring themes that are unique to her. It is particularly important that the client develop her identity distinct from being "an anorexic," along with the capacity to have relationships with others that are based on autonomy and independence.

The sessions in stage 3 are less structured. At this point, the client is able to follow more abstract instructions. The therapist moves less and watches more, as the client initiates movement under her own direction. The therapist's role is to encourage the client to explore her own specific movement preferences and creativity. The therapist may move with the client, but only at the client's request or based on the therapist's clinical judgment. The role of "witness" to the client as "mover" is an important one. By observing the client's exploration of her own movement themes, the therapist can attest to the client's separateness and capabilities. The therapist provides the initial metaphor, while the client expresses herself in movement and generates her own interpretation of these expressions during the discussion. The following are techniques we use to address issues in stage 3:

Theme-Centered Exercises. These exercises are used to expand a client's limited repertoire of movement and emotional expression along a particular theme. They also can provide a framework for exploration and interpretation of life's experiences. Typically, the therapist suggests a theme that is relevant to the client, based on material from previous sessions. Often the specific assignment is based on a dichotomy, and the client is encouraged to explore the range of possible expressions between the poles or extremes. Examples include, "Find a way to explore the concepts of 'open' and 'closed' through movement," and "Explore the concepts of 'active' and 'passive' through movement." "Push–pull" and "fall–recover" are other dichotomies.

Balance. This exercise is designed to enhance a client's belief in her body's ability to balance itself—in other words, to trust her body and its reflexes. The client is asked to lean forward and let herself catch her fall. She is then asked to try the same exercise leaning sideways and then leaning backward. If this is too frightening for the client to do standing, it can be done sitting or kneeling.

TREATMENT PLANNING

In developing a treatment plan, we tend to work through the above three stages in the order listed, regardless of the number of sessions. We do at least one or two of the exercises from each stage. Treatment planning involves careful selection of exercises that are appropriate for the particular client. We base our decisions on several factors, including severity of the illness, the client's strengths and weaknesses in movement, the rigidity or flexibility of her body, the client's basic sensory capabilities, and her preferences and motivation for doing movement work.

As mentioned earlier, both assessment and education of the client occur in the initial session. We focus our questions on the client's experience of her body and her perceptions of influences on the development of her body image. We may educate a client about anatomy and kinesiology.

We find it most informative to ask a client to demonstrate something in movement, rather than to talk about it. For example, we may ask a client to show us anything she enjoys doing with her body. In addition, we try doing the activity ourselves, following her instructions. We pay particular attention to how our bodies feel; what body parts we are aware of; whether the movement is comfortable or uncomfortable, painful or enjoyable; and whether certain body parts are held or released. We may share with our clients how we feel doing their movements, as a way of building empathy. We find that the act of duplicating even simple movements, such as a client's walk, gives insight into her internal experience. For example, the therapist may understand empathically what it is like for the client to walk around with a retracted pelvis, holding back this center of sexual energy.

In addition, we address specific body concerns that the client presents. If indicated, we may refer her for a medical consultation or recommend that she speak to her physician. We may prescribe between-session assignments, such as a focusing exercise, as a structured way for the client to practice what she is learning in sessions. The following sessions emphasize movement expression.

A number of factors are considered in determining whether treatment will be short-term or long-term. First, body image work is usually adjunctive to the primary therapy. The primary therapist may refer the client for work on a very specific problem or on more general body image issues. Second, the client's readiness to work on body image material, her degree of discomfort with her body and movement, and the severity of her illness (e.g., degree of distortions) must be considered. Third, the dance/movement therapist must assess how well the modality suits the particular client.

In long-term dance/movement therapy, more time can be spent on each exercise, with fewer activities included in a session. The work typically becomes less problem-focused and more exploratory as treatment progresses. Dance/movement themes generally emerge from the client's verbalizations in the session. Metaphors can be created for real-life situations that the client is dealing with, and the client can explore these situations through movement.

CASE STUDIES

Case 1: Short-Term Dance/Movement Therapy

Jodi was an eighteen-year-old high school senior, diagnosed as having anorexia nervosa. She was referred to me (J. B. R.) by her primary therapist for a brief consultation, in order to deal with an impasse in Jodi's therapy. The consultation consisted of three sessions. In the initial session, Jodi stated that she felt fat all the time and was unwilling to wear shorts or a bathing suit. Jodi exhibited shallow breathing, a soft voice, and a rigid trunk. Since we agreed to three sessions, the focus of her treatment was primarily educational, with body exercises assigned for practice between sessions.

During our first session, I explained the concept of body image. I asked Jodi questions about her body, such as how she would describe herself physically, her likes and dislikes, her physical activities, her physical symptoms, and so forth. I decided to use the chair exercise as a quick, relatively easy method to assess—and concretely demonstrate to Jodi—her body image distortion. Not surprisingly, Jodi discovered how distorted her body image was. She looked stunned and found it hard to believe to what extent she distorted.

As we continued talking, Jodi's contracted breath and rigid, upright posture were apparent to me. I asked her to show me some of her favorite movements. She launched into an elaborate aerobics routine and quickly became winded. I stopped her and demonstrated diaphragmatic breathing, as I do with most clients. (Proper breathing helps with stress and tension problems and can be an indirect approach to working on stomach movements, which threaten many anorexics.) When I asked her to try this breathing, Jodi stated, "It will make my stomach stick out." I suggested an experiment to test her assumption. Laying on the floor with her hands on her stomach, I asked Jodi to be aware of the outward and inward movements of her rib cage as she breathed. She practiced breathing and slowly was able to allow more movement in her chest and stomach area. I asked Jodi to stand and repeat the aerobic movements, this time focusing on her breathing. Together we worked out a breathing pattern to go with her movements. As a result, her movements slowed down and became less frantic. Her breath became more rhythmic, and her stomach muscles were able to release and contract more freely. I asked Jodi to practice this breathing before our next session and to notice instances when she held her breath.

Jodi came to our second session having practiced her breathing daily. Exhibiting greater awareness of her breathing patterns, she reported that she held her breath when she felt watched or judged. Upon further discussion, Jodi realized that this occurred most often with her mother. I asked Jodi to do the mother's body exercise. Jodi described her mother as slim and precise. Jodi imitated her mother's characteristic posture by crossing her arms over her chest and holding her legs close together. As she moved as "Mother," Jodi took small, confined steps, with little active weight. Mother's arm gestures were directional and spoke-like, lacking curving flow.

After the exercise, Jodi talked about the strong, negative, nonverbal messages that she internalized from her mother. She realized that she assumed her mother's crossed-arms posture when she felt challenged. We worked for the rest of the session on discovering new postures for Jodi to develop a stronger sense of her own movement repertoire and define how her body differed from her mother's. I reassured Jodi that it was permissible to be different from her mother, with the implication that differentiation and separation were appropriate goals.

For Jodi's last session, the goal was to have Jodi experience good ways of moving in her body, to balance the unpleasant experiences she had typically had prior to therapy. I asked her to lie on the floor, continuing her diaphragmatic breathing, and to find ways to move that felt good. Jodi closed her eyes, and I observed her movements in the role of "witness." (I had explained to Jodi that I would be watching, not judging.) Jodi moved for about twenty minutes (which is the length of time I have clients move during stage 3 exercises). When she was finished with the exercise, we talked about her experience. Jodi stated that she felt like she was under water. She described images associated with water—"warm, pleasant" sensations—and mentioned that water was calming to her and gave her a sense of freedom. I had noted that her movements had free flow and more force, and her body "molded" more easily, than, for instance, during the aerobics. I shared this observation with Jodi, and she reported that she felt a difference, more relaxed and slower. I instructed her to continue to practice moving daily in ways that felt good to her, using her recent movement experiences to give her clues to what she liked.

Acknowledging the termination of her work, we discussed what she had learned in sessions and how she could apply this new knowledge in her life. Jodi came up with the idea that she could use deep breathing when around her mother. Jodi also noted that she was more aware of her physical responses and now had an inkling that her body could have more pleasurable experiences. I reminded her that, since she was able to experience pleasure in the session, she could have this experience at other times as well.

Case 2: Long-Term Dance/Movement Therapy

Ellie was a 23-year-old woman who was anorexic for 5 years and was an incest survivor. She was referred to dance/movement therapy by her primary therapist, as Ellie was unable to verbalize her internal experiences in psychotherapy. I (J. B. R.) worked with Ellie for nine months, once a week. Ellie continued to work with her primary therapist weekly during this time.

In the first session, I observed that Ellie's movement patterns were marked by a frozen pelvis, little spatial clarity, and arm gestures with bound flow and limited dynamic range. Ellie focused on her somatic complaints, which included constipation, generalized fatigue, headaches, and intermittent back pain. I listened to her detailed explanation, to establish a bond and to reinforce that she was the expert on her body. I also validated Ellie's perceptions by acknowledging the reality of her complaints, for example, that stomach and bowel discomfort can be physical side effects of anorexia.

Ellie and I agreed that one treatment goal would be to increase her body awareness. I then taught her about diaphragmatic breathing, explaining that this would help her to sense her body in a new, safe way. Due to her fearfulness and resistance to moving and being seen, I had Ellie continue to sit in her chair as she worked on diaphragmatic breathing.

Within a few sessions, we decided to focus on awareness of sensations in specific body parts, given Ellie's general mistrust and dislike for her body. Ellie was cut off from most body sensations, and it seemed more manageable to work on each of the puzzle pieces separately, before putting them together. Progress was made over subsequent sessions. Her pelvic region, which was like a frozen block, was particularly problematic, and we spent a considerable amount of time on this area. I began with education about the anatomy of her pelvis area, and we did a variety of movement exercises in order for Ellie to explore movement in that region. Tentatively, Ellie allowed herself to experience sensations in her lower trunk.

During the course of her treatment, while working on the pelvic region, Ellie's experiences intensified in both verbal and dance/movement therapies. She started to have flashbacks to early incidents of incest and became suicidal; she was hospitalized in order to provide her a safe place. Making use of this safe environment, we worked during her hospitalization on a body map that specifically recorded parts of her body that had been abused. We then worked with this information with the goal of reclaiming these body parts. For example, Ellie practiced touching these areas of her body, stating "This is my leg, and I can choose who touches it."

After her hospitalization, we worked with movement to integrate the frozen body parts into Ellie's body image. First, we identified these parts. Then we worked on moving them and initiating movement in them. Finally, we worked on reintegrating these parts into her body image using whole body movement.

Another issue Ellie worked on was touch and being touched. Ellie practiced touching herself—then she would say "stop" and cease touching herself. As she became more comfortable, acquiring the experience of having limits respected by herself, Ellie practiced with me touching her and responding to her limit-setting. (Touching occurred on the hand, foot, and sometimes cheek.) Through these exercises, Ellie was learning to use other senses, in addition to sight, to become more aware of her world.

After Ellie had a sense of her body, the next goal was to enclose that sense within spatial boundaries. The safe space/bubble exercise helped her to clarify her personal space boundaries. At first, Ellie's bubble imagery contained an open unlockable door, which left her vulnerable; perhaps it symbolized the incest. After she worked on boundaries, she gained control over her body, as symbolized in her imagery; Ellie's image now included her having the key to the door, which had a dead bolt on it as well.

Ellie responded favorably to movement involving tactile stimulation. She reported enjoying the rolling exercises, which served to increase her sense of full body integration. Perhaps the child in her enjoyed rolling. Ellie stated that it made her feel playful yet sad for the childhood that she had never had. In subsequent sessions, rolling served as a warm-up, so Ellie could start with something guaranteed to be a pleasant body experience, setting the stage for further movement work in the session. We added rolling over each other's bodies, to give Ellie a sense of how strong and resilient her body was. Starting on our stomachs, she would initiate with her hips and roll over me. Then I would initiate with my hips and roll over her. Ellie discovered that her weight was not so powerful that it crushed me, as she had feared, even with her increasing weight.

At times, Ellie regressed to earlier stages, as manifested by fear and rigidness. We would then return to the safe bubble/space exercise to allow her to regain control by experiencing clear boundaries and a sense of autonomy within her bubble. While in her space, Ellie would often initiate a gentle rocking motion. During our discussion, I suggested that this motion was a return to a time when she felt safe in her body, probably prior to the abuse. Ellie agreed that the rocking meant safety to her. Ellie wanted to find an "adult" way of experiencing the safety of rocking that she felt in sessions; subsequently, she requested a rocking chair for her birthday.

After 3 or 4 months, Ellie's movements were consistently stronger and clearer. She appeared less resistant and timid, both in and out of sessions. She started dating again. As her body boundaries became clearer and she was more accepting of her body, she began to wear clothing that was brighter and more close-fitting.

At this point, Ellie was ready for the third stage of body image therapy. She identified several personal issues, including her fear that assuming a feminine role would deprive her of newfound strength and autonomy. To address this concern, she explored "masculine" and "feminine" movements and worked at finding her own solution to integrating these two movement styles. For example, she learned to include punching and floating movements within her repertoire.

Ellie also voiced the fear of becoming fat and not being able to control her increasing weight. To address this fear, we returned to her old body map and recorded her new outline at 5-pound increments, using different colors. This allayed Ellie's fear; she could see the tiny changes in size that resulted from a 5-pound weight gain.

As Ellie reached her weight goal, and was completing her stage 3 goals, she was able to bring themes to our sessions and to work through them using creative movement. For example, one day she described an incident of being slighted by a friend. She was able to recognize her internal physical cues of anger and to validate her own feelings. Furthermore, she was able to contain her intense feeling and to express anger in a manner that suited her and the situation.

In another session, Ellie complained that the dance/movement therapy room was "too small," a symbol that she was getting healthier and needed more space for self-expression. It was becoming clear that termination was appropriate.

During our last session, Ellie and I moved together for a while; then I instructed Ellie to find a way to move away from me. Ellie created an opening rising movement, which she explained was a symbol for her of the freedom that a bird experiences. As she discussed the free expansiveness in her body that her movements gave her, Ellie mused that she could repeat this particular movement phrase in the future to remind herself of her own special spirit.

DISCUSSION

Dance/movement therapy is uniquely suited to clients with anorexia nervosa, for whom the body is the battleground on which they have chosen to fight their internal struggles. To ignore body image issues is to align with the client's denial and misuse of her body.

Considerations

There are several issues for a therapist to consider when deciding to use dance/movement therapy in the treatment of a particular client. First, it is important to assess a client's medical status before initiating treatment. Generally, we ask clients if they have had a recent physical examination. If not, we ask them to do so before the second session. It is particularly important to know if heart arrhythmias or electrolyte imbalances exist, in order to plan exercises that will not be strenuous for the client or deplete her energy. In addition, potassium deficiency can result in muscle weakness, fainting, and mental confusion, which are particularly problematic for dance/movement work. At times the dance/movement therapist is the first health professional to hear about a client's laxative or ipecac use. The dance therapist must respond to this with sensitivity to her role in the client's treatment. For example, if the client has a primary therapist, the dance therapist would obtain the client's consent to share this information with the primary therapist and to consider appropriate steps for medical evaluation.

Related to this health issue, the movement therapist must also be aware of the activity level that is possible for the client. A client with anorexia nervosa may need to be restrained from demanding physical activity if she is unaware of her body cues indicating fatigue and pain. Initially, she may need to learn basic self-care, such as knowing when a part of her body hurts and how to tell when to stop. She may need to learn to utilize the strength in her body, as well as to "unlearn" abusive attitudes toward her body.

Second, many clients have severely abused their bodies through starvation, excessive exercise, purging, and other means. In addition, some clients have a history of physical and/or sexual abuse. If the body abuse has been severe, the amount of time spent on learning and practicing self-care often needs to be lengthened. The reason for this is that intensely punitive thought and behavior patterns that have typically developed along with the abuse require more active, lengthy intervention.

A third consideration has to do with the use of touch, which is involved in a number of dance/movement techniques. Touch is a very potent tool as it occurs on a close, personal level, and it must be used respectfully. "When you touch the body you touch the soul" is an important guide that we use when employing touch. For some clients, merely talking about body image is seen as an intrusion or body violation. With these clients, it is best initially to avoid using touch or rigorous movement. For others, however, particularly clients who experience dissociative states, touch is a primary way for them to become grounded during a session. Therapists are advised not to touch a client if they feel uncomfortable doing so. It is our experience that clients tend to personalize the therapist's discomfort. It is also important that the therapist be clear about his or her own body boundaries (e.g., differentiation of self from others, privacy of various body parts, appropriate ways of touching) and trust his or her clinical judgment as to whether touch is appropriate at that particular time for the client.

Generally, clients with anorexia nervosa do not fare well in a group in the initial stages of treatment. Tendencies toward perfectionism are often exacerbated by competition with other group members. Clients may detrimentally compare their own body weight and appearance to others in the group with antitherapeutic results. As the client becomes healthier and more autonomous, the therapist may consider the benefits of group treatment.

In working with anorexics, we have found that any focus on the body is helpful for these individuals who have become so split off from their bodies. However, the therapist should be competent in terms of sensitivity to body movement and body issues and must have a respect for the power of movement to evoke strong feelings and defenses.

Movement therapists can serve in a variety of roles: as primary therapist, as part of a team approach, and as adjuncts to traditional, verbal psychotherapy. As in all collaborative ventures, it is important that the therapist and client be clear about the role of dance/movement work in the client's overall treatment plan.

Countertransference Issues

The therapist should be clear about personal feelings regarding his or her own body in order to deal effectively with the client's body issues. The therapist should be aware of personal reactions, such as comfort level with touch, feelings about various body parts, attitudes about fat and body weight, concerns about closeness and maintaining appropriate boundaries, among others. He or she should also try the techniques to be used, in order to have an idea of what it is like to experience the exercise.

We have found our clients with anorexia nervosa to be very sensitive to body cues from others. As mentioned earlier, these clients often pick up on a therapist's unease about his or her own body and personalize the discomfort (e.g., "My body caused her to feel uncomfortable"). If a therapist is personally uncomfortable with body issues, or reacts uncomfortably when with a particular client, then it is recommended that the therapist refer the client to dance/movement therapy.

Therapists may be asked how much they weigh by clients during dance/movement work. For some clients, this question reflects their difficulties in accurately assessing their own and others' body size; for others, it may reflect issues of competition. Regardless, it is helpful to answer questions regarding body size, weight, and shape accurately and openly, which also includes disclosing to the extent that one feels comfortable. The therapist can model positive valuation of his or her own body, which is particularly important since many clients initially rely on the therapist's healthy ego and body image to learn to accept themselves.

CONCLUSION

Dance/movement therapy is a relatively new and pioneering field. The potential for its effectiveness in the treatment of anorexia nervosa lies in the central position of the body in both the disorder and this treatment modality.

REFERENCES

American Psychiatric Association. (1987). *Diagnostic and statistical manual of mental disorders* (3rd ed., rev.). Washington, DC: Author.

Bartenieff, I. (1980). *Body movement: Coping with the environment.* New York: Gordon & Breach.

Bernstein, P. (1972). *Theory and methods in dance-movement therapy.* Dubuque, IA: Kendall/Hunt.

Bruch, H. (1962). Perceptual and conceptual disturbances in anorexia nervosa. *Psychosomatic Medicine, 24,* 187–194.

Bruch, H. (1973). *Eating disorders: Obesity, anorexia and the person within.* New York: Basic Books.

Chaiklin, H. (Ed.). (1975). *Marian Chace: Her papers.* Columbia, MD: American Dance Therapy Association.

Dell, C. (1970). *A primer for movement description.* New York: Dance Notation Bureau Press.

Dulicai, D. (1984). *Heightening diagnostic skills in analysis of movement: A special intensive course in dance/movement therapy.* Workshop presented in Kansas City, MO.

Espenak, L. (1981). *Dance therapy: Theory and application.* Springfield, IL: Charles C. Thomas.

Fletcher, D. (1979). Body experience within the therapeutic process: A psychodynamic orientation. In P. Bernstein (Ed.), *Eight theoretical approaches in dance-movement therapy* (pp. 131–154). Dubuque, IA: Kendall/Hunt.

Freud, S. (1961). The ego and the id. In J. Strachey (Ed. and trans.), *The standard edition of the complete psychological works of Sigmund Freud* (Vol. 19, pp. 3–66). London: Hogarth Press. (Original work published 1923)

Kestenberg, J. (1965a). The role of movement patterns in development: I. Rhythms of movement. *Psychoanalytic Quarterly, 34,* 1–36.

Kestenberg, J. (1965b). The role of movement patterns in development: II. Flow of tension and effort. *Psychoanalytic Quarterly, 34,* 517–563.

Kestenberg, J. (1967). The role of movement patterns in development: III. The control of shape. *Psychoanalytic Quarterly, 36,* 356–409.

Lowen, A. (1971). *The language of the body.* New York: Collier Books.

Mahler, M. S., & McDevitt, J. B. (1982). Thoughts on the emergence of the sense of self, with particular emphasis on the body self. *Journal of the American Psychoanalytic Association, 30*(4), 827–848.

Mahler, M. S., Pine, F., & Bergman, A. (1975). *The psychological birth of the human infant.* New York: Basic Books.

Reich, W. (1949). *Character analysis.* New York: Orgone Institute Press.

Schilder, P. (1935). *The image and appearance of the human body.* London: Kegan Paul.

Schmais, C. (1985). Healing processes in group dance therapy. *American Journal of Dance Therapy, 8,* 1–36.

Siegel, E. (1979). Psychoanalytically oriented dance-movement therapy: A treatment approach to the whole person. In P. Bernstein (Ed.), *Eight theoretical approaches in dance-movement therapy* (pp. 89–110). Dubuque, IA: Kendall/Hunt.

Siegel, E. (1984). *Dance-movement therapy: Mirror of ourselves.* New York: Human Sciences Press.

14

Art Therapy and Anorexia: Experiencing the Authentic Self

Mari M. Fleming

Hilde Bruch (1985) considered anorexia to be characterized by an underlying disturbance in the development of the self, an identity, and autonomy. She spoke of her work with anorectic patients as helping them "to discover their creative and human potential, and to give up the hateful, unlovable, empty, and defective self-image that underlies the illness" (p. 18). Art therapy with the anorectic individual can provide a means of addressing underlying deficits in the organization of the self.

This chapter presents a developmental model for using art in therapy with the anorectic patient. This model emphasizes the creative process as a means to experience the true or authentic self, leading to establishment of new internal structures. In this chapter, I use concepts from object relations and self-psychology, focusing on the model developed by Goodsitt (1985). In his application of self-psychology theory to the understanding and treatment of anorexia nervosa, Goodsitt emphasized that effective therapy with the anorectic individual requires an active role for therapists in filling the deficits in the patient's self.

This chapter addresses developmental tasks in the treatment of the anorectic patient from the perspective of art therapy theory and the role of art in normal development, based on the following ideas:

1. The art process can be used to address deficits in the client's structures and functions, related to needs for soothing, protection from stimulus overload, and mirroring (Lachman-Chapin, 1979).
2. The art product serves as a transitional object, leading to the grad-

ual internalization of a sense of self and a feeling of well-being (Kramer, 1979).

3. The art process provides experiences of mastery leading to increased self-esteem (Kramer, 1979).

4. Art making as a creative process provides a means of initially tolerating unacceptable feelings and aspects of the self and experiencing the self as a whole (Fleming, 1982).

I first discuss the theoretical issues in the organization of the self, relating each stage to art therapy theory. Second, I describe the role of the art therapist in each stage of therapy and how the role changes as the client develops and changes. In the chapter, the goal of the therapist in each stage of therapy is related to appropriate art materials and methods. A case study is provided to illustrate the integration of theory, the therapist's role, materials, and methods. Finally, I discuss implications for treatment, including application of the model to individual treatment, training of therapists, and other concerns in using art with the anorectic patient.

THEORETICAL ISSUES

Theoretical issues are addressed primarily from the standpoint of the stages presented in Goodsitt's discussion (1985) of development of a self-structure in the treatment of anorexia. These concepts are then related to art therapy theory.

Goodsitt described Kohut's use (1971) of "self" in a broad sense. The self is a cohesive unit that includes id drives, ego interests, and superego values; an experiencing self; and a self-regulatory structure. The self is formed through relationships with others and initially contains an idealized parent image and a grandiose self.

Selfobject Functions

In order to develop a cohesive self that can tolerate separation, an individual must have internalized certain mental functions and structures. Important among these are "the capacity to provide one's own cohesiveness, soothing, vitalization, narcissistic equilibrium, . . . tension regulation, and self-esteem regulation" (Goodsitt, 1985, p. 61). The mother initially provides these functions through empathic selfobject mirroring (Kohut, 1971). A "selfobject" is Kohut's term for a person experienced as part of the self and used in service of the self. In mirroring, the selfobject empathically responds to the child's grandiose self.

Lachman-Chapin (1979) related the role of the art therapist, in the provision of empathy, soothing, tension modulation, and reflecting of the client, to that of the mother as the selfobject. The art therapist fulfills these functions through the choice of art materials and the therapeutic relationship. He or she mirrors the client by verbal reflection and repetition of movement and themes in art.

I propose that the art product provides a similar function. The child's use of art materials is in response to early developmental needs; this use of art records the child's own choices and movement. The sensory qualities of fluid and smeared art material can be soothing; the imprint of hand and gesture on the page mirrors the touch and gesture of the artist. The field of sensuous color and texture has been suggested by Fuller (1980) as re-creating the experience of oneness with the soothing, mirroring mother. As in the mother–child interaction, the mirroring of the anorectic patient through art confirms the individual's uniqueness.

The Transitional Object

In normal development, the holding and mirroring functions are gradually transferred from the mother to a transitional object such as a blanket. This object, which the child can manipulate, provides a sense of security and comfort and represents the mother. It is cognitively perceived as external, but it is experienced as part of the self (Goodsitt, 1985). With appropriate selfobject response, the need-gratifying aspects of the transitional object are gradually internalized into a sense of self, aiding the development of self-esteem.

Winnicott (1965) theorized that the unique value of art in human development and society is in its function as a transitional object, external to the individual but imbued with meaning. Edith Kramer (1979), who developed much of the theoretical base for the use of art as therapy with children, stated that while art does function as a transitional object, art products are *new* configurations invested with meaning; these art products are not found, but *made.*

To make art, one must initiate action. The artwork made within the treatment process stands for its meaning to the artist and for the relationship with the art therapist. In its function as transitional object, art can provide a corrective experience leading to gradual internalization of soothing and confirming functions.

The Developmental Use of Art

Kramer (1979) differentiated five ways in which art is used at any stage: (1) exploration of materials; (2) expression of impulses and feelings, which can lead to loss of control; (3) art used in the service of defense; (4) pictorial communication; and (5) formed expression, which incorporates sublimation. In artistic sublimation, unacceptable feelings and impulses are expressed and transformed into an acceptable form without loss of drive energy. These feelings may then be integrated as aspects of the self. Like play, making art allows trial action and can lead to experiences of mastery; these experiences increase self-esteem and further strengthen the boundaries of the self.

The Role of Creativity in Development

During adolescence, the themes of separation and individuation re-emerge as the adolescent struggles to define her own identity, separate from internalized selfobjects. This period of increased instability may bring about regression to early wishes for selfobject merger, mirroring, and idealization, particularly when the individual does not have a secure foundation for a cohesive self (Blos, 1962). This regression, however, presents the possibility of reworking early unmet needs, thus allowing the adolescent to reintegrate disowned or inadequately integrated aspects of the self. This process is referred to as "regression in the service of the ego" (Kris, 1964).

Shaw (1981) proposed that creative endeavors are engaged in more often during adolescence than at any other time. He suggested that the creative act provides the adolescent who mourns the loss of the internalized selfobject with a means of safely handling anxiety, tolerating opposing feelings, and exploring alternative solutions. Art gives form to chaos and provides a means of productive functioning, a way to "work through" the struggle. Additionally, experiencing the self in art supports self-cohesion over the course of time. Thus, as creativity operates in the service of maturation in development, it also serves as a therapeutic element in art therapy.

Art Therapy with Anorectic Patients

Art therapists have used art with eating-disordered patients to increase the patients' awareness of unrecognized and unacknowledged feelings, as an outlet for expression, to increase self-control, for mastery over impulses and fears, and to incorporate the art therapist as a selfobject (Haeseler, 1982; Wolf, Willmuth, & Watkins, 1986).

The art process can also provide a means for the anorectic individual to integrate an authentic self within a stable self-structure. As the art therapist assists the anorectic patient in developing self-regulatory structures, he or she modifies materials and techniques to meet the patient's needs at each stage of development within the process of treatment.

THE THERAPEUTIC PROCESS

The Role of the Art Therapist and the Use of Art Materials

The art therapist, in working with the anorexic, provides and protects safe conditions. He or she serves as a model of ego functioning and as an auxiliary ego who acts on the patient's behalf, supporting the patient's ego.

Goodsitt (1985) proposed that the therapist must maintain a flexible stance. The art therapist supports the patient's independent functioning, yet is always ready to provide more active structuring. As does the "good enough" mother, the art therapist supports the patient's risk taking and solution finding. The art therapist also respects the patient's need to retreat for comfort and soothing by providing structured use of art materials.

The art materials recommended in each stage of treatment are those used by children and adolescents as they proceed through developmental stages in art. For example, materials used in beginning exploration of art by children are used in the beginning stages of this therapeutic model. Within this framework, the therapeutic goal in each stage of therapy is presented with the corresponding modifications in the therapist's role, as the therapist adjusts to the patient's changing developmental needs. Art materials and procedures appropriate to the developmental stage and goals of treatment are discussed.

Beginning Therapy

In the initial stages of therapy, the therapist assesses motivation for treatment. The main issue is often the anorectic individual's reluctance to be a patient and the disavowal of her illness. Goodsitt (1985) felt it important to make contact with the part of the self that experiences pain.

To help the patient tolerate experiences of discomfort and pain, the art therapist initially must provide a nonthreatening holding environment. In beginning therapy, the art therapist develops an empathic understanding of the patient's experience and actively mirrors the patient's art expression.

Familiar and nonthreatening art materials such as pencils, markers, and crayons help reassure or calm the patient. These materials tend to encourage cognitive responses. Since intellectual abilities are a strength for many anorexics, cognitive responses can feel familiar and certain, and they can help to maintain a protective stimulus barrier for affects that may feel threatening.

Beginning art activities focus on comforting images or experiences of safety, then move to depiction of the patient's presenting problem and concerns. A drawing of somatic concerns can be used as a bridge to feelings (Fleming & Cox, 1988). Returning to materials or activities that are perceived as safe, such as making a collage or placing a border around the paper, is encouraged if the patient becomes apprehensive.

Mid-Stage Therapy

Once an initial transference is established, the patient begins to work through repressed needs and wishes, re-enacting her defenses. The patient's needs and demands are experienced and mirrored. Through manageable frustration and internalization of aspects of the therapist, the patient gains mastery, and, gradually, a fully functioning self is integrated (Kohut, 1971).

The art therapist, through confirming and mirroring the patient's expression, serves as the selfobject. He or she supports investment in the art work and preserves and protects it in its function as a transitional object. The therapist accepts but does not encourage stereotypic responses and/or defensive work. Regressive use of materials is reflected by the therapist and related to life events; self-soothing is taught and encouraged. Acting as an auxiliary ego, the art therapist assists the patient in overcoming frustration or regression, which may follow perceived loss or failure of empathy by the therapist. The therapist reinforces experiences of mastery, supporting self-esteem. As the patient progresses, she is recognized for her growth and supported in her awareness of personal rhythms and her acceptance of herself.

Materials such as soft pastels, oil pastels, and paint promote the expression of affect, encouraging self-investigation. Thick paint may encourage regression because of smearing, running, or its similarity to body fluids. Clay can also invite regression; however, its cohesive qualities support reintegration. Once again, returning to materials that the patient has experienced as safe or soothing is encouraged in response to patient anxiety.

Tasks begin with exploration of the physical self or presenting problem. Feelings concerning the physical body are related to feelings and experiences of the (psychological) self. Art activities next explore experiences within the context of family and society. Aspects of the self are pictured, and integration of part-selves is supported by placing images within a container or a shape such as a circle. Depiction of memories may precipitate mourning for unmet needs. As the patient develops increased self-awareness and acceptance, she is encouraged to choose materials and themes. A dictionary of feelings in color and line can assist the patient in exploring similarities and changes in her work, developing a sense of consistency.

Throughout treatment, the patient is supported as the authority concerning the meaning and interpretation of her art work. Idealization of the therapist is de-emphasized.

Termination Stage

In this final phase of therapy, issues of loss and possible regression to early needs must be worked through (Goodsitt, 1985). Separation anxiety, rage, and guilt are explored and related to previous experiences and art work. Self-understanding and a cohesive sense of self are supported.

The art therapist maintains consistency. He or she emphasizes the patient's self-investigation and understanding of herself and her work. The therapist also supports the patient in constructive defenses.

Returning to materials used in the beginning stage of art therapy can provide soothing and assist in closure. Control over the art materials provides a substitute, or outlet, for wishes of control previously manifested in eating behavior and preoccupation with body image.

Tasks emphasize expression of feelings and depiction of memories of early losses. A review of the artwork together with drawings and discussion of the patient's changes during hospitalization assist in closure.

The following case study allows us to see how this theoretical model is incorporated into art therapy treatment. I have chosen to discuss Crystal, a restrictive anorexic, because she possessed some initial availability for treatment that was mobilized through art therapy. Crystal did not identify herself as an artist and had not used art materials. Her response to the art process demonstrates how this model can address the needs of the patient with a deficit in the self-structure.

Art therapy treatment took place within a milieu that included individual, group, and family therapy as well as nutritional and medical management. This case study demonstrates the importance of effective collaboration. Case conferences and problem-oriented records provided daily communication among staff members. I used treatment issues as indicators of developmental needs; these became themes for art therapy group sessions. Memories, needs, and feelings that surfaced in art therapy were often brought by the patient to her individual therapist and verbally explored. The therapies meshed and supported each other and the patient.

CASE STUDY

Crystal, a 21-year-old anorectic patient, was admitted to the eating-disorders unit of a small private hospital. Her treatment occurred in an art therapy group that focused on issues of self-image. The art therapy group included from two to six bulimic and anorectic individuals at varying stages of treatment. The group met two or three times each week.

Crystal's eating disorder began when she was 13. Her older sister and brother had also experienced eating problems in adolescence. Crystal lived at home while she attended college. She was a good student, majoring in a helping profession. As her last year in college approached, her eating problems worsened, and she became anorectic. Crystal became aware of her need for help through her coursework, and she sought treatment. She was immediately hospitalized. On admission, she expressed a wish to be better but conveyed fears of showing her private self and of losing her eating disorder.

At 5'9" in height, Crystal's maximum weight had been 146 pounds approximately $1\frac{1}{2}$ years before admission. Since that time, she had severely restricted food intake and exercised two–three hours per day. Her eating problems had resulted in major weight loss and amenorrhea. On admission Crystal weighed 97 pounds, with 14% body fat. Her ideal body weight was 139 pounds. She was dehydrated, with general weakness, chest pain, and palpitations. The first week or two on the unit she responded with mute and angry behavior to intravenous hydration and supplements administered to stabilize fluid and nutritional status. Crystal's physical weakness, and the fact that she responded to medical intervention with withdrawal, reflected her severely restrictive style.

Beginning Therapy

In beginning treatment, the major emphasis was on the establishment of trust. Art was used as a way for Crystal to communicate her distress and bypass her fears of accepting help.

At the first self-image group three days after admittance, Crystal looked like a shy deer. She was thin and quiet and appeared withdrawn. Sensitive to her apparent nervousness, and seeking to build trust, I suggested to the group that they imagine a color that helped them feel peaceful or whole. Crystal was able to tell the group she had pictured sunlight; she added that in her life she had never felt seen or understood.

Crystal came to the next group visibly upset about medical interventions. For a nonverbal way of communicating feelings in relation to the physical body, I suggested that group members draw a life-size body outline and place within it a symbol to represent their physical self. Crystal became increasingly disturbed as she drew and tore up her first attempt. Her second drawing showed a slim, child-like figure with a tiny golden sun inside her brain. Five large hands reached to grab her "yellow essence," which she had drawn inside her heart (Figure 14-1).

As became her pattern, Crystal showed this picture to her individual therapist after the group session. She told him about the helplessness and discomfort she felt when her parents drank and fought. Crystal said she

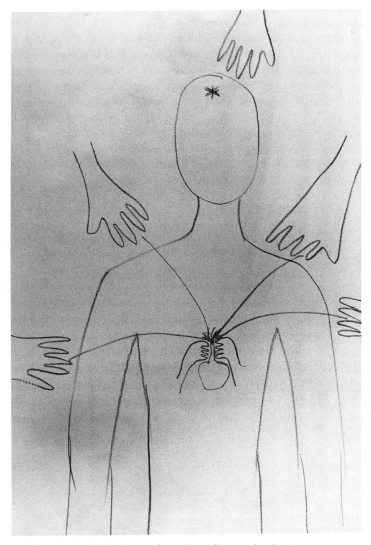

Figure 14-1. This picture shows Crystal protecting her "essence."

resented her parents for wanting her to give them happiness when she had never gotten happiness from them. This suggested that Crystal had not experienced an empathic and responsive early environment.

Because of Crystal's fears of intrusion and loss of her fragile yellow "essence," I asked her to construct a "Self-Box," a technique developed by Keyes (1974). In this technique, the patient pastes pictures and materials on the outside and inside of a cardboard box to make an image of herself. The inside images are used to depict the private or inner self; the outside portrays the self as shown to the world. The project provides permission to cover or hide the inner self; this allowed Crystal to portray her feelings of isolation and need.

Crystal chose a picture of a child reaching out for a man who turns his back on her. She said, "I only occasionally feel this way—I'm not creative," as she attempted to defend against her feelings. Encouraged to place the picture somewhere on or in her Self-Box, Crystal pasted it on the inside back of the box. She cut out the word "caring" and pasted it above the figure. On either side of the word, Crystal pasted flowers with yellow streamers that touched the little girl (Figure 14-2).

In an attempt to support self-soothing, I asked Crystal if, as a little girl, she had ways of making herself feel better. She said she had made herself feel better by focusing on nature and small beauties.

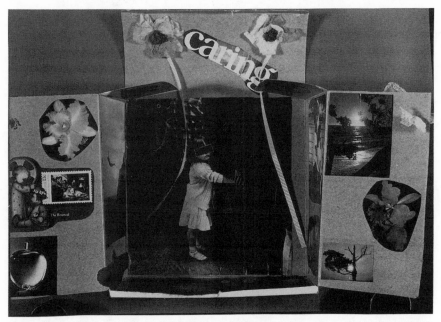

Figure 14-2. The inside of Crystal's Self-Box shows her protected, hidden self. (Child's face obscured by publisher for privacy.)

Crystal placed the closed box on an open shelf in the art room; it became a transitional object for her. Over the next several weeks, Crystal regularly checked her box and put new words and pictures inside it, including a picture of a glass apple filled with light.

Crystal used these images to tell her individual therapist that she felt little and precious, but she said she wanted to get away from self-exploration. During a subsequent staffing, the therapist told the staff that he felt these images showed that there existed in Crystal some sense of self that was fairly unharmed and thus predictive of a positive prognosis.

In this beginning stage of therapy, art therapy topics and materials, with nonintrusive discussion, had been used to build a safe, nurturing environment. Once given permission to protect and care for herself within this empathic environment, Crystal was able to acknowledge feeling threatened and needy, yet special. Drawing and collage materials had supported and reflected her cognitive strengths. Crystal's ability to depict childhood needs and strivings indicated she could mobilize an observing segment of her personality in order to take on the work of therapy.

Mid-Stage

In the next stage of therapy, the goals were to help Crystal get in touch with her repressed needs and the ways in which she had defended against them. In the process of art therapy, exploration of the self moves from the external physical self—the symptom focus—to internal self-perception, to the self in the family. My role as therapist now was one of confirming and mirroring, acting as the self-object. Through manageable frustration and working through developmental processes arrested in childhood, Crystal could begin to internalize aspects of herself and develop an inner structure in order to comfort, mirror, and maintain her own tension reduction.

Experiencing Part-Selves

The group was asked to picture liked and disliked aspects of their bodies. Crystal pictured her "worst parts," the sexualized pelvis and breast areas, in black. Shoulders, neck, lower arms, hands, and feet were pink, representing "satisfactory parts." My hypothesis, based on an earlier study (Cox & Fleming, 1987), was that Crystal's use of black to represent negative body feelings indicated possible early loss or separation. Later in treatment, Crystal confirmed that she had experienced an early separation: Her mother was repeatedly hospitalized when Crystal was a child.

We used these body drawings to explore early influences on her beliefs about a woman's body and a woman's roles. Crystal said her mother felt "It's a man's world," and "Men only want one thing." Her grand-mother, however, felt that, as a woman, you should "Keep your figure and be self-sufficient." These views were reflected in Crystal's identification of her sexual areas as negative and her hands and feet as acceptable.

Other group members shared similar images and stories of adolescent maturation, which helped to lessen Crystal's sense of isolation and supported her emerging separateness. In other aspects of the program, however, Crystal stated she was upset and didn't want to talk about feelings. She increasingly focused on her body and fears of gaining weight. She told her therapist she wanted people to read her mind.

At the next group meeting, Crystal was asked to use clay to make animals to symbolize two opposing aspects of her self, a beginning step to accepting part-selves experienced as negative. Clay can be manipulated and modified. The patient's touch shapes the image; gentle touch can be experienced as soothing. Animal themes can provide a relatively non-threatening way of beginning to experience repressed aspects of the self.

Crystal created a deer. She identified it as good and described it as smart, quiet, and hidden. She said, "The deer will defend the helpless with her life." The "bad animal self" was "a shark . . . brute strength . . . stupid . . . grabbing and killing to eat!" Crystal said, "I'm afraid this is what will come out of me."

Crystal could "talk" through her "silent" animals. Making art had encouraged self-perception and communication. Through the visual images, she clearly depicted her conflicting needs and "false self" adaptation. Her concern for others seemed to negate her own selfobject needs. Eating was associated with bad and consuming needs. Crystal needed to experience the origin of these feelings; art tasks focusing on the family seemed an appropriate next step.

The Self in the Family

In the next art therapy group, "picturing an important family relationship and your needs within it" was suggested as a theme. Crystal responded by staring at her paper. Finally she wrote words she would like to say to her mother and hid them as she wrote. She was able to read these to the group. "Why did I have to mother *you*? Why didn't you ever hold me? Why have I been old since I was born? Why did you ever have me?" She rocked her body back and forth as she read these desperate cries.

I asked Crystal about her rocking, and she said she had always rocked herself and still rocked herself to sleep at night. Then Crystal remembered that her mother had frequently been sick when she was a child. She described staying home from school to nurse her mother and said she was never able to be a child.

As Crystal's grief and guilt for having her own needs surfaced, she regressed and displayed early ways of self-soothing, such as cuddling her teddy bear or feeling a need to binge, outside of art therapy. She became negative and withdrew from activities when the dietitian increased her calorie intake.

In order to reduce Crystal's distress to a degree that she could begin to manage, in the next session I returned to a focus on the physical self and the use of clay, a previously soothing medium. Crystal used clay to form images of her early self, herself on admission to the hospital, and a future self, a task devised by Wooley and Kearney-Cooke (1986). Crystal sculpted her early self as a tall stick, representing her family's focus on her height. Her before-admission sculpture demonstrated that she felt like a huge blob with a tiny head. She then created her future self as a block-like shape with many protrusions and indentations. This image indicated increased complexity of self-concept and openness to the interior. I reflected to Crystal that she was in the process of forming and changing.

In her future figure, Crystal experimented with self-containment, allowing the outside to reach in and herself to reach outward. These three figures, representing different periods in her life, were made out of a consistent material in order to support integration of her self-concept. Modifying body image in clay also provided experiences of control which reinforced boundaries in a way that was not food related.

As these variable self-images were discussed in the art therapy group, Crystal reported she had stopped eating with her parents years ago, leading to feelings of exclusion and emptiness. She was able to modulate her distress in response to these feelings, which indicated an increasing capacity to regulate herself. Therefore, in the next group, we returned to the feelings around herself within the family. I asked the group members to draw abstract family portraits. Using soft pastels, they each pictured the personalities and relationships of family members with colors and symbols (Figure 14-3).

Crystal described her mother, represented in this picture by red lines circling the page, as intense and angry. Her mother surrounded the whole family and isolated it from others. Crystal said only she could see her mother's vulnerability (a yellow line under the red). Crystal said her older sister (a red star-shaped figure in the upper right) was like mother, but reaching out. Crystal described her father (a blue planet, lower right), as being intense and closed in. She told the group her brother (a green planet with yellow center, far right) was similar to her father, but had some vulnerability (yellow) and was tentatively reaching out to other family members. Crystal drew herself as a yellow sun (lower left) touching her mother's lines and with yellow lines extended to her father, sister, and brother. She described herself as vulnerable, which seemed to imply a wish for closeness.

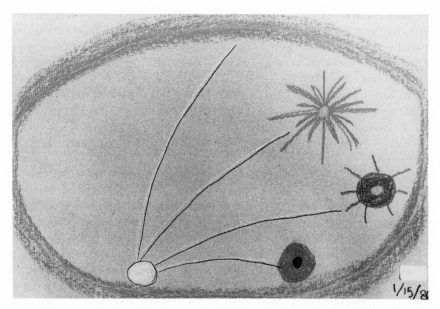

Figure 14-3. In this abstract family portrait, Crystal's isolation and caretaking are seen. Lines were reinforced for photographic reproduction.

Crystal's use of yellow was compared with her original essence and the "caring" streamers on her Self-Box. Crystal identified her role as "vulnerable and sick." She also commented that she had nothing to offer others unless they were also sick.

Crystal's needs, strengths, and anger were reflected, talked about, and owned in this abstract family portrait. The soft smearing qualities of pastels had encouraged affective communication. The consistent use of yellow to symbolize herself, her needs, and her provision of comfort seemed to indicate some beginning internalization of self-soothing.

Regression in Response to Perceived Loss

In response to her hospital roommate being discharged and her psychiatrist leaving on vacation, Crystal felt abandoned and angry. She retreated to a focus on weight.

In the next art therapy group, members talked about roles in their families. It was suggested that they draw family members and their personal space, including boundaries. Crystal felt unable to draw, but as she thought about this idea, she realized she had not been allowed privacy in her family. She told the group she was not allowed to go to her room and shut her door; she also described her mother retreating to her own bedroom and locking Crystal out. As she remembered these experiences Crystal realized she had "made my own place—in my own room. I have a ritual for eating." She also said that sometimes she would vomit and later feel euphoric. She talked of her reluctance to have others see inside her: "It feels just like my mother knowing my every thought." Crystal then negated her feelings by saying she wanted to take her parents' pain: "I'm strong enough to keep their pain and protect them!"

Secrecy and ritual had been a way for Crystal to confirm her separate identity and provide self-soothing in the face of perceived abandonment by her mother. As she now experienced abandonment by both her roommate and her therapist, she again retreated. Following this group session, Crystal was able to admit that she had been purging on the unit when she was not able to restrict food intake. She recognized that she needed to accept staff help.

As she became more "visible," Crystal experienced diffuse anxiety. In verbal groups and family meetings she acted helpless and distracted others from focusing on their own concerns. Her role as a distractor was clarified as her own anger was addressed; she refused to use art materials or participate in discussion for three group meetings. She said she felt abandoned and angry.

I introduced thick fluid paints to provide an experience of sensory gratification, encouraging Crystal to express her underlying feelings and to develop empathy with herself, leading to self-soothing. I suggested that Crystal experiment with the paint, testing which strokes, colors, and images felt right to her. Crystal drew a plant. Then I gave her a larger piece of paper. She dipped her finger in yellow paint and began to gently smear it, creating flower-like shapes. She added red and then other colors. As she expanded the shapes and then attempted to cover over or soften the intense colors, Crystal experienced her need to cover her intense or negative feelings. She finally placed playful finger prints of red, blue, and yellow over the page (Figure 14-4).

By creating this image, through the caressing and soothing experience of paint Crystal nurtured herself after feeling needy and depleted in response to her therapist's absence. Through art, Crystal practiced reaching out and meeting her own needs; the group's acceptance and positive response encouraged her. As Crystal re-created an early experience of being loved and nurtured—her yellow vulnerable self—she also mourned the lack of "good enough" mothering in her childhood.

Crystal came to the next group stating she was desperately trying not to cry. In a meeting with her family that morning, she had cried as she asked for their help. Her parents had told her to handle it herself, that they had sacrificed so much. Crystal asked for paint; she had learned that using flowing materials helped her soothe and gratify herself. As she painted, she said she felt like crying. She was afraid that if her feelings came out they'd "destroy the world." Using art materials, and with the

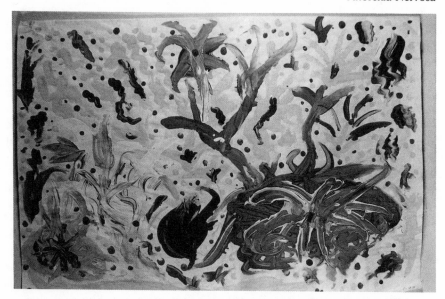

Figure 14-4. This picture demonstrated sensory exploration and mirroring in paint.

therapist's support, she was increasingly able to tolerate and experience her feelings of emptiness.

Crystal reported feeling like she was "putting up a wall"; this phrase was then used as a theme for visualization. In this visualization, group members were encouraged to explore the wall and see if there might be a way to enter or see what was beyond it. Crystal did not want to draw this image; she said she was afraid of "looking like a child, and not doing it right." Crystal remembered when, as a little girl, she had begun to do things on her own, and her mother had called her "bad" and "dirty." As she re-experienced her parents' lack of empathic support, Crystal said, "Something went wrong in my process of growing up."

Reintegration

Since Crystal seemed to need more time to experience and integrate her emerging feelings of separateness and resulting sadness, I suggested that she return to her Self-Box as a way of reinforcing her boundaries. This transitional object had come to represent her first experiences of safety and trust in art therapy. The three-dimensional material had supported her in her growing ability to manipulate the environment (Bell, 1986) and convey her feelings. In response to my suggestion, Crystal tied the doors shut, using a lace ribbon. Then she wanted to smash the box because "it was made up of what others had created." For Crystal, the words placed on the outside of the box reflected the exterior that she showed to others; destroying the box symbolized destroying this "false self," not *her*.

Encouraged to listen to her own needs for safety and comfort, Crystal reported to the group that her parents had said that she had never told them how she felt. It seemed useful at this point for Crystal to begin to experience empathy and connection with others, beyond the art materials and therapist. Therefore, I proposed a communications drawing task. In this nonverbal exercise, group members are paired. The partners take turns drawing and responding to the each other's line or color. During the discussion following the exercise, Crystal noted that she felt understood and supported by her partner, suggesting that she was able to experience mirroring from and a positive connection with another patient.

As Crystal experienced greater comfort with her emerging sense of self, I encouraged her to choose materials and themes that interested her. In the next group, she experimented with colored tissue paper, making an image of nature which she found comforting. This brought to awareness her memories of love and acceptance as a small child while vacationing with her grandparents in Hawaii. The picture was colorful, and she related it to herself as full of life. Crystal then talked about how new it was to say what she felt.

At the next art therapy group, Crystal requested an imagery exercise. She recalled a 10-year-old playmate and the playmate's family, who had welcomed Crystal into their home. This memory seemed to reflect Crystal's feeling of being accepted by her therapeutic family. She said, "Everyone needs a place to be crazy sometimes" and engaged spontaneously with the others in the group, painting a free abstract painting. Crystal said she felt about 10 years old; she wanted to read children's books.

These experiences of good memories and playful exploration showed increased mastery as Crystal integrated new internal structures. Crystal's psychiatrist returned from his vacation, and she was able to see a relationship between her feelings about his absence and her eating behaviors.

At the next group, Crystal brought photographs of herself and her family. She talked about her wish for nurturing, but she still blamed her lack of it on her not being "cuddly"—she was "too independent." "Picturing your needs" was suggested as a theme. Crystal drew small specific symbols of her needs for love, care, and "flowering." She then asked me if I would draw her portrait. As we talked about her wish to be important to me, she recalled her jealousy when her older sister was anorectic and received all of her parents' attention. Through these interactions, Crystal began to modify the needs of her grandiose self and internalize emotional nurturance.

This period of integration and self-acceptance was threatened by Crystal's family and by my vacation. Crystal experienced feelings of loss, jealousy, and anger, which affected her eating—she gained only 1 pound during this period. Still having difficulty tolerating her jealous and angry feelings, Crystal talked in group therapy about the relationship between needing to please her mother and her eating; *not* eating was related to denial of dependency. Now more aware of her wish that her mother would give her a sense of self-esteem, she chose to paint a rainbow and flowers, thus giving *herself* pleasant feelings.

On my return, Crystal told me she felt more and more like a child, shy and sometimes playful. She voiced her feelings of vulnerability, accepting them as a sign of her growing sense of self. She began to gain weight.

To support Crystal in being more able to appreciate herself, I asked her to picture aspects of herself that she wished to keep. Crystal drew her family, a warm sun, and peaceful nature, circling them in yellow. She drew a yellow chick peering out of a shell and said it symbolized shyness. Crystal drew a teddy bear, representing her playful child-self, and she labeled a mountain as strength, then added simplicity. She drew teardrops for her sadness.

During discussion of this picture, the group noted that Crystal's perception of her size in the pictures varied with her feelings. This observation was related to her earlier discovery, with the clay figures, that her body image reflected her self-image. In addition, Crystal's yellow color, previously hidden within or experienced as the caretaking of others, now was shown encircling images of love and comfort. This seemed to reflect Crystal's increasing sense of self, that is, she could let her vulnerability, her essence, be seen.

As Crystal began to integrate good aspects of herself, she became more aware of the other patients and members of her family as separate individuals. She could increasingly tolerate silences in the groups without needing to take care of the other patients. She could talk about her wish for a strong father, newly aware that he was chronically depressed. She explored new ways of relating to her mother. Her dreams and imagery grew stronger.

Termination Stage

During the termination stage, I needed to take a medical leave. At the next meeting I told the group I would be there for only 2 more weeks. I encouraged them to use materials to explore their reactions to my absence. Crystal was flooded with memories of her mother's illness. She recalled that her mother had been near death when she was a small child, and she had been left to the care of her father, his mother, and his sister, who "didn't understand about children. They expected me to be an adult and didn't hear me—I feel like all my life I've been screaming 'I'm trying as hard as I can!' "

Crystal covered her paper with dark clouds and hazy lines surrounding a dropped ice cream cone (Figure 14-5). A heavy black line surrounded red and blue shapes, which she identified as anger and sadness. This picture, of an incident when her caretaker assumed that she had deliberately dropped the ice cream and her father's mother believed the caretaker, symbolized her wished-for but nonexistent closeness with her mother.

Crystal's mother, alternately intrusive or withdrawn due to illness, could not meet Crystal's early needs for empathic mirroring and provision of regulatory functions. Crystal had been unable to develop an internal structure that provided self-soothing, tension regulation, and self-esteem regulation. Her mother's hospitalizations had threatened Crystal's inadequate sense of self, and Crystal had retreated to taking care of both her ill mother and depressed father.

In response to my imminent departure, as with other losses, Crystal became generally unresponsive, although she said she was "trying to be good." To provide a framework for exploring her feelings, I suggested that the group make personal dictionaries of colors and symbols. A feeling word (e.g., "calm," "anxious") was given, and each person in the group represented the feeling, using color and a line or symbol. This feeling symbol was then used as the basis for a second, personalized drawing.

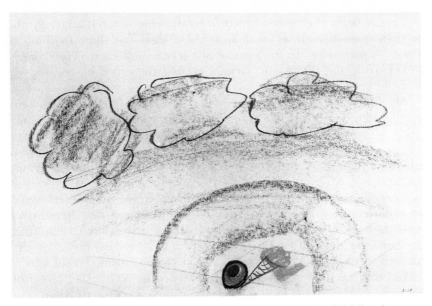

Figure 14-5. This picture evokes the lost, uncared-for self of childhood.

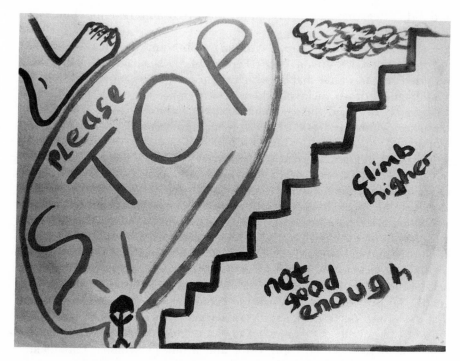

Figure 14-6. Crystal's rage at parental expectations is seen here.

Crystal began her second picture by drawing her red anger symbol. She then drew herself as small with short legs—too short to climb the stairs of expectations. In the picture, she screams, "Please STOP" (Figure 14-6). During the discussion, Crystal related these feelings of anger to parental expectations.

My illness and perceived abandonment appeared to have reawakened Crystal's memories of early loss of her mother and being watched by non-responsive caretakers. The primitive, childlike drawing conveys Crystal's feelings of abandonment and resulting rage; these feelings are consistently experienced by children who have suffered early losses (Fleming, 1982).

Crystal talked in her individual therapy about the intense feelings she had experienced while drawing this picture. She and her therapist discussed the costs of repression versus the costs of expression. Crystal feared that "letting it out will make me weaker, and I need all my strength to deal with it [separation]." She said she felt she was a small child and was shocked to look at her body and realize it was the body of a 21-year-old. Her therapist encouraged Crystal to tell me about her overwhelming child needs.

Yet Crystal did not come to art therapy; she stated that I was abandoning her. The next day, however, she worked with art materials in her room and drew her feelings. She pictured her needy split-off child-self inside a large fat body. The child is yelling, "Let me out!" (Figure 14-7). Crystal then drew a second picture, of me leaving, with herself as a little child, unprotected facing a voracious mouth and grabbing arms.

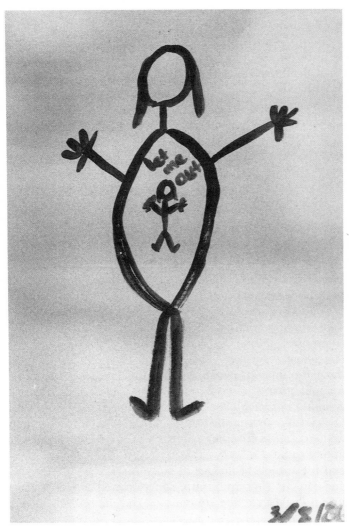

Figure 14-7. This shows Crystal's response to her therapist's illness; her split-off child-self is trying to come out.

Following this expression of her feelings, Crystal began to initiate activity, to eat, and to gain weight in the 2-week interval before I left.

Crystal showed me these pictures on my last day with the group. We reviewed her artwork as a visual document of her experiences and changes since her admission to the hospital. Crystal's personal dictionary was used to understand her feelings as expressed in her artwork, particularly her fears that her voracious needs and resulting depression would overwhelm her in my absence.

As Crystal was helped to see her consistent use of color and symbol in representing her feelings during her hospital stay, a sense of herself, consistent over time, was supported. She saw that her vulnerable self, which she had sought to hide and protect, was increasingly pictured as able to move out in the world and experience a wider range of feelings. In this way, art had been used by Crystal to practice going out into the dangerous world of needs and feelings.

My absence initiated Crystal's concerns about termination. During my absence, the art therapy group met once a week, led by the nurse who had been my co-therapist. Themes and materials were used to provide experiences of safety and soothing, providing a structure for reviewing the course of treatment and planning for the future.

To address termination, the therapist suggested that each patient picture the road of her life, using colors and symbols to review life and the period of hospitalization. Crystal called her picture "Change." She began with a black spiral which changed to red and then softened to blue tears. The line flowed into a green plant shape. She said the black symbolized feelings of self-hatred and being trapped. This line became the red of her anger, which had gradually changed to mourning; the green pictured the new life and hope that she was beginning to feel.

During another art group, Crystal remembered the relief she had experienced when restricting food, and she drew an iridescent, pale-pink, soothing emptiness. Now, she said, she could also bring peace by talking about her feelings.

As discharge time approached, trial visits home precipitated fears and concerns about eating. Crystal felt out of control. She expressed fears about her mother's intrusiveness and about her lack of protection for her possessions and her space. She was encouraged to talk to her family about these fears and found that her parents were trying to develop new ways of responding to her.

Crystal used internal images of sunshine and peace to comfort herself. In her last art therapy group, she returned to her initial image of self within an enclosure. She commented that herself was now protected by her own caring hands. Arrows represented movement outward. Her wish to be open was now as strong as her former need to remain hidden and protected (Figure 14-8).

Crystal was able to use art as a self-, or transitional, object, which

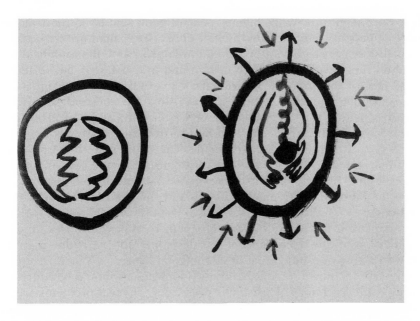

Figure 14-8. In her final painting, Crystal showed her mourning self protected by a safe enclosure and her own comforting touch. Arrows symbolize her wish to move toward others.

stood for our work together and allowed her to express her needs and fears instead of restricting her eating in response to guilt. The process of creativity within an art therapy group had supported her beginning awareness of rejected and internalized feeling and part objects. Crystal could now experience and contain her feelings within a better-integrated self.

Crystal menstruated for the first time in more than a year during the final week of her stay. Discharged after 3 months of treatment at the agreed weight of 115 pounds, she was able to say good-bye appropriately to staff and fellow patients. She was discharged to ongoing individual psychiatric treatment and family therapy once every 2 weeks. Although she experienced some setbacks during the next year of treatment, 1 year later she had graduated from college and was living successfully away from home.

DISCUSSION

This model of using art in a group setting was developed as part of an intensive treatment program in a small eating-disorders unit in a general hospital. Both bulimic and anorectic individuals were admitted and included in the groups. While bulimic patients generally stayed for 1 month, anorexic patients remained on the unit until achievement of their agreed-upon discharge weight. Approaches developed for bulimic individuals, based on their readiness to both take in and to expel, may be ineffective in the face of the anorectic individual's fear of taking in or of intrusion. The restricting anorexic, with an impoverished self and undernourished body, has neither the energy nor the self-esteem available for investment in artwork and self-exploration. Refusal to participate in artwork or wishes for merger with the idealized therapist may precipitate defensive withdrawal or attempts to please the therapist. Our art group, containing both anorectic and bulimic patients, necessitated constant recognition of the anorectic patients' developmental issues and the need for individual adaptations.

Adaptation for individual or outpatient treatment requires minimal modification of this model since it was developed for use within a group, but with a focus on individual developmental concerns. When treatment is not part of a milieu, physical and nutritional issues should be addressed through the art. Issues of trust and presenting physical problems are focused on until additional weight allows, and often precipitates, awareness of intrapsychic concerns.

To use art with the anorectic patient, the therapist needs to have familiarity with the creative process as well as an understanding of the dynamics of the anorexic individual. The registered art therapist (ATR; American Art Therapy Association) trained in the diagnostic use of art and in the art process may require additional training in the dynamics of eating disorders. The trained eating-disorders professional who has a respect for the art process or a personal involvement in creativity may incorporate these techniques into treatment. Without art therapy training, the emphasis should be on the patient's own interpretations and self-understanding.

The collaborative process is vital in treatment of the anorectic patient. She will often first present her central concerns in art therapy sessions. These issues can then provide a focus for treatment in individual or group therapy. A reciprocal sharing of information provides optimal therapeutic benefit. Art can also provide visual evidence of the patient's strengths and progress, providing hope and encouragement to team members in this often long and difficult work.

Concerns in using art with the anorectic individual generally focus on loss of control. However, art is more often used as a defense by these patients. Empty or stereotypical art is a particular danger in work with anorectic patients as they seek to please others or intellectualize their reactions. This defensive use of art, however, may be encouraged for therapeutic reasons when the patient is threatened by feelings that seem out of control. Chaotic discharge, while less likely with the anorectic patient than with the bulimic patient, is feared by the anorexic. Easily controlled materials and themes that are reality based or support pleasant experiences can provide safety. As trust increases, the patient is invited to experiment with fluid materials and experiences of losing and then imposing control.

CONCLUSION

Many of the specific techniques discussed in this chapter have been used by others in treating eating-disordered patients. This art therapy model emphasizes an awareness of the patient's developmental needs, with appropriate modifications of therapist interactions, art materials, and methods to meet the needs of each anorectic patient.

Art used in therapy may provide the first experiences of safety and the first expression of pain. Projected images often escape internal censorship, bypassing customary verbal defenses. Art has ready access to inner feelings and early experiences. Experiences of mastery support self-esteem.

Through the art process and the relationship with the art therapist, the empty and unlovable self can be safely experienced. In its function as a transitional object, the art product helps the gradual incorporation of self-soothing and mirroring.

Creativity in normal adolescence provides a model for the use of art with the anorectic patient. Just as creativity allows the possibility of handling anxiety so that unacceptable feelings can be tolerated and the self experienced as a whole, this art therapy process can provide a means to experience and develop a cohesive, fully functioning, authentic self.

REFERENCES

Bell, M. (1986.) *An art education curriculum for a child with learning problems: A rationale for the use of three-dimensional materials.* Unpublished master's project, California State University, Sacramento.

Blos, P. (1962). *On adolescence.* New York: Free Press.

Bruch, H. (1985). Four decades of eating disorders. In D. M. Garner & P. E. Garfinkel (Eds.), *Handbook of psychotherapy for anorexia nervosa and bulimia* (pp. 7–18). New York: Guilford Press.

Cox, C., & Fleming, M. (1986). *Somatic distress: Report on results of study from the 1983 Conference workshops.* Unpublished manuscript presented at the Sixteenth Annual Conference of the American Art Therapy Association. Los Angeles: CA.

Fleming, M. (1982). Early object loss and its relation to creativity as expressed through art therapy. In A. Di Maria (Ed.), *Proceedings of the 13th annual conference of the American Art Therapy Association* (pp. 53–57). Philadelphia: American Art Therapy Association.

Fleming, M., & Cox, C. (1988). Engaging the somatic patient in healing through art. In H.

Wadeson, J. Durkin, & D. Perach (Eds.), *Advances in art therapy*. New York: John Wiley and Sons.

Fuller, P. (1980). *Art and psychoanalysis*. London: Writers and Readers Publishers Cooperative.

Goodsitt, A. (1985). Self psychology and the treatment of anorexia nervosa. In D. M. Garner & P. E. Garfinkel (Eds.), *Handbook of psychotherapy for anorexia nervosa and bulimia* (pp. 55–82). New York: Guilford Press.

Haeseler, M. (1982). Why are patients with anorexia nervosa responsive to art therapy? In A. DiMaria, E. Kramer, & L. Regner (Eds.), *Art therapy: A bridge between two worlds*. Falls Church, VA: American Art Therapy Association.

Keyes, M. (1974). *The inward journey: Art as therapy for you*. Millbrae, CA: Celestial Arts.

Kohut, H. (1971). *The analysis of the self*. New York: International Universities Press.

Kramer, E. (1979). *Childhood and art therapy: Notes on theory and application*. In collaboration with L. Wilson. New York: Schocken Books.

Kris, E. (1964). *Psychoanalytic explorations in art*. New York: Schocken Books.

Lachman-Chapin, M. (1979). Kohut's theories on narcissism: Implications for art therapy. *The American Journal of Art Therapy, 19,* 3–9.

Shaw, J. (1981). Adolescence, mourning and creativity. In S. Feinstein & P. Giovacchini (Eds.), *Adolescent psychiatry* (pp. 60–77). Chicago: University of Chicago Press.

Winnicott, D. (1965). *The maturational process and the facilitating environment*. New York: International Universities Press.

Wolf, J., Willmuth, M., & Watkins, A. (1986). Art therapy's role in the treatment of anorexia nervosa. *The American Journal of Art Therapy, 25,* 39–46.

Wooley, S., & Kearney-Cooke, A. (1986). Intensive treatment of bulimia and body-image disturbance. In K. Brownell & J. Foreyt (Eds.), *Handbook of eating disorders: Physiology, psychology, and treatment of obesity, anorexia, and bulimia* (pp. 476–502). New York: Basic Books.

15

Music as a Therapeutic Tool in Treating Anorexia Nervosa

Alice Ball Parente

Since anorexia nervosa was first described by Morton (1869), diversified attempts have been made to understand as well as treat this problem using a variety of therapeutic modalities (Bruch, 1973; Crisp, 1970; Garner, Garfinkel, & Bemis, 1982; Masterson, 1977; Minuchin, Rosman, & Baker, 1978; Selvini-Palazzoli, 1978). Although a considerable amount of work has been done through music therapy, very little has been written about the use of music in treating persons with anorexia nervosa. Since substantial evidence exists demonstrating music to be an effective tool in treating a multitude of mental, physical, and emotional disorders (Carter, 1982; Gaston, 1968; Priestley, 1975; Tyson, 1981), the application of music to the treatment of anorexia would seem a likely extension.

This chapter presents both a theoretical model and a practical model for the use of music in therapy. The theoretical model presents music therapy as a discipline. It also describes the three basic processes of music therapy and how they can be used to address the specific issues of anorexia. The treatment model presented is a music therapy program that serves chronic or severely anorectic women; it is also a resource for other community members.

THEORETICAL MODEL

Music Therapy Defined

Music is the art and science of organized sound (Cooper, 1974). Its existence is noted in every major culture; its origin as an accompaniment to ritual predates science. "Music" (from the Greek *mousike tekhne* or "Muses' art") has also been described as human behavior (Michel, 1979). It is produced by humans with sounds from various sources, including themselves, and the sounds are put into a system that humans label "music." As such, music can be thought of as various behaviors, such as blowing, striking, or picking on some sound-producing source, which together are called music or musical behavior.

When used in therapy, music can benefit people with problems, helping them to change their behavior by acquiring new or more adaptive behaviors (Gaston, 1968). Occasionally, music alone elicits behavioral changes. Most often, however, music is a therapeutic tool used either directly or indirectly, under the guidance of a trained therapist, to bring about desirable changes in client behavior.

Music therapy is defined by the National Association for Music Therapy (NAMT), Inc. as the systematic application of music or music activities to attain therapeutic goals (NAMT, 1980). Music is a tool used by the therapist as a means of attaining predefined goals and assisting clients in lengthening the amount of time they engage in constructive and desirable behaviors. In discussing the therapeutic use of music, the term "music" may refer to any of four designations: the music itself, listening to music, having music in the environment, and the making of music.

Music therapists have a unique medium with which to work. Persons unfamiliar with the possibilities of accomplishing dynamic change through the use of music may view music therapy as either professional music performance, music education, or music appreciation. Because of music's association with recreational and leisure-time activities, music therapy can be mistakenly viewed as a nice break from the stress of "real" therapy. Music, however, is a pervasive, pleasurable, and sometimes even undesirable and inescapable part of our society. It is a powerful influence in everyday life, and, in the hands of a skilled music therapist, it is a powerful therapeutic tool for accomplishing significant therapeutic change.

Music therapy can be utilized in any treatment setting, including medical hospitals, psychiatric hospitals, outpatient clinics, inpatient clinics, and state hospitals. Some music therapists also have private practices through which clients are treated.

Clients may come to music therapy through self-referral, referral from another member of the treatment team, or as a requirement of the particular treatment program in which they participate. For example, if music therapy is part of the treatment strategy used in an inpatient psychiatric unit, the client may be required to participate.

Music therapy is most often defined as an experiential treatment, that is, a treatment in which a person engages in some activity, looks back at the activity critically, abstracts some useful insight from the analysis, and puts the result to work (Pfeiffer, 1985). Experiences in music therapy are organized to aid clients in dealing with their present situation, that is, their behaviors, attitudes, beliefs, and lifestyles. Clients' pasts are used only to help them learn to explain and understand their present. The emphasis is then placed on changing the present to ensure a healthier, more rewarding future.

Music therapy offers clients the opportunity to "do something musically." Having experienced the activity, the chosen follow-through is usually to have each client then share what she saw, heard, and/or felt during the musical experience. Clients use their musical experiences to examine their cognitive and affective reactions during these experiences. It is then the responsibility of the music therapist to process with the individual her reactions and observations derived from the musical experience and to help her generalize them, that is, determine how they might be applied to everyday life outside the music therapy session. The music therapist might suggest some applications to the individual client or group; ask each client to, as part of the session, construct her own applications of the musical experience to her "real world"; or end the session after the musical experience has been processed, leaving each client to generalize the experience on her own.

Music therapy, in general, utilizes three basic processes through which music is used to elicit positive behavioral change and client improvement: experience within structure, experience in self-organization, and experience in relating to others. This chapter describes these three music therapy processes and discusses their systematic application to the specific issues of anorexia nervosa.

Experience within Structure

Experience within structure refers to those behaviors required of the client that are a natural part of the musical experience. The structure discussed here refers to that inherent in the music. For example, structure can come from melody, harmony, rhythm, form, style, and the precise way they all work together to create a particular musical piece. The structure of the music itself demands experiencing, and, thus, it contributes to the uniqueness of music as a therapeutic tool.

Within the music therapy session, the client comes to terms with and manipulates a part of her environment, a musical part in this case. She may come to understand the environment as a place with a definite purpose (e.g., to create, study, and/or perform music) where she can effectively interact and experience control. Music elicits participation in a way that is nonverbal, nonthreatening, and even pleasant. Though "externally influenced," the client feels more free and able to expand her "self," to discover her own potentialities, and to govern herself.

Through experience within structure in the music therapy sessions, specific goals can be accomplished with anorectic clients by addressing three clinical issues: control, reality orientation, and stress reduction.

Control

The need for structure and for control within that structure are characteristics of anorectic people discussed extensively in the literature (Bruch, 1973; Garner & Bemis, 1982; Garner *et al.*, 1982; Masterson, 1977). Rigid attitudes and behaviors (related not only to weight control and other interpersonal issues, but also to careers, sports, and/or studying), inability to face reality (e.g., dangerously low weight, self-destructive eating behaviors), and irrational decision-making (e.g., accepting all responsibility for problems belonging to others) are found to be typical in clients with anorexia (Sandbek, 1986). Such problems illustrate the perceived lack of control, noted in all areas of anorexics' lives—physiological, emotional, mental, and behavioral.

A major goal of psychotherapy with anorectic patients, then, involves assisting them in achieving realistic self-control and experiencing such control through beliefs, mainstays, and behaviors not related to weight issues (Garner *et al.*, 1982). A client may enter music therapy fearful of this new environment, focusing only on ways she can burn energy and remain thin (as a means of maintaining control) and concentrating on her low weight as her immediate source of strength and self-fulfillment. The music therapist's role is to utilize the structure of the music to temporarily take the client's attention away from her thinness and compulsive energy-burning, and enable her to experience strong feelings of satisfaction and fulfillment through influence over the music and the musical environment. At all times, the focus is placed on the reality of the *music* and what the client achieves *musically*. This is accomplished by helping the client learn to relinquish herself to the music and to experience success in doing so.

The unique structure of music allows the client to commit herself to the musical experience only to the extent she desires. Although music demands time-ordered behavior—participation and involvement at the rate and in the sequence dictated by the music itself—the client is free to "let go" to the music only as much as she chooses and only for the length of time she desires. Music is a moment-by-moment experience that cannot be interrupted without losing its overall scope. However, the time the client "gives in" to the music can expand from a phrase to a measure to an entire piece, leaving her free to begin at her own level of tolerance.

As music is studied, played, composed, or sung, the client learns how to let go to the music and to let it direct her. She can experience security and safety in the supportive, nonthreatening music therapy environment. From this supportive base, a client and music therapist might work together in the music session to help the client examine and learn to manage disruptive feelings. Examples include confronting fear by discussing musical participation requirements so that all elements of the situation become objectified and "safe"; reducing anxiety by reviewing what to expect from upcoming musical activities, thus reducing fear of the unknown; coping with depression by reviewing musical accomplishments through verbal critique and tapes of music session, thus enhancing self-esteem; and overcoming helplessness by accomplishing any sort of musical response and demonstrating accepted responsibility, such as setting up the tape recorder for the music session. The client can then parallel these accomplishments with her work in psychotherapy—for example, development of a reasonable perspective on weight or realistic life values.

Reality Orientation

Correction of their distorted sense of reality is another major aspect of psychotherapy with anorectic clients (Garner *et al.*, 1982). This requires correction of both their faulty thinking and the beliefs they apply to themselves and the world around them. Music can help change these misinterpretations of reality through its capability of bringing about certain pictures or ideas. The association-provoking quality of music can be used to reinstate or teach the client with anorexia healthy images, standards, and forms of behavior and to desensitize anorectic clients to antagonistic ideas, images, values, beliefs (e.g., healthy weight, self-acceptance, trust in self and others). For example, soothing music can be played as clients study pictures of "fattening" foods, discuss their ideal weight, and visualize themselves as heavier. Pictures of average-weight persons enjoying themselves as they eat and play can be viewed in accompaniment with favorite musical selections. Music—with its structure, stability, and security—can generate feelings of peace and relaxation in anorectic clients as the therapist and client discuss and continually review healthy values, ideals, and behaviors as well as faulty perceptions of reality.

As another means of identifying, evaluating, and changing faulty thinking patterns and erroneous beliefs, music can demand reality-ordered behavior (Gaston, 1968). In musical situations the client experiences a variety of objective elements ("realities"). Specifically, these include aural stimuli, both musical and verbal; musical instruments; musical scores; a conductor's or therapist's directions; and the client's own body and its parts that are involved in the musical event, such as fingers, hands, and/or mouth. The client's responses can then be evaluated for their appropriateness to the "real" stimuli of the music. For example, the music therapist and client might evaluate whether her hand-clapping to a soft piece of music or her weak, inhibited tambourine playing in accompaniment to a John Philip Sousa march truly matched the mood of the music.

Specific songs, with their extramusical ideas and associations, can be used to discuss and promote a healthy orientation to reality through ideas such as the following:

1. Being free from food obsessions and fear of fat (e.g., Big Jim, the slave, singing to Huck Finn in "Free At Last" from the stage musical *Big River*).
2. Moving into the future with health, confidence, and control (e.g., "Move On" from the Broadway show *Sunday in the Park With George*).
3. Facing the reality of a world which often challenges fulfillment of personal goals (e.g., in *Pippin,* the main character sings of finding his own "corner of the sky" and making his life something more than just existing, despite obstacles presented to him by life and by others.

The music therapist might encourage a client to use these songs, with their lively tempos and upbeat philosophies, as motivation when by herself. Such songs can be used during times of trouble (e.g., panic attacks or depression) or when doing homework and working to change her beliefs.

Stress Reduction

In addition to their need for structure and a nonthreatening environment, anorectic clients also demonstrate a strong need for stress reduction (Sandbek, 1986). Strober (1984) found that persons with anorexia typically suffer $2\frac{1}{2}$ times the magnitude of life stress experienced by their peers. Additionally, stress among anorexics has been found to be most often self-generated. For example, teenage girls with anorexia may pressure themselves far more than their friends to achieve good grades, be thin, run for office, and be cheerleaders. Such excessive stress can contribute to the client's loss of self-control and her inability to control her environment. Sandbek (1986) proposed that stress must be reduced or even eliminated before anorectic thoughts and behaviors can be effectively confronted.

Appropriately chosen music can be an effective tool in influencing and changing the behavior and internal states of individuals and/or groups (Gaston, 1968). Therefore, music may be indicated as a means of reducing stress. Music can easily contribute to an internal sense of well-being and thus a more focused, relaxed, and secure mind and body. Slow tempos, smooth (legato) lines, simple harmonies, and little dynamic change (i.e., changes in loudness or softness) are characteristics of music that tends to reduce or sedate physical arousal and may even enhance reflection and relaxed thought-focusing. For example, "Jesu, Joy of Man's Desiring" by Bach or a Scarlatti sonata might be used for this purpose. In contrast, fast tempos, detached (staccato) lines, complex and dissonant harmonies, and sudden dynamic changes can increase or stimulate physical activity, resulting in tension reduction and reduction of unwanted mental activity. Appropriate musical examples include Stravinsky's ballet, "Firebird Suite," or Smetana's "The Moldau," given that the latter piece paints a musical picture of an angry, raging river.

Additional examples of the therapeutic use of music for the purpose of stress reduction in clients with anorexia might include the following:

1. Engaging in deep, natural breathing to the slow tempo of Barber's "Adagio for Strings."
2. Playing a flute or singing an aria from Handel's *Messiah* as a means of practicing breath control.
3. Accompanying muscle-relaxation exercises with peaceful pieces such as Respighi's "Pines of Rome" or Debussy's "Claire de Lune."
4. Generating positive, pleasurable memories and associations that are realistic, which create an internal sense of well-being and promote deep relaxation through the use of favorite musical selections.

Through such activities, the client can establish positive associations between specific musical selections or activities and stress-reducing behaviors. She is then able to take the instrument or musical selection (and its associations) away from the therapeutic setting, practice on her own, and work to reduce stress in other situations outside the musical setting. As an illustration, one client in a hospital music therapy group used Pachelbel's "Canon in D" to practice both her natural breathing and progressive relaxation. Now, whenever she hears the piece, she is able to achieve a rapid state of relaxation, peace of mind, and a sense of security.

The music therapist must, of course, be alert to possible unique associations that individual clients may have with a particular piece or style of music. For example, if the music therapist is working on achieving muscle relaxation with an anorectic client and plays a piece that reminds her of her mother—who belittled her every action—true relaxation cannot occur, and another piece should be chosen.

Experience in Self-Organization

This second process of music therapy is concerned with a client's attitudes, interests, values, appreciations, and personal regard for self and life (Gaston, 1968). At this level, clients may come to establish their own personal identity, find their own ways of living, and find ways to value and appreciate themselves and their lives. Experience in self-organization deals primarily with inner responses that may only be inferred from behavior. Through the music therapy session, a number of specific clinical issues for anorectic clients can be addressed, including self-esteem, external belief systems, negative thinking, affective expression, and gratification.

Self-Esteem

Using music to provide experiences in self-organization parallels the therapeutic strategies outlined by Garner et al. (1982) for changing and improving the negative and underdeveloped self-concept of the client with anorexia and eliminating the need for weight control as a reference for self-evaluation. The anorectic client who suffers from lack of self-esteem and who typically uses weight control to alleviate self-doubts and to establish her personal essence can be helped in this area by first having specific, successful musical experiences structured for her. The permissive atmosphere of most musical group activities provides a continuum of opportunities for success, ranging from mere presence within the group to a position of prominence. The client can feel needed by others, as her musical contribution is both important and required in order for the musical experience to occur at all.

Whether she is a musical leader or a simple participant in structured musical situations, the client experiences personal success and accomplishment through something other than weight control. She can also experience the esteem of others for the music she creates. She can then use these experiences to further develop her own personal feelings of self-worth and her belief in her capabilities outside of music therapy.

External Belief System

Many anorectic clients are reported to rely primarily on acceptance from others as their criterion for positive self-evaluation before turning to the weight and exercise standard (Garner et al., 1982). Rotter (1960) referred to this as an external locus of control or orientation to life: the rewards and punishments of life are believed to be controlled by sources outside oneself (e.g., luck, chance, fate, the intervention of other people). For instance, music therapists report that persons with anorexia rarely offer a suggestion when asked what music they would like to hear. Rather, they respond, "Whatever you would like." They typically do not volunteer to sing a solo ("There must be all kinds of singers better than I am!"), nor would they turn on a radio for musical enjoyment if they thought it might bother someone ("How selfish!").

Music has many unique attributes that can be utilized effectively in helping clients with anorexia develop an internal orientation to life. Music is flexible and versatile, that is, capable of being changed (in rhythm, dynamics, tempo) according to the desires of each listener, performer, or participant. Music is nonverbal and is generally nonthreatening. Music has no set societal restrictions, no absolutes, no "shoulds," all of which are found in external belief systems. For instance, in the movie version of *Cabaret*, the main character lyrically expresses a yearning that her luck hold and her latest boyfriend stay with her. As song lyrics can illustrate belief systems, these lyrics can be used in music therapy to generate a discussion on external locus of control ("Fate, luck, chance determine whether a man remains in a relationship with me.") compared with internal locus of control ("I am a wonderful person. I am capable of creating my own happiness. I do not require a man's love and attention to convince myself I am valuable and worthwhile.").

The music therapist seeks to build and reinforce an anorectic client's slow discovery of her own opinions and perceptions and also gently challenges her feelings of self-worth, which are dependent on others' expectations and evaluations. The client might become involved in independent activity, such as selecting group musical numbers, orchestrating ensemble pieces, conducting performances, or any musical activity requiring her to state personal preferences and musical opinions. Personal critiques of her performance and musical accomplishments, using only positive statements and without input from others, can contribute toward her own positive, personal evaluation of self.

Psychotherapeutic techniques used with anorexics must also work toward encouraging self-acceptance despite poor performance and human fallibility. Care is therefore taken by the music therapist that the client's self-evaluation remain disconnected from her evaluation of both her musical and her everyday performance. A client who shares successful musical experiences with others, who makes mistakes with others, and who learns with others can learn to accept the esteem and the criticism of herself, her peers, and her leader. She is taught that reaching excellence (in this case, through music) is not the requirement for self-acceptance.

The music therapist might also explain to clients that musical activities are therapeutic tools and can be helpful when carried from the session and used independently for purposes of self-help. For example, a group activity in music therapy might be to listen to the song, "I Am What I Am," from the musical, *La Cage Aux Folles,* and to have each client list her strengths, attributes, and positive personal characteristics. (If she has trouble doing this, the therapist can ask other group members to generate lists for her.) As a follow-up homework assignment, the music therapist could ask the client to independently listen to the song and copy her list generated in therapy as she listens. Long-term goals might include memorizing (and thus internalizing) the list and learning to play "I Am What I Am" to reduce feelings of depression when they occur.

The music therapist can also encourage clients to use music and musical events as leisure-time activities. These may include listening to music, attending concerts, singing to records, joining a chorus, and taking piano lessons. The therapist can ask the client to discover her personal interests and preferences and to pursue them without seeking the input of others.

Negative Thoughts

The destructive thoughts that negate the anorexic's value of self, and that are the basis of underlying faulty assumptions (Garner *et al.*, 1982), often occur quickly, habitually, and powerfully (Sandbek, 1986). In order to change the powerful influence negative thoughts have on the behavior of anorexics, therapeutic techniques providing the client with concise, constructive responses to negative thoughts and with positive statements concerning self and life would seem appropriate and effective.

Affirmations, which are strong, positive statements about herself that may initially seem unbelievable to the client, can be used to change destructive, recurring thoughts and to establish self-control. To be successful (i.e., internalized and believed), however, affirmations require excessive repetition, which can lead to monotony and boredom. Finding affirmations stated in songs, writing songs with strong affirmations, and listening to music whose personal associations generate the thoughts and feelings stated in affirmations can all add intrigue and variety to the affirmation process. Songs such as "I Am Woman," or lyrics about "learning to love yourself" from "The Greatest Love Of All" (sung by Whitney Houston), can be used effectively here. A client whose assessment indicates poor self-esteem, and whose therapeutic goals include enhancement of feelings of self-worth through experiences other than weight control, might choose an affirmation such as, "Even though I have faults and make mistakes, I still love myself." Writing such a statement 100 times can assist with development of feelings of self-worth and can be further internalized by listening to the song, "I've Gotta Be Me." From evaluations by the client and her therapists, the music therapist can determine the success of the affirmation/music process.

Affective Expression

Garner *et al.* (1982) noted that anorectic patients frequently experience a serious deficit in the area of affective recognition and expression. A crucial component of psychotherapy with most anorectic clients, therefore, involves assisting them to accurately identify their internal feelings, to accept these feelings, and to reduce their discomfort. Sandbek (1986) referred to this as changing "destructive" emotions (e.g., depression, irrational fear, helplessness) to "constructive" emotions (e.g., sadness, rational fear, weakness). Because music has been found to evoke affectively ordered behavior (Gaston, 1968), and because of its adaptability, music provides avenues for self-expression of affective states. Through performance and listening, music offers socially acceptable ways of expressing negative feelings, which may reduce the need for expression through symptomatic behavior, such as excessive weight control. In music therapy, clients may be asked to find pieces or create music expressing various emotions, perhaps beginning with those identified by the therapist. As clients become comfortable with such activities, they may then feel more inclined to use the music to express their own personal feelings. As Bruch (1973) discovered, the anorectic client benefits most when she is allowed to discover her inner feelings and "say it first." The client can next be encouraged to express musically her "unacceptable" emotions with the music therapist; she can then learn that this expression does not lead to retaliation or rejection. Finally, the therapist can introduce methods of expressing appropriate, constructive feelings openly through musical activities. For example, if a client chooses to make a musical statement expressing her depression, the music therapist might lead a discussion comparing the destructiveness of depression ("I'm so rotten, there is no point in trying to change") with the constructiveness of sadness ("It's sad that I have this problem, but there are definitely ways I can help myself").

Gratification and Rewards

As has been previously noted, experience in self-organization has to do with, among other things, a person's interests, sense of identity, and meaning in life. Self-organization is a result of what is commonly termed gratification (Gaston, 1968). Music can be used to achieve self-organization (pride in accomplishment, enjoyment in listening, excitement over expression of internal affective states) due to its capacity to provide personal gratification within the aesthetic experience and because nearly all people like some kind of music.

Music can also provide opportunities for socially acceptable rewards, such as applause and verbal praise. The adaptability of music allows both immediate and delayed reinforcement. For example, listening to a favorite musical selection might be an immediate reward for an anorectic client following a discussion on handling depression. Giving a public recital after months of practice could provide intrinsic rewards such as pride in self, sense of accomplishment, or feelings of happiness. A client might reward herself with attendance at a Friday night concert, if she maintains recommended nutritional guidelines over a specified period of time.

Experience in Relating to Others

This third process of music therapy refers to the individual's behavior in relation to other individuals. As no person can effectively function in isolation, learning to relate to others is imperative. Gaston (1968) wrote of the individual's need of others for ultimate fulfillment. In general, this first requires development of the self, provided in music therapy through experience in self-organization. Participation in more significant groups, or more significant participation in the same groups, is then possible in music therapy. Gaston stated that, in therapy, music can be used as a socializing agent to "increase the size of the group in which the individual can successfully interact . . . and to provide experiences that will help him relate to noninstitutional life" (p. 41).

Music, by its very nature, draws people together, whether for purposes of listening, playing, or creating. Music provides an environment comprised of sensory, motor, emotional, and social components in which, for the most part, participants share. It unifies the group for common action, and it is the musical setting that elicits or changes many extramusical behaviors. The music is the reason for the group experience, and the client can feel accepted as a musician. Roles may include being a chorus member, a member of a dance troupe, or an instrumentalist in a band. In the case of the client with anorexia, the goal in music therapy is to teach the client to behave effectively and interact with others in group musical situations. Relating to others may involve interaction with one other person or with a large ensemble. Whatever the nature of the group, she is generally accepted and needed by others. Musical situations provide opportunities to identify strengths, weaknesses, and successes. The individual can also perform "reality checks," such as "Am I behaving/thinking 'normally'? Do I look healthy, or do I appear sick?"

Specific issues for anorectic clients are addressed in music therapy by providing experiences in relating to others. These experiences include self-directed behavior in groups, individual choice of response within groups, and communication with others.

Self-Directed Behavior in Groups

The person with anorexia experiences little confidence or trust in the validity of her own thinking, feeling, and perception (Selvini-Palazzoli, 1978), and she usually displays an overreliance on external frames of reference in an attempt to organize her own internal experiences (Garner et al., 1982). Although self-organization can be achieved by a client working individually (e.g., in individual therapy, at home), unless newly obtained skills such as positive thinking, control of emotions, using an internal belief system, and demonstrating pride in self are transferred to and used within group situations, the anorectic individual's functioning may be limited.

Music provides a client with anorexia a wide range of group experiences and levels of achievement that demand self-organization within a group. Examples include learning to evaluate her own performance without input from others; continually attending music therapy groups despite insecurity regarding whether others like her; offering critiques of music without fear of rejection from others; taking responsibility for creating melodies within the group experience and risking the criticism of other group members; openly communicating with other group members between musical activities; and sharing herself on a personal level. Through such group musical experiences, the client gradually assumes even more responsibility for directing herself and her life. Progress, both musical and personal, can be attributed to her own efforts; it is not achieved for her.

Individual Choice of Response within Groups

In order for any musical group to function best, optimum performance and commitment by each musician are important. Each group member, however, is free to choose her own level of involvement. For the client with anorexia, this freedom of choice can be more important than the choice itself. By providing opportunities for individual choice within a group, music can help build the necessary personal autonomy and independence stressed by Crisp (1980). The client is helped to make her choices based on her own internal experiences, to accept those choices, and, through music, to present them to the group.

Communication with Others

Music is a medium widely used for social communication and social intercourse (Michel, 1979). In therapy, the anorectic client sometimes finds it easier to talk more freely when music is playing in the background. She may also express, in music or through musical preferences, feelings not otherwise expressible, thus helping herself to relate to others more easily. Music can often speak where words fail (Gaston, 1968).

A MODEL FOR USE OF MUSIC IN THERAPY

Moreno (1975) stated that an important part of the therapeutic process involves assisting clients in transferring behaviors, feelings, and thoughts from life into the therapeutic setting and back from the therapeutic setting into life. In teaching emotional self-help skills to clients with anorexia, however, therapists have found that such learning, especially effective confrontation and handling of reality, is less likely to occur within the client's everyday environment, where stresses and cues for negative thinking and behaviors are present. "Reality learning" is best tested and practiced within an artificial setting, where emotional self-help skills are introduced, learned, practiced, and reintegrated within the framework of psychotherapy modeled after life itself. Process Theatre, Inc., a music therapy program dealing specifically with transfer of learning from therapy to everyday life, is a model of such a psychotherapeutic environment.

As previously established in this chapter, anorexics have difficulty with reality testing, coping skills, self-actualizing, and independent functioning. It is therefore an important part of the therapeutic process to teach them skills (i.e., reality confrontation, self-help skills) within protective setting (e.g., hospital, clinic), away from the client's everyday environment and cues for negative thinking and behavior and to develop a maintenance program for them, by allowing clients to practice their skills in settings similar to their "external" setting. Process Theatre has developed a music therapy program to assist anorectic clients in these two areas.

Through the therapeutic work of Process Theatre, music has been found to be effective in helping clients transfer the self-confidence, organization, and sense of well-being experienced during music sessions into life at home, at work, or in the hospital. One of my clients once described herself as "a piece of human flypaper" because of the impact she allowed others' comments and outside influences to have on her feelings, thinking, and behavior. However it is precisely this personal capacity that enables clients to "absorb" music and to transfer its messages and its associations in and out of the music therapy setting as a self-healing tool. Through mental imagery, clients can take their music, with its self-help and self-control messages and associations, with them wherever they go, using it in healthy, self-enhancing ways. As an illustration, a very musically oriented client traveled to Mexico, where—due to the change in environment plus the fun and excitement of the trip—she was able to let go, eat many new foods, eat more than usual, and sit on the beach without worrying about fat and lack of exercise. While there she bought an album of songs sung by a very popular Mexican performer. Upon returning home, she found that playing the songs while she ate meals created positive memories, feelings, and associations. This enabled her to experience eating as a more relaxed, enjoyable, and productive experience.

Description of Process Theatre

The goal of Process Theatre is to use the universal medium of theatre as a setting, and music as a tool, in improving the quality of life of persons with problems in living (e.g., anorexics) and community members. Theatre troupes are formed so that each participant works to achieve personally specified learning goals and objectives through participation in professional musical productions. Productions and performances by these troupes also strive to educate and enlighten the general public through high-quality artistic entertainment. Process Theatre differs from other music therapy approaches in that the product (that is, a musical performance) is a vital aspect of therapy. Whereas very few music therapists stress product or musical outcome, in Process Theatre, the therapy (or learning process) always results in a final product.

The name "Process Theatre" was chosen for two reasons. First, "process" emphasizes the experiential component—the therapeutic element for each participant is learning by doing and being involved. Each participant identifies personal needs and plans for meeting those needs through preparation, rehearsals, and performance of a musical production. A final product (the musical production) always results, but it is not of primary importance for the participant. Second, "process" also refers to reintegrating, or integrating, people who have experienced problems in living (for example, anorexia) into society in an enhancing way for both the participants and other members of their community, such as their families and friends. The music, the theatre, and the production all work to change the image that the participant, her significant others, and audience members in general have of the performer's worth and ability to function in society.

Because of its therapeutic emphasis, community approach, and use of a social system (i.e., the theatrical community), Process Theatre is a form of milieu therapy, or the "therapeutic community approach." As defined by Daniels (1975), the "therapeutic community approach" attempts to make maximum use of a social system (e.g., hospital, psychiatric ward) and its constituents (e.g., personnel, therapists) to modify a patient's behavior, so that she can manage her life and personal relationships in a more constructive fashion. Some of the principles and practices under which the therapeutic community operates include the following: (1) communication is open and direct between therapist and client; (2) clients are encouraged to participate actively in their own treatment; and (3) the therapeutic community remains in close contact with the outside community, and there is frequent communication and interrelating between them.

As an illustration both of a specific model of music therapy and of Process Theatre as a therapeutic community, this chapter discusses in detail how Process Theatre uses musical theatre in helping anorectic clients.

Background of Process Theatre and Anorexia

In June 1982, eight women recovering from eating disorders, graduates of a 16-week group therapy outpatient treatment program at the California Clinic in Fair Oaks, CA, were organized into a theatre troupe for purposes of continued self-help and personal growth. Through the clinic, these women had learned how to manage their anorectic thoughts, behaviors, and emotions and were next challenged with living independently and maintaining their progress. Upon returning to the community, however, a significant number of clients returned to self-abuse and overly restrictive eating. Support groups and/or transition programs led by recovering anorexics (graduates of the clinic's program) and centering on verbal discussions of everyday problems had met with limited success. Group members complained that meetings resulted in "symptom swapping" and focus on problems without adequate discussion of solutions. I learned of this situation, and received the clinical director's approval to offer Process Theatre as an alternative to his recovering anorectic clients. The theatre troupe, "Companions," was thus formed as a means of helping chronic and more severe anorexics bridge the gap to return to the community.

Participants for Companions were recruited by both the music therapist and the director of the clinic. Opportunities for potential participants included a different form of self-help, enjoyment, challenge, personal fulfillment, friendship, support, and the assistance of a trained music therapist. Auditions were held. Each woman was required to sing a musical selection of her choice, create a simple dance or movement sequence to a Broadway show song, and improvise the dialogue of a suggested scene. Additionally, potential participants all completed questionnaires about their background in both music and treatment of anorexia plus their current personal issues, goals, and objectives. The women selected for the troupe were those whose needs, interest, and willingness to work were evaluated by the music therapist as being most urgent. Musical talent was given minimal consideration.

At first, cast members and the director—music therapist held numerous discussions of key issues concerning their anorexia and problems in everyday life. Discussions centered around feelings of shame regarding the label, "anorexic"; excessive and self-destructive personality characteristics; lack of control; and self-esteem and control gained by reducing fear of fat and obsession with weight control. The content of the troupe's discussions was incorporated into a musical, *COMPANIONS—A New Review*, which deals with fear and coping.* The songs and dialogue of the show were written to communicate the particular issues of the actresses' lives as well as demonstrate the experiential element of these issues (e.g., the racing thoughts, the distorted thinking, the lack of self-esteem, the dependence on others' opinions for self-approval).

While *COMPANIONS* helped educate the cast members' community

---

COMPANIONS—A New Review was written by Joseph Parente, co-director of Process Theatre.

of friends, family, and others, the primary accomplishment was the cast members' increased self-acceptance, gained through the sharing of the internal experience of their anorexia with others. For example, one cast member stated that singing about her limitations and weaknesses to an entire audience of people and receiving applause for doing so was emotionally cleansing, helped her with self-acceptance, and gave her "enormous personal strength."

Cast Selection

Process Theatre now maintains an ongoing theatre troupe called "Companions & Company." Each cast member is required to take an active role in her own treatment and to use her theatrical experience adjunctively to further her growth.

Each anorectic client interested in Companions & Company is required to "audition." As part of the audition process, potential cast members are asked to (1) sing, dance, and improvise a suggested scene, (2) complete a written assessment stating their personal treatment history (medical and psychological), at least three current personal objectives, and five reasons for wanting to become part of the troupe; and (3) be personally interviewed by the director–music therapist.

Members of the troupe are chosen according to the following criteria, listed in order of priority: (1) personal need for a community support group; (2) personal interest in joining a community support group with a music therapy/theatrical basis; (3) support of significant others (family members, psychologist, doctor); and (4) musical talent. Once individuals have auditioned and been chosen as members of the company, they remain until they no longer feel the need or interest. Commitment to the group requires attendance at weekly rehearsals for 3 months and performing in two performances given for the community at the end of the rehearsal period.

Director

Companions & Company is directed by a board-certified registered music therapist. Outside consultants in theatre, dance, stress reduction, and mental health sometimes work adjunctively with the group.

As with milieu therapy, communication is open and direct between the music therapist and each cast member. Both the amount of self-help/theatrical work completed and the rate of progress in accomplishing personal objectives is directed by each participant. Both areas are also closely monitored and guided by the counseling and direction of the music therapist, through individual meetings and group discussions.

Treatment Collaboration

Because of the continuing medical needs and problems of women with anorexia, and because music therapy with anorexics is an adjunctive treatment, each member of the troupe is required to maintain periodic contact with a medical doctor and to have received or be currently receiving treatment from a clinical psychologist or psychiatrist. Companions & Company is a support group whose work begins following the crucial treatment period. One of the primary purposes of the troupe is to assist cast members in establishing and maintaining control over their own community functioning. Each cast member decides the extent to which the troupe's director maintains contact with other members of the client's team to emphasize choice making and personal control. The music therapist contacts the primary therapist and/or the doctor only if given permission to do so by the actress.

Therapeutic Elements and Methods

In milieu therapy, the therapeutic environment needs to feel secure to clients and also needs to resemble the outside community (Daniels, 1975). Rehearsals for Companions & Company are therefore held in classrooms or rehearsal rooms adjacent to the theatre where the group will perform. The space is confined and "belongs" to cast members to use as they wish for their own self-improvement. The setting helps each individual work with issues of control, reality testing, and stress reduction through the music therapy by practicing control of fears and phobias through the music and the show, rather than through weight control; working and sharing within a "normalized," community-oriented environment (i.e., a chorus, choir, musical production); and broadening artistic/musical opportunities (i.e., learning vocal techniques, dance movements, theatrical relaxation exercises).

For example, a cast member striving to stay around others for more than 5 minutes without physically or verbally withdrawing might use the rehearsal setting as a practice situation. She may practice supportive self-talk, such as "I want to do this show, and I don't want to disappoint myself, my co-performers, or my family. I can stay in this room and practice for 1 hour without losing control."

Here, too, relaxation for purposes of reducing performance anxiety can be practiced. Relaxation exercises are regularly done in Companions & Company with musical accompaniment, utilizing natural breathing, progressive relaxation, and mental imagery. The group has devised a series of "Stress Coping Statements," which cast members use as part of the production process. Cast members then adapt these statements to situations outside rehearsals and performances. The statements listed are intentionally forceful, strong, and "black/white" in order to combat the overwhelming helplessness and distorted thinking typically experienced by cast members.

1. *During and between rehearsals*
   I am going to be all right.
   I won't let negative thoughts bother me.
   What exactly do I have to do for each song?
   I will just jump right into each song and have fun.
   I CAN do it.
2. *Before going on stage*
   Take it song by song. Don't rush.
   I can do this. I am doing it now.
   Any tension I feel is normal.
   I am not alone on stage ever.
   It is OK if I make a mistake.
3. *While on stage*
   Relax now!
   Just breathe deeply.
   I will keep my mind on each song.
   I will not lose control!
   Singing will help lessen my fear.
4. *After the performance*
   I did it!
   I'm a star!
   Next performance, I won't be as nervous.
   I am able to relax away my nerves!
   I can't wait to tell all my friends what I did!

Within the theatrical setting, reality can also be faced and discussed. This is done by focusing on audience members: "What do audience members (i.e., "normal" people) want to see? What do they eat before a show? What do they think about themselves? What do they do to find meaning in life?"

Finally, within the theatrical community setting, cast members and community members are able to use labels such as "actor" and "performer" rather than "anorexic," "client," and "patient." These labels serve as symbols to the cast members that they are moving on, having made substantial progress toward taking healthy control of their lives.

Members of Companions & Company, because of the chronic and severe nature of their anorexia, are continually recovering: they engage in ongoing struggles; work to maintain control over their thoughts, emotions, stress level, and behavior; and struggle to use an internal locus of control as their approach to life. They function most effectively by continually setting goals and reconfirming objectives over time. Each cast member of Companions & Company is required to make daily, weekly, monthly, and yearly objectives for herself and thus be continually responsible for her own ongoing improvement.

As a means of utilizing the basic music therapy process of providing ongoing experience in self-organization, Companions & Company assists each cast member in the following:

1. Taking care of herself—including getting proper nutrition, adequate sleep, and necessary relaxation—in order to have enough physical and intellectual energy to last through rehearsals and performances.
2. Learning to substitute personal responsibility, communication with others, appropriate response to internal affective states, and healthy self-care behaviors for negative thoughts, helplessness against overwhelming emotions, withdrawal from others, lack of commitment, and excessive response to others' advice and opinions.
3. Improving self-confidence and self-esteem in musical, personal, and interpersonal skills.

The troupe has developed several affirmations relevant to assisting each troupe member with self-organization. Again, all are stated strongly and extremely in order to combat the powerful negative thoughts experienced by cast members. Also, actresses seem to respond best if affirmations are clear-cut (i.e., black/white) statements.

1. I am strong and can control myself on stage.
2. I am not trapped, because I choose to be on stage.
3. No matter what I do on stage, I am a wonderful, delightful, and lovable person.
4. I will just think about now and what I have to do on stage. I will do my best and have fun doing it.
5. Just by being in this show, I am doing wonderful things for myself and for others. I am taking control of myself and my situation.

As a means of providing experience in relating to others, Companions & Company asks cast members to share their objectives with each other during discussions or with the director on an individual basis. Here the focus is on developing and strengthening meaningful friendships; supporting self and others within musical ensemble; and experiencing enjoyment and excitement through performance of songs.

DISCUSSION

As stated in most theoretical perspectives (Bruch, 1973; Garfinkel & Garner, 1982; Selvini-Palazzoli, 1974), anorexia nervosa represents an attempt to solve the psychological or concrete issues of life through direct, concrete manipulation of body size and weight. Regardless of the type or nature of the issues involved, which vary greatly within a group of anorectic clients, learning to resolve conflicts and effectively face psychological challenges without the use of weight control is the essence of therapy for these clients. To accomplish this, anorexics must learn to divorce their eating from their other difficulties; stop using food as a tool for problem-solving; face their problems; and believe in themselves as the best source for solving those problems. Music therapy is a dynamic means of persuading clients to accept themselves and their ability to control their lives, without the obsessive use of weight control, and to interact effectively and fearlessly with others.

Many health professionals have acknowledged the difficulty of engaging the person with anorexia in therapy, and music has been found to work well here. Through its nonverbal, nonthreatening, creative characteristics, music can provide a unique, experiential way to help clients acknowledge psychological and physical problems and resolve personal issues.

Music therapy is one of the behavioral sciences; it is a scientific approach that uses research to study human behavior. The music therapist uses not only the results of his or her own research but also the research results of others on the treatment team, or other experts dealing with the same disorder, to set therapeutic goals and design therapeutic procedures. The objective analysis of the outcomes of music therapy, then, is used to pinpoint the efficacy of the specific techniques, activities, and approaches used in music therapy sessions and to plan future therapeutic strategies. Music therapy is thus a substantial form of treatment, based on theory and research.

The education and training of music therapists is unique in that it provides a thorough study of music as well as psychology, sociology, physiology, and special education. These areas of study are then interrelated through courses on acoustics and the influence of music on behavior. The therapist acquires a bachelor's degree in music therapy and then completes a 6-month, 1,040-hour clinical internship. Upon registration with the National Association for Music Therapy, Inc., the therapist is granted the title "Registered Music Therapist" and, after passing an examination given by the Certification Board of Music Therapy, can become a Registered Music Therapist, Board Certified (RMT-BC).

Accomplishing changes in anorectic behavior and beliefs demands a concerted effort by both the client and trained individuals. The music therapist often serves as a member of a treatment team for the client which at a minimum includes a doctor and a mental health professional. Other members of the treatment team might include a nutritionist, occupational therapist, art therapist, exercise physiologist, drama therapist, dance therapist, and nurse. The music therapist consistently maintains close contact with other members of the client's treatment team, continually sharing and reviewing assessments, goals and objectives, treatment programs, and evaluations.

The music therapist and the anorectic client are able to form a relationship other than that of therapist–client. Together they work to play, create, appreciate, and/or perform music. The music therapist is the conductor, musical director, or producer, guiding an experience where the focus is on the music and not directly on the client herself.

As a regular part of most music therapy programs, each client's musical background, training, skills, interests, and musical preferences are assessed. This can be done through written assessment, personal interview, or both. Many music therapists also conduct both individual and group music therapy sessions prior to setting goals as a means of assessing the anorectic client's behavior when alone and with others. Current therapeutic objectives and goals, along with client background, can also be learned through team meetings and/or facility records. Music therapy, whether used in the hospital, clinic, or community, usually occurs once or twice each week, with the average treatment being 3 months.

How and why clients are referred to music therapy is often important for their treatment plans. For instance, a self-referred client may be more motivated to work in music therapy and may be more ready for challenging objectives than a client "assigned" to music therapy. If a music therapist learns from a particular client's primary therapist that she has demonstrated a greater capacity for relaxation when listening to music, the music therapist could use this knowledge and begin with music and relaxation, which is already familiar to the client. Music could then be used to provide successful experiences in other key areas (e.g., improving self-esteem).

In dealing with the anorexic's difficulty in recognizing and expressing internal feeling states, as described by Bruch (1973), music can be a valuable tool for eliciting internal feeling states and attitudes. Music is an expressive medium and has a quality of expressiveness that words lack. Clients with anorexia can use music as a bridge to verbal therapies. Feelings, attitudes, and perceptions can be recognized, acknowledged, clarified, and tested through music before exploring them in verbal therapy.

In the case of the client with anorexia, objective documentation and evaluation of treatment progress are often difficult to accomplish. Difficulties include factoring out the impact of music therapy intervention when several therapies are being applied at the same time; being subject to clients' decisions to continue/disrupt their treatment; dealing with clients in medical hospitals who are admitted based on life-threatening physical problems and released when their physical condition has improved; and not having opportunity to observe the client's overt behavior following the session. Additionally, little is known about what exactly happens to a person when she is engaged musically. The music therapist must therefore rely on more subjective means than directly controlled research, including reports from clients at the next session or reports from other members of the treatment team, in order to study the efficacy of music therapy. Sometimes, however, noting even subjective responses is impossible, and the music therapist must use his or her own interpretations and conclusions regarding the therapy's effectiveness.

CONCLUSION

This chapter has presented the diverse field of music therapy and how music therapy can be applied to the treatment of people with anorexia nervosa. The understandings of the disorder and the knowledge of music therapy presented here are derived both from the experiences of the author and from the literature.

Anorexia involves many overlapping, multifaceted dimensions of disturbed functioning including deficiency in self-esteem, confused perception of reality, and fear of social involvement and responsibility. Because these are all interrelated areas of human functioning, successful amelioration of their effects on the anorectic client's thinking and behavior has been found to require overlapping, multifaceted treatments. Music therapy, although requiring further investigative research and experimentation, may provide assistance to therapists and clients, dealing with this complex disorder.

REFERENCES

Bruch, H. (1973). *Eating disorders: Obesity, anorexia nervosa and the person within.* New York: Basic Books.
Carter, S. A. (1982). *Music therapy for handicapped children: Mentally retarded.* Washington, DC: National Association For Music Therapy.
Cooper, P. (1974). *Perspectives in music theory.* New York: Dodd, Mead.
Crisp, A. H. (1970). Premorbid factors in adult disorders of weight, with particular reference to primary anorexia nervosa (weight phobia): A literature review. *Journal of Psychosomatic Research, 14,* 1–22.
Crisp, A. H. (1980). *Anorexia nervosa: Let me be.* London: Academic Press.
Daniels, R. S. (1975). The hospital as a therapeutic community. In A. M. Freedman, H. I.

Kaplan, & B. J. Sadock (Eds.), *Comprehensive textbook of psychiatry* (pp. 1190–1995). Baltimore: Williams & Wilkins.

Garfinkel, P. E., & Garner, D. M. (1982). *Anorexia nervosa: A multi-dimensional perspective.* New York: Brunner/Mazel.

Garner, D. M., & Bemis, K. (1982). A cognitive-behavioral approach to anorexia nervosa. *Cognitive Therapy and Research, 6,* 123–130.

Garner, D. M., Garfinkel, P. E., & Bemis, K. M. (1982). A multidimensional psychotherapy for anorexia nervosa. *International Journal of Eating Disorders, 1,* 3–46.

Gaston, E. T. (Ed.). (1968). *Music in therapy.* New York: MacMillan.

Masterson, J. F. (1977). Primary anorexia nervosa in the borderline adolescent: An object-relations view. In P. Hartocollis (Ed.), *Borderline personality disorders* (pp. 475–494). New York: International Universities Press.

Michel, D. (1979). *Music therapy: An introduction to therapy and special education through music.* Springfield, IL: Charles C. Thomas.

Minuchin, S., Rosman, B. L., & Baker, L. (1978). *Psychosomatic families: Anorexia nervosa in context.* Cambridge: Harvard University Press.

Moreno, J. L. (1975). Psychodrama. In A. M. Freedman, H. I. Kaplan, & B. J. Sadock (Eds.), *Comprehensive textbook of psychiatry* (pp. 1891–1908). Baltimore: Williams & Wilkins.

Morton, R. (1869). *Phthisiologia—or a treatise of consumption* (2nd ed.). London: Smith, 1720.

National Association for Music Therapy. (1980). *A career in music therapy.* Washington, DC: National Association for Music Therapy.

Pfeiffer, J. W. (1985). *Reference guide to handbooks and annuals.* San Diego: University Associates.

Priestley, M. (1975). *Music therapy in action.* London: Constable Press.

Rotter, J. B. (1960). Generalized expectations for internal versus external control of reinforcement. *Psychological Monographs, 80* (1), no. 609.

Sandbek, T. J. (1986). *The deadly diet.* Oakland, CA: New Harbinger Publications.

Selvini-Palazzoli, M. (1974). *Self-starvation: From the intrapsychic to the transpersonal approach to anorexia nervosa.* (P. Tauser, Trans.). London: Human Context Books.

Selvini-Palazzoli, M. (1978). *Self-starvation: From individual to family therapy in the treatment of anorexia nervosa* (2nd ed.). New York: Jason Aronson.

Strober, M. (1984). Stressful life events associated with bulimia in anorexia nervosa. *International Journal of Eating Disorders, 3,* 3–7.

Tyson, F. (1981). *Psychiatric music therapy: Origins and development.* New York: Creative Arts Rehabilitation Center.

Index